Poisoned Relations

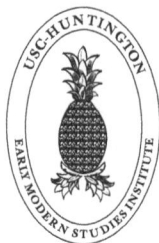

THE EARLY MODERN AMERICAS

Peter C. Mancall, Series Editor

Volumes in the series explore neglected aspects of
early modern history in the western hemisphere.
Interdisciplinary in character, and with a special
emphasis on the Atlantic World from 1450 to 1850,
the series is published in partnership with the
USC-Huntington Early Modern Studies Institute.

A list of books in the series is available
from the publisher.

POISONED RELATIONS

Healing, Power, and Contested Knowledge
in the Atlantic World

Chelsea Berry

PENN

UNIVERSITY OF PENNSYLVANIA PRESS

PHILADELPHIA

Published by
University of Pennsylvania Press
Philadelphia, Pennsylvania 19104–4112
www.pennpress.org

Printed in the United States of America on acid-free paper
10 9 8 7 6 5 4 3 2 1

Hardcover ISBN: 978-1-5128-2649-4
eBook ISBN: 978-1-5128-2650-0
A catalogue record for this book is available
from the Library of Congress.

To Mr. Aube, Mr. Willis, and Mr. Divis,
who taught me to look closer

CONTENTS

Contents

A Weapon of the Weak or an Abuse of Power?

Consider the following: a paper packet containing herbs and a root buried under a path; a healing substance given from one enslaved person to another without the knowledge or consent of their enslavers; pouches of unknown "drugs" distributed from plantation to plantation and suspected of being capable of causing languishing illnesses; and small pieces of a certain stone mixed into a chocolate drink intended to change an enslaver's behavior.[1] Which of these was "poison"? The question is a trick. They all were, or at least they all were investigated as such. European enslavers were deeply anxious about healing practices among the enslaved and considered "taming" efforts—like the stone in the chocolate—as malicious acts of poisoning to be punished. However, the activities of these same healers composing powerful substances, hidden or otherwise, were also viewed ambivalently within communities of African descent as the possession of power always contained the potential abuse of that power. People of both European and African descent conducted investigations to get to the bottom of what they saw as dangerous "poisoning" events and the "poisoners" in their midst, but the two groups held different ideas on what these terms meant.

There is a danger in uncritically imposing a singular definition of "poison" onto the past without thinking through what it meant to whom and when and what they did about it. This book explores this capacious category of "poison" in the Atlantic world—a space of intense cross-cultural interaction and contestation of ideas—from the late seventeenth to the mid-nineteenth century. It asks how the different actors involved in poisoning cases—enslavers and the enslaved; practitioners and clients; accused, accusers, witnesses, and judges—perceived and understood these "poisoning" events. The meanings of "poison" were not only numerous but contested; people in the Atlantic world struggled with each other over differing interpretations that, especially in the context of trials, could have deadly consequences. There were also places and moments where gaps in ideas between people in enslaved communities and slaveholders operated as "dialogues of the deaf" and facilitated investigations into alleged poisoning events.[2] I track the history of the relationships between ideas about "poison" and the people who held them in the geography of this contested Atlantic world.

From 1680 to 1850, courts in Virginia, Martinique, the Dutch Guianas, and Bahia tried hundreds of free and enslaved people of African descent for "poisoning." As events, poison accusations were opportunities for the contestation of ideas about health, healing, and the use of power. Many of these cases centered on the activities of healers of African descent. For example, in 1749, several residents of a neighborhood in Salvador de Bahia complained to the Inquisition about the deaths allegedly caused by Paulo Gomes and Ignacia, both free health practitioners. They were well known to their neighbors, who called them "*feiticeiros*" (sorcerers) and claimed that they could both inflict and treat illnesses caused by *feitiços* (charms, sometimes used interchangeably with "poison" in the eighteenth century). Seven years earlier in Suriname, an enslaved man named Goliath was convicted and executed for making *vergift* (poison) from the burial grounds, hiding it in his house, and allegedly using it to kill other enslaved people. The trials of the enslaved men Jean François in Martinique (1742) and Tom in Virginia (1744) each revolved around the suspect and possibly poisonous nature of their drugs, powders, and remedies.[3] These four cases unfolded in four very different colonies, yet each shared a set of associations: healing practitioners of African descent connected to poison accusations and practices of alleged "sorcery." These practitioners are the key to understanding poison accusations; even though they were only involved in about a third of the total cases, their activities (and colonial officials' concern about their activities) shaped legislation and slaveholders' ideas on the relationship between poison and healing practices. Legislation and familiarity through public knowledge of investigations and trials helped expand and perpetuate poison accusations, but these laws were reactions to existing practices from plantations to urban streets. Practitioners as potential healers and inflictors of affliction had ambivalent relationships with enslaved communities and enslavers who both valued and feared their services; they were also crucial to the development and justification of narratives about poison.

This book explores changes in ideas about poison through waves of cases over this 170-year period and the many different people who were bound up in them. I have analyzed over five hundred investigations and trials in Virginia, Bahia, Martinique, and the Dutch Guianas (including Suriname and the former Dutch colonies Berbice, Demerara, and Essequibo that later became British Guiana)—each a vastly different slave society that varied widely in its conditions of enslaved labor, legal systems, and histories. It is these differences that make the shared patterns I have discovered in key concepts and (mis)understandings of poisoning events so intriguing.

"Poison" was a cultural construction. Western Europeans and Atlantic Africans had developed significantly different cultural idioms and understandings of poison, particularly in relation to power. Europeans discussed poison as a gendered "weapon of the weak" through the lens of demonology, while Africans discussed it as an abuse of power by the powerful through the lens of political morality. Though distinct, both idioms centered on fraught power relationships. When translated to slave societies, these understandings of poison sometimes clashed and sometimes converged through contemporaneous interpretations of alleged poisoning events. The social and relational nature of ideas about poison meant that the power struggles that emerged in poison cases, while unfolding in the extreme context of slavery, were not solely between enslavers and the enslaved: they also involved social conflict within enslaved communities. The forced intimacy of plantations in the Americas created spaces that were not necessarily harmonious but could instead be spaces of uncertain trust filled with fear of attack from within.[4] Healing included communities of both the living and the dead. Relationships with both were crucial to understanding and curing afflictions as these illnesses were embedded in webs of social context and conflict.[5] The violence and fraught power relationships of slave societies also influenced the ideas surrounding alleged poisonings. Over time and through the development of self-perpetuating legal regimes for trying poison cases, European enslavers and their descendants developed and solidified key misunderstandings of diasporic African thought.

The gendered discourse of poison as a "weapon of the weak" that undergirded European interpretations of "poisonings" had a particular history and was not a universal norm. Uncritically assuming European normativity obscures the ways that people from other regions of the world thought about poison; understanding how people thought is crucial to understanding how and why they acted. The methods of historians of Africa can assist with the challenge of developing a comparable archive on the history of ideas between Europe and Africa, despite significant differences in their source bases.

Comparative historical linguistics made it possible for me to build such a history of ideas for West Central Africa, a region of intensive cross-cultural interaction with Europeans after the 1480s that also, and relatedly, became the region of embarkation of nearly half of the African captives who were forced across the Atlantic in the centuries that followed.[6] Together with ethnographic information from early modern sources on West Africa, this analysis of Atlantic African moral philosophy brings insight to some of the range of ways that Africans and their descendants in the Americas understood and dealt with "poisoning" as a critique of powerful individuals.

Examining ideas across a wide geographic and temporal scope—with four very different colonies as case studies—clarifies the significance of Atlantic African thought for understanding these waves of poison cases. Existing studies of these cases have predominantly trained their focus on single colonies or empires without expanding their analyses to contemporary cases. Good work has been done, particularly in the French imperial context, examining waves of poison cases and their local contexts.[7] Understanding both the fine-grained local conditions and the particular laws that shaped poison trials is crucial for grounding any comparative analysis. However, by limiting their studies to specific locales, these works have missed important connections between cases, especially in the expressions of ideas on health, healing, and power within enslaved communities—which conducted poisoning investigations of their own. A geographically discrete approach cannot fully embrace the phenomenon because poison cases and the dynamic ideas that shaped them were not unique to any one location: they spilled beyond imperial and linguistic boundaries. Several collaborative works have brought together cases of spiritual practices and their criminalization in the Caribbean. When there has been comparative work done on poisoning, it has usually centered on famous mid-century poisoning events in Jamaica and Saint-Domingue—the "jewels" of their respective empires.[8] Yet the comparison of isolated cases—especially the most famous cases—alone misses their position in a wider context of poisoning trials and African and European discourses about poison.

By focusing on the cultural construction of "poison" and the transmission and transformation of both European and Atlantic African ideas in the Americas, this book aims to complicate analyses of poison as a "weapon of the weak" and an assumed tool of resistance against enslavers. Much of the analysis in the literature of alleged poisonings committed by enslaved people has been conducted through the framework of resistance.[9] These works have made significant contributions to historians' knowledge on these cases and on the violence deployed by slaveholders—from plantations to courthouses to legislatures—to address them. There is no question that enslaved people resisted their enslavement, and these works have been a valuable corrective to older views on the passivity of enslaved people. However, there is a danger in taking enslavers' fears and ideas on poison at face value; to do so is to adopt the assumptions and perspectives of these slaveholders—though with a very different interpretation on the morality of these alleged acts. As Marisa Fuentes has noted, a rigid framework of resistance can obscure both the full weight of violence on enslaved people and their "messy and contradictory behaviors."[10] This book contributes to an ongoing conversation in the intersecting fields of the history of slavery, criminal justice, and medicine critiquing this resistance-focused approach, a conversation that is finding a way forward through a critical examination of how knowledge and ideas about poison or arson or *obeah* practices were constructed by multiple groups of actors involved in these cases.[11] These works have also highlighted relationships—both "predictable antagonisms and unexpected alliances," as historian Randy Browne has put it—and the negotiation of these relationships within infrastructures of colonial power.[12]

Histories of medicine and healing in the context of slavery in the Americas have predominantly analyzed the topic through the lens of power relationships—and rightly so.[13] Pioneers in the field have largely discussed the efforts of enslaved people to control their own bodies and healing practices as a struggle rooted in the relationship between enslavers and the people they treated as property.[14] In slave societies, enslavers held enormous power over the lives of the enslaved. Violence was a central component of slavery, and slaveholders could and did use force to impose their preferred medical treatment on enslaved people.[15] Studies have examined the negotiation and contestation of medical treatment between enslavers and enslaved people, as well as that in the relationship between healing practitioners of African descent and the enslavers who both relied on and distrusted their services.[16] However, a focus on the struggle between enslaved people or practitioners with slaveholders alone can miss the relationships of power *within* enslaved communities—along with the accusations of harm caused by abuses of extraordinary powers originating from inside these communities.[17] Untangling the webs of social relationships among the enslaved is necessary to understanding both poison accusations and efforts to diagnose and treat illnesses. The living quarters of the enslaved were potential sources of both solidary and fear.[18] Fraught relationships—not only between enslaved people and enslavers but also within enslaved communities—were at the heart of both poison accusations and healing.

Poison accusations were community-wide processes that were emotionally fraught and embedded in these webs of social relationships. The vast literature on witchcraft and witch hunting in both Europe and Africa has been useful for understanding these social and emotional dynamics and their relationships to power. This history is necessarily intertwined with the history of healing, as both Europeans and Africans have perceived malevolent practices through damage to personal and communal health—affliction rendering a person powerless. As with accusations of "witchcraft" in early modern Europe, the personal stakes involved should not lead historians to assume that "poison" was merely a cover for some other "real" conflict. A turn in European literature on witchcraft since the 1980s has insisted on taking an emic approach—attempting to understand how early modern Europeans understood witchcraft—rather than thinking about witchcraft belief as an indication of ignorance or superstition.[19] Works on ideas about witchcraft in early America have likewise sought to understand the ideas of Africans, Indigenous Americans, and Europeans on their own terms while exploring how cross-cultural interactions altered and reshaped these ideas.[20] In African history, communication with and manipulation of spirits for either communal or selfish ends has not been code for political power; rather, it was central to conceptions of power, and that power was relational. This insight—not so much that spiritual power is political but that politics is a form of spiritual power—has been influential for thinking about relationships of power in Atlantic Africa and the African diaspora in the early modern period.[21] In terms of poison cases, these durable and widespread ideas about the morality of power centered on intent and use help us understand why enslaved communities sometimes critiqued and accused healers of African descent for allegedly abusing their powers.

Alongside exciting new works on the intellectual history of the Black Atlantic—whether focused on rituals of diplomacy or attitudes toward water culture or practices of bloodletting—this book explores diasporic African thought and practices on their own terms in addition to tracking their complex interactions with European ideas.[22] I build on scholarship from the past decade that seeks to move past old creolization debates on change versus continuity from the African past to examine what practices and rituals of diverse peoples "did" and how they interacted in contexts of power.[23] An analysis of the cultural construction of "poison" is also at its heart an analysis of the relationships between health, healing, and power in the African diaspora, as many of those accused were healers. Healing interactions between Africans and Europeans and regionally between Atlantic African societies form an essential context for understanding ideas and practices in the Americas.[24] A deeper understanding of durable concepts surrounding poison enriches our conversations on the intellectual Black Atlantic, not because of any assumed static continuity but rather for insight on the ideas that healers in the Americas drew on and how they resonated with their diverse clientele.[25]

Communities—of free and enslaved people of African descent, of enslavers, of colonial officials and natural philosophers—were also essential for constructing narratives about alleged poisoning events through ritual ordeals, trials, letters, and books about poison. These narratives reveal assumptions about what different observers expected to see, as well as the circulation and amplification of "common knowledge" and key (mis)understandings about poison. The concept of "dialogues of the deaf" from anthropologist Wyatt MacGaffey is useful for understanding the ways that these constructed narratives from multiple communities converged and slipped past each other.[26] My work also draws on therapy management and public healing from scholarship on health and affliction in African history to better understand the actions of communities of African descent involved in poisoning events. At its core, therapy management focuses on the social relationships that have shaped medical knowledge and action.[27] Parallel to the turn in European medical historiography, the emergence of the framework of therapy management has expanded the negotiation and interpretation of affliction to a wide group of actors, each with their own perspectives, and focuses on the therapeutic process rather than on single events. Public healing is a framework developed by Africanists for understanding the relationship between politics and broadly defined social illness and cures.[28] In the conception laid out by historian Steven Feierman and anthropologist John Janzen, healing and health need to be understood as relational and fundamentally rooted in historically changing social orders. Succinctly, whoever has had the power to diagnose illness has had the power to define cultural conceptions of evil and harm in the wider public.[29] In its relationship to conceptions of afflictions as public threats, public healing has been intertwined with the responsibilities of powerful people to cure. Public healing is useful for thinking about poison cases both for the way it connects healing to political power and for the emphasis it places on the need to first understand social relationships in order to understand the diagnosis and curing of affliction.

Terms, Locations, and Sources

This book brings together sources from multiple languages and archives. While its expansiveness of scope is what allows for the book's core arguments on African and European ideas, it also poses a problem for terminology. In short, this book is written in English when a central argument is that the idioms and durable themes regarding "poison" are culturally constructed in ways revealed by language. The logic of English words—and of ideas expressed in a range of European languages generally—does not quite fit a range of African concepts relating to health and empowerment. "Poison" as both a verb and a noun is a key example. It is the primary term used across my sources whose forms—poison, *empoisonner, vergift, feitiçaria* (which eighteenth-century Portuguese speakers could use to describe both "sorcery" and "poison")—appeared in colonial trials where narratives about affliction and power were contested. When a twenty-first-century English speaker says "poison," they usually mean a substance capable of causing illness or death; the first image that may come to mind is perhaps a little bottle of liquid, maybe even with a skull and crossbones on the label. This image is not necessarily wrong, but incomplete; it is only one of a kaleidoscope of possible meanings that have each been constructed in historical context. I do not offer a precise definition for "poison" in this book because my point is that it was culturally contingent and did not have a universal or permanent transhistorical meaning. Fully aware of the faults of the term, I have chosen to use "poison" throughout the book precisely to highlight its constructed and malleable nature.

The English language also poses problems for discussing accusations against the alleged activities of so-called "poisoners," "witches," or "sorcerers." There are problems inherent with using the terms of the accusers, as doing so can lead to an uncritical assumption of their perspective on whom the accused were and what they allegedly did or did not do.[30] However, these terms of accusation are still important for what they can tell us about the ideas and perspectives of the accusers. I strive throughout the book to be clear on who accused whom of being or doing what. At the same time, whenever possible, I refer to the accused by the terms they used to describe themselves,

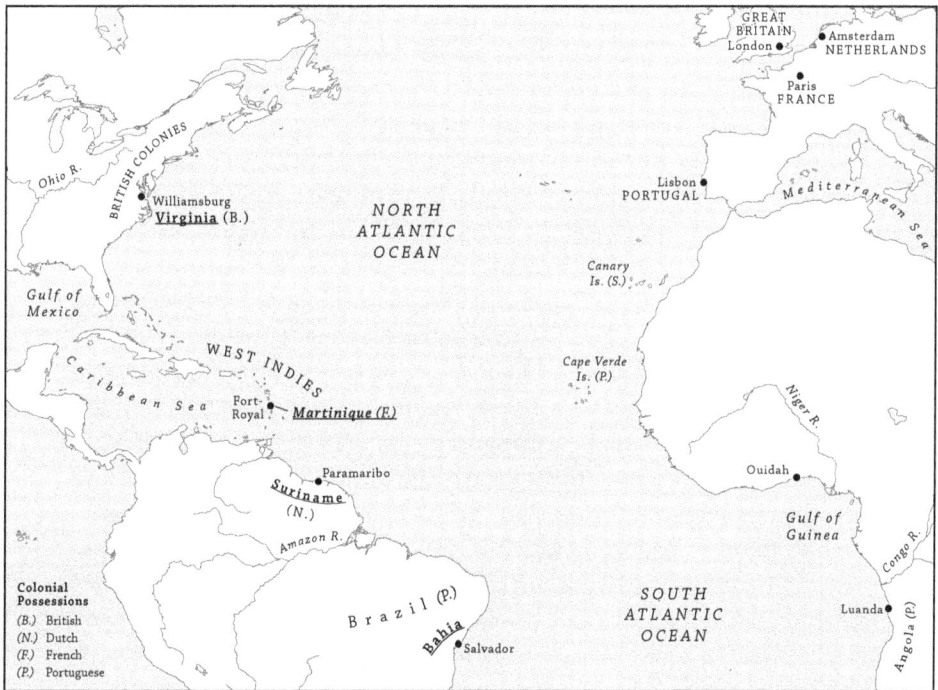

Figure 1. Map of the Atlantic world, c. 1760. Erin Greb Cartography.

often a vernacular variation on "doctor." Historians of medicine have critiqued and analyzed the ways that terms rooted in western biomedicine—like "medicine" and "doctor"—shape discussions on legitimacy in the West due to the history of modern medical professionalization; for this reason, they generally prefer terms such as "healing" and "health practitioners" to get past that discourse. While I note whenever I found usage of African terms such as *nganga* (expert, healer-diviner), most of the surviving information we have about these cases—including testimony by people of African descent—was spoken and recorded in European languages. Most often, I use the term "practitioner" to keep the focus on practices that could include actions perceived as healing or harmful by different historical audiences depending on their perspective.

The four political jurisdictions I chose for this study—Bahia, Martinique, Virginia, and the Dutch Guianas—are not necessarily an intuitive grouping and require explanation. All four locales were slave societies; by the late seventeenth century in Virginia, Martinique, and the Dutch Guianas—and significantly earlier in Bahia—their respective economies, social relations, and legal structures revolved around slavery. However, they were not all the same. They each were a part of different empires: Bahia in the Portuguese and later Brazilian empire, Martinique in the French, Virginia in the British and later the United States, and the Dutch Guianas split and changing hands between the Dutch and the British. Bahia as a slave society was significantly older than the other locations, and Virginia had several dramatic differences in the lower proportion of enslaved people in the general population, the higher proportion of creoles (American born) in the enslaved population, and the main system of enslaved labor revolving around tobacco rather than sugar production.[31] There were also significant cultural and religious differences between the Catholic Portuguese and French and the Protestant Dutch and English in power in these respective locations. I chose these four very different locations for my study precisely because of their legal, demographic, cultural, and economic divergences; these differences highlight the striking patterns I found in poisoning cases. Ideas about poison were transimperial and inextricably bound with the power relationships of slave societies and the ideas of the Africans forced into them. These discourses on the morality and use of power had an impact on poison cases in each colony, even though the internal context of each slave society was different.

I do not wish to imply that these were the only four slave societies in the Americas with the kinds of cases connected to healing practitioners of African descent highlighted in this study; historians working on these locales and others—such as Saint-Domingue, South Carolina, the British West Indies, and the Spanish Caribbean—have also discussed similar cases and tropes about "poison."[32] Nor were these the first major poisoning trials in the Americas. In the sixteenth and seventeenth centuries, several recurring tropes and themes of the later waves of poison cases—for example, concerns about poison as the "weapon of the weak," the activities of healing practitioners in a diverse marketplace, and the creation of narratives about causes of and solutions to affliction through rituals and trials—appeared in Spanish colonies in the Americas.[33] Spanish institutions mapped their idea of weakness and susceptibility to manipulation from the devil—so prevalent in European gendered discourse about women, witchcraft, and poison—onto their ideas about Indigenous peoples and religions in the Americas.[34] While Indigenous practitioners came up frequently in testimony given to the seventeenth-century Mexico City Inquisition—for complex reasons that included the

Inquisition's lack of jurisdiction over *indios*—they appeared but rarely on the edges of the poison cases I examined from Bahia, Martinique, the Dutch Guianas, and Virginia, which were each demographically different from New Spain.[35] Still, the core European idea of the "weapon of the weak" resonated even when applied to different alleged practitioners. Seventeenth-century Cartagena offers particularly salient precedent for later eighteenth-century cases, as the practitioners of African descent who numerically dominated the city's competitive marketplace of health practitioners were also susceptible to accusations of "poison," especially during a wave of "witch-conspiracies" in the 1620s and 1630s.[36] Although the eighteenth-century records I examined did not explicitly reference these Spanish precedents, the Atlantic world was an entangled space where knowledge—including assumptions, (mis) understandings, and tropes—could and did flow between imperial borders.[37] Many of the ideas that surfaced in these earlier cases continued to do so in later centuries because the problem of how to survive and concerns about the morality and use of power only intensified with the expansion of slavery and the transatlantic slave trade.

However, the four locations I chose each had comparable runs of surviving trial records with chronological overlap that allowed for large-scale comparative quantitative and qualitative analyses that were not always available for other locations. For example, while evidence from other sources points to cases of alleged poisoning in eighteenth-century Jamaica, the only surviving pre-1770 regular slave court records for the British Caribbean is a spreadsheet-style summary from 1834 of cases tried before the St. Andrews parish slave court from 1746 to 1782.[38] Even this summary contains more information than the surviving fragments of Barbados cases in eighteenth-century council meeting minutes.[39] Due to their differences, the four locations from four empires offer a broad sampling of the wider phenomenon of poison trials and highlight the significance of shared Atlantic African ideas about poison. While the focus of this book is on ideas, I have included a quantitative examination of my dataset along with a geographic and chronological overview of poisoning trials as Appendix D.

Trials form the backbone of this project; it is necessary to critically examine the context of their production. Michel-Rolph Trouillot has influentially highlighted the many moments of silencing in historical production, from the creation of the sources that form the basis of archives to their interpretation and use by historians.[40] Historians must critically contend with the epistemic violence of the archive, considering who appeared in documentary records—and who did not—and in what particular contexts. The traces of the past that make up colonial archives were produced in specific contexts of violence and power in slave societies, and the purpose of these trials was to police and control people of African descent; they are by their nature fragmentary, distorted, and limited.[41] Historians seeking to write histories of marginalized people in the Atlantic world have demonstrated both the violence embedded in the creation and preservation of these sources and ways forward for critical analysis.[42] For example, Sophie White's recent social historical work using trial records from French Louisiana productively and critically mines courtroom testimony by enslaved people and the parallel narratives they created in a range of cases.[43]

With the limitations of trial records in mind, comparative analysis of trials can yield important insights on the demographics of the accused and the relationship between cases and legislation. For most of the court systems, I was able to collect information on individuals from all social groups tried for all alleged crimes, allowing me to place poison accusations in a wider criminal context and track changes in this context over time.[44] My analysis of this data is also informed by close readings of various laws and local ordinances on poison; trials only made sense in the context of the laws under which courts tried them. Changes in laws yield insight into shifting relationships of power through the ability to define crime. Poison legislation marked these relationships through attempted boundary drawing for what constituted the legitimized practice of healing and the limits of an enslaver's power—at least in theory—to judge and wield violence toward enslaved people.[45] In addition to discussions where relevant in each chapter, I have included an overview of legal changes over time in Appendix D. Correspondence between colonial officials and various metropoles both enriches the context for poison trials and laws and, in some cases, helps bridge gaps in trial data. Personal correspondence written by slaveholders involved in poison cases also offers an expanded view of their interpretation of poisoning events. Together, the trials, laws, and correspondence weave a large tapestry through which we can see the expression of ideas on poison, healing, and power.

The trials are valuable sources not only as data but as scenes of action where people articulated multiple perspectives on poisoning. Courtrooms were not only sites of slaveholding power and violence but also potential sites of contestation over the meaning of alleged poisoning events.[46] Our ability to observe these contested ideas is mediated through these problematic surviving sources.[47] All trial records must be handled with caution, as individuals were highly unlikely to be speaking freely—especially when forced to defend themselves. This caution is particularly necessary for working with cases from legal contexts that allowed for torture to extract confession, including the Lisbon Inquisition, the Suriname Court of Policy and Criminal Justice, and the French *Ancien Régime* tribunal and appeals courts.[48] However, records with testimony are still valuable as rare contemporary recordings of Africans and people of African descent in their own words—at least as recorded by clerks—and the stories that defendants chose to present to try to survive their cases.[49] Historians can use their words, and the questions asked by the courts, to identify different assumptions and perspectives undergirding ideas about poison in particular cases, as well as the manipulation of these ideas.

An additional word of caution is necessary on discrepancies in the level of detail provided by documents originating from different court systems—especially in relation to testimony from enslaved people. Both the surviving Virginia county court records and the eighteenth-century Martinique Conseil Supérieur records are case summaries: very useful for collecting demographic information on the accused but often lacking in extensive detail about the affliction an alleged target suffered; how the case first came (or was brought) to the attention of enslavers; or how suspicion landed on the individual being tried. The summaries from Martinique sometimes identified enslaved witnesses testifying in cases against other enslaved people; in Virginia, while enslaved people were legally allowed to testify in such cases, they were rarely identified beyond a maddeningly terse note of "divers witnesses." For Virginia, many of the records from "burned counties" did not survive the Civil War, rendering any quantitative efforts to tally poison trials suggestive rather than definitive. The functioning of the Lisbon Inquisition is also important for understanding the context of the production of information on alleged poisoning practices. As part of their discreet initial investigations following private denunciations—which were sometimes launched by free and enslaved people of African descent—Inquisitorial commissioners in Bahia often cast a wide net in interviewing community members, including enslaved people, who might be able to shed light on the accusations. These records were detailed but were also shaped by the questions commissioners asked. The trial records from Suriname have by far the most detail about enslaved people in the orbit of poisoning events as they contain transcripts of questions and answers of both defendants and witnesses. However, even in the Suriname cases, there was significant variety in the manner enslaved voices appeared in each case. Sometimes courts recorded enslaved witnesses delivering testimony in the courtroom; in other cases, their statements were collected as depositions to be read, or summarized and likely filtered by an enslaver or an overseer when making their own deposition or testimony to the court. The distinct and distinctly fraught contexts of each form of testimony need to be considered when handling these cases. Trial records from these four locations, with their many limitations, nevertheless do contain significant information. Wherever possible, I have corroborated evidence from trials with information from plantation papers and personal and official correspondence.

Understanding the multifaceted phenomenon of poison cases in the Americas requires a multifaceted approach. This book is a social history of ideas: tracking the transmission, transformation, and interaction of ideas about poison while never losing sight of the people who created, shaped, and lived them. It is also an intellectual history that looks beyond elites to see what Rhiannon Stephens and Axel Fleisch describe as "the intellectual work of ordinary people."[50] Multiple languages and methods have made it possible for me to approach my sources from multiple angles. Social historical analysis of the demographics and content of poison trials has yielded insights on large social patterns over time and connections between my research locations. Thick descriptions of individual poison cases and close attention to the perspectives of the various actors within them, borrowed from anthropology, have assisted my efforts to understand how people involved in these cases saw and comprehended these events themselves. Finally, my training in the use of comparative historical linguistics grounds ideas expressed in poison cases in deeper changes over time and has allowed me to expand my field of inquiry to oral societies beyond (predominantly European-created) written records.

One of the major challenges of doing African history, and especially of doing comparative work between African and European history, is the difference in source bases. Most societies in early Africa—indeed, most societies in the pre-modern world—were orally based, and, with some important exceptions, there are relatively few surviving documents created by Atlantic Africans before circa 1450.[51] I am indebted to several important works in history and anthropology in the past decade that have brought together ideas on extraordinary powers to heal and harm from Europe and Africa to trace their influence in the Americas.[52] However, by being forced for their sections on Africa to rely on predominantly European-created observations from the early modern period—or, in the case of anthropologists, ethnographic work from the more recent past—these scholars have not been able to give a deeper history of how Africans discussed and changed their ideas *before* Europeans arrived.[53] I am also indebted to the close attention and valuable insights Robert Slenes and others have drawn from linguistic connections between Atlantic Africa and the African diaspora, for example, on the use of Kimbundu words in colonial Brazil or Kikongo in Saint-Domingue. However, what the comparative method of historical linguistics does that these works do not is develop a deep history of change over time by reconstructing words across an entire family of languages and dictionaries rather than connecting words recorded in the Americas to single African languages.[54] It is this deeper history that shows how fraught discussions about the work of practitioners of African descent involved in poison cases were part of a two-thousand-year critique of healing and healers as institutions of power. Early African history is inherently interdisciplinary; historians who use comparative historical linguistics also work closely with anthropologists and archaeologists, as the recent culmination of the Kongo King Project on a new history of the Kingdom of Kongo can attest.[55] Embracing Africanists' interdisciplinary methods can lead to a much richer and deeper understanding of the ideas and durable idioms of Africans and their descendants in the Atlantic world.[56] I have included more in-depth discussion of the history, methods, uses, and limitations of comparative historical linguistics as Appendix A.

*   *   *

This book has six chapters divided into two sections that first explore the development of key concepts about "poison" in Atlantic Africa and Europe and then trace the ways these ideas resonated and interacted in the waves of poison cases in eighteenth- and nineteenth-century slave societies. The first two chapters together are a conceptual history tracking long-term changes over time in Atlantic African and European thought and cultural idioms about poison. I use historical linguistics to analyze reconstructed African word roots, complementing philological work in published and manuscript European sources. With both, I track movement and changes in key ideas about poison and power. Chapter 1 focuses on long-term roots and development of these key ideas up to the emergence of the Atlantic world, while Chapter 2 examines cross-cultural interactions and the interplay of these ideas in Atlantic Africa and Europe. In tandem with these cross-cultural interactions, Europeans and Africans brought ways of discussing illness, healing, and extraordinary powers with them across the Atlantic and translated them to new circumstances.

The bulk of this book, in Chapters 3 through 6, combines a social historical analysis of the trials and close readings of individual cases to examine four key ideas about "poison." The third chapter focuses on contested views of poisoning as a weapon of the weak versus an abuse of power by the strong. Europeans and their descendants transformed their gendered associations of weakness and poisoning into racial ones in the context of slavery in the Americas. This framing of weakness also illuminates the anxiety and loss of control experienced by enslavers in the face of what they saw as illicit usurpations of power. However, while the idea of the "weapon of the weak" has had a long impact on abolitionist discourse and historiographic treatments of poison, I argue that it was not the only contemporary interpretation by focusing on the ideas of people of African descent involved in these cases. Drawing on a long history of African moral philosophy on power and healing, we can see discussions of poison centered on the use and abuse of power within enslaved communities. Chapter 4 homes in on the relational and emotional aspects of poison accusations and explores multiple perspectives on the idea of "taming"—connecting Atlantic African idioms of cooling and calming with practices commissioned by enslaved clients to alter the behavior of their enslavers. Chapter 5 explores the idea of power as binding or tying for a range of healing and harming effects. It does so through a close analysis of both the material culture of healing objects and the composition of networks of knowledge by the practitioners of African descent who frequently found themselves at the center of poisoning accusations. Finally, Chapter 6 examines ways in which people of African and European descent constructed narratives about poisoning through ritual practices, treatises, and the trial records themselves that serve as the primary source base for this book. These forms of narrative building could be both contested and collaborative, as communities containing diverse ideas about "poison" could come to suspect the same individuals for different reasons.

Ideas are not free floating; humans create, adapt, and act on them, and it is humans who live with the consequences of these actions. While this project is in some senses an intellectual history—tracking how ideas about poison, health, and power became intertwined and changed over time—my primary concern is the lives of the people who articulated and constructed these ideas. For the people involved in these poisoning cases, the stakes could not have been higher. For members of enslaved communities banding together to support an afflicted relative from a perceived malevolent attack; for enslavers who imposed violent terror on plantations while grappling with fears of being poisoned by the people they considered to be their property; and for free and enslaved practitioners of African descent who continued cultivating practices of healing and harm in the face of high risk of arrest and execution, poison cases were matters of life and death. This book explores how these diverse people thought about and acted through these cases.

CHAPTER 1

Pre-Atlantic Poisoning Cultures

When Heinrich Kramer and Jacob Sprenger linked witchcraft with women in their 1487 witch-hunting manual *Malleus Maleficarum*, they were not breaking new intellectual ground in Europe. The idea of women as weak and power hungry—and therefore prime targets for demonic seduction—rested on a gendered assumption of weakness that by the fifteenth century was already commonly accepted.[1] Poison and witchcraft were intertwined in European thought as weapons of the weak: tools to invert the natural order of things.[2] By the early modern period, Europeans spoke of poison as a gendered crime committed by the weak against the strong: wives poisoning husbands, servants poisoning masters, cowardly men and effeminate courtiers resorting to poison to defeat stronger rivals.[3] This idea is so firmly rooted in western discourse that European-descended observers of eighteenth-century poison cases in the Americas, including antislavery activists, approached poison through this framework, focusing on enslaved people who allegedly poisoned their enslavers and describing them as usurpers of power and poison as a tool of the weak.

However, the link between poison and weakness was neither timeless nor universal. Consider, for example, the Kikongo concept of *kindoki*, the power to curse or protect—an extraordinary power held by both kings and "witches"—distinguished morally by how individuals *used* that power.[4] Or consider the political title *ndembu* some communities in the Kwanza River valley began giving their leaders after about 1000 CE, a word that meant both "lord" and "medicine" and that shared a root with "harmful sorcery."[5] In contrast to Europeans, people in West Central Africa by the emergence of the Atlantic period had built their discourse of poison around the idea of abuses of power committed by people with extraordinary spiritual abilities—the strong.

Much of the scholarly work on poison cases in the slave societies of the Americas has been conducted within a framework of resistance, implicitly drawing on the idea that enslaved people primarily used poison as a means to fight those in a more powerful position than themselves.[6] When we focus exclusively on poison as a "weapon of the weak," we are in danger of uncritically adopting the perspective of Europeans and missing the fuller and much more complex picture of how different people in the Atlantic world understood poison and poisoning cases. We need to examine how Africans and Europeans discussed and thought about poison, healing, and power, and how they changed their ideas over time, in order to understand how people in the Atlantic world transformed, wove together, and created new ideas.

Africans and Europeans developed different ontologies of "poison" centered on this issue of who could—and should—wield power and the moral responsibilities that came with it. Across these frameworks there were areas of convergence around ways of understanding "poison," for example, on the significance of tying and binding, that later facilitated translations and misunderstandings during the Atlantic period. This chapter will explore the discourses on poison in West Central Africa and Western Europe before contact in the fifteenth century, while the next chapter will examine how the ideas of Africans and Europeans interacted and transformed during the Atlantic period.

Roots

A deep chronology of the roots of ideas about "poison" is necessary for three reasons. First, change in language use is often slow and only visible from a significant distance. More recent changes and interactions between speakers of African and European languages from the mid-fifteenth century onward cannot be understood without examining what words meant to language speakers before those interactions. Second, in order to understand later cross-cultural contacts, one must first understand previous regional changes and histories of interaction between language speakers that continued to have an impact into the Atlantic period. Finally, the work of comparative historical linguistics requires going to the roots of a language family, to the protolanguage from which the relevant languages in an area descended, to understand their relationships to each other and how speakers changed the words they used over time (see Appendix A for greater detail). The comparative method uses the "skeleton" of these family trees to look for usage and nuances in word roots across a range of related languages; only then is it possible to reconstruct words rather than imposing definitions from extant languages onto earlier times.[7]

Classification trees in Appendix B show how the language families I work with in this chapter developed over time, including the Romance and Germanic languages in Western Europe and the Njila languages and Kikongo Language Cluster (KLC) in West Central Africa. I chose the Njila language family as it includes many (though not all) of the languages spoken by peoples involved in and affected by the transatlantic slave trade in the region, including well-known languages like Kimbundu and Umbundu. Speakers of the root, or mother, language, Proto-Njila, overlapped in time with speakers of Latin in Europe—allowing for a loosely comparable periodization. A list of word roots for each language family that I work with can be found in Appendix C. Reconstructed words are commonly identified as a "star" form with an asterisk, with hyphens isolating the root from prefixes or suffixes.[8] Noun class prefixes are an important feature in Bantu languages. Each noun class and its regular plural correspond to a semantic domain that can give historians valuable information on how a word was used and on categories of past thought.[9] For example, words in noun class one (and its regular plural, noun class two) fall in the semantic domain of human beings, proper names, and kinship terms.[10] For European word roots, I use the forms as they are given in etymological dictionaries.

Speakers of Romance languages in the Middle Ages and early modern periods—as well as English speakers, by way of French loanwords—drew from two very different inherited Latin roots to discuss poison, roots that Latin speakers respectively used to connect poison to drinking and to "sorcery." The noun *pōtiō*, root of the French *poison* and Portuguese *peçonha*, had several meanings: the act of drinking, especially wine; a drink; a potion "given as a medicine"; and a potion "given to procure death" or enchantment.[11] The connection between these potions to heal or kill—the word "potion" itself being derived from the same root—was that they were substances consumed by drinking, as the noun *pōtiō* itself came from the verb *pōtō* ("to drink, to swallow"). Latin speakers also used a root noun *uenēnum* ("a potent herb or other substance used for medical, magical, etc. purposes; a magic or supernatural influence; a poison; the use of poison, poisoning as a criminal offense").[12] From *uenēnum*, Latin speakers developed a whole suite of words, including a transitive verb *uenēno* ("to bewitch, enchant; to imbue or infect with poison"), a noun *uenēficum* ("the use of magical arts, sorcery; the act of poisoning; a potent or poisonous substance"), and the practitioner noun *uenēficus* ("sorcerer, poisoner—male or female").[13] Romans in the late republic were concerned enough about the actions of *uenefici* to develop a law in 81 BCE against *uenēficum* as an action causing sudden or unexpected death through hidden means of poison or sorcery, or both.[14]

The linguistic descendants of Latin speakers continued to elaborate and layer meanings onto *uenēnum* and *pōtiō*, while also innovating new words from Latin roots. French and Portuguese speakers continued to make the connection between sorcery and poison with *uenēnum* words well into the early modern period. Speakers of Old French made a significant innovation in their usage of *pōtiō* words in the twelfth century. While maintaining both medicinal and harmful connotations in the noun *puison*, by circa 1130 they created the verb *empoisonner* (to kill by poison). By the end of the thirteenth century, Old French speakers had further developed a new noun *empoisonneur/euse* (person who poisons). Both the earlier *poison* (n.) and the Old French innovations spread across the channel. In the fourteenth century, Anglo-Norman speakers had adopted *empoisoner* the verb, changing it to *poison* (v.), and developing their own practitioner noun by adding an extension, *poisoner* (person who poisons).[15] These innovations are significant for what they reveal about the concerns of speakers of Old French and Anglo-Norman. Both the verb and the practitioner noun had exclusively negative connotations—one would not use the verb *empoisonner* to mean "to give medicine," even if in Old French *poison* still had older connections to drinks that could be either healing or harmful—and the fact that people felt the need to create a word to describe individuals who poisoned suggests that they were a topic of particular concern.

In West Central Africa, several key roots to discuss a wide semantic web of health, healing, misfortune, and malevolence proved highly durable as speakers in the Njila and KLC families continued to pass down and make use of them. One of the most widespread and central of these roots was **-gàng-* (to tie up), with the major derivative nouns for the substance of healing **-gàngà* (medicine) and the practitioner **-gàngà* (expert, healer-diviner). These roots were *old*: the verb and derivative nouns were used by Proto-Bantu speakers thousands of years before their Proto-Njila-speaking descendants entered the river valleys of West Central Africa. They were also widespread: the core idiom linking health and affliction to the idea of tying/untying can be found expressed in words from this root across Bantu-speaking Africa, and I found attestations in most of the Njila and KLC languages I studied. When speakers of a language inherit and pass down word like *-gàng-, it tells a story of continuity; numerous people across a very wide area found this root useful, and so they continued to use it.

Durable does not mean unchanging: generations of language speakers layered on new meanings and creatively expanded semantic webs by developing new words from a shared root. A shared ancestor of Proto-Njila and Proto-KLC speakers made several key innovations to their inherited words on health and healing.[16] From a root verb *-bánd- (to split), they innovated a new verb "to heal, to cure" and noun "healing, curing."[17] They made a new semantic connection by layering "to be in good health" onto the verb *-kód- (to be strong, hard).[18] They also made a significant innovation to the verb *-dèmb- (to be tired, be weakened), layering on a new dominant meaning "to calm, sooth, pacify, tame," while also making several innovations with *-kác- (to dry up, coagulate, be hard) in the semantic domain of tying/untying and tightening, building on a similar knotty metaphor connecting this idea to affliction and healing made in the ancient root *-gàng-.[19]

The histories of words can paint a picture of the lives and cares of the people who used them and the inheritance that their descendants, such as Kimbundu speakers, worked with. Proto-Njila speakers living at the border between the savanna and equatorial rainforests of the Middle Kwilu River region around 500 BCE worried about people with access to extraordinary powers and their actions, layering a new meaning "to poison by means of nkisi spirits" to their inherited verb *-dòg- (to bewitch, to curse).[20] They spoke of *-gàngà expert healer-diviners as people who could tie or untie others and of healing at a most basic level as the act of tying or untying. Being metaphorically caught, tied up, and perhaps captive, those who suffered from malevolent afflictions were bound—endangering their strength and good health. Crucial as well to the maintenance of good health was the ability to *-dèmb- (to calm, tame, or, in a new meaning innovated by Proto-Njila speakers, "to beseech" angered ancestors).[21] As Proto-Njila speakers began moving south and west into the savanna, they also innovated a word for a new kind of specialist practitioner in healing craft. While continuing to discuss *-gàngà experts, they used a new noun *-bàndà (healer, diviner) incorporating the new meanings their linguistic ancestors had forged from the verb *-bánd- (to split). Just as people used the root *-gàng- to discuss both tying and untying, the use of *-bánd- could have entailed the metaphorical resonance of both splitting and binding.[22] As attestations for such a practitioner noun are absent in KLC but present in other branches of the Bantu family from more recent divergences, this noun was likely innovated after the split of the KLC branch from the Bantu tree.[23] The fact that Proto-Njila speakers felt the need to use this new specific title suggests that this kind of healing and divinatory work was important to them and required considerable expertise and likely specialization.

The changes speakers of Njila languages made to their vocabularies of healing and the timing of those changes—identified using sound change patterns and semantic distributions read through a classification tree—reveal a social history of ideas.[24] The construction of this history is intertwined with the history of Njila settlement: the spread of Njila languages across the West Central African savanna from circa 500 BCE to 1000 CE.[25] Beginning between approximately 500 BCE and 100 CE, Proto-Njila speakers who were the farthest apart from each other to the north and south came into less and less frequent contact, gradually developing their own idioms, innovations, and eventually their own languages. This process of divergence and the subsequent divergences between the descendants of Proto-Njila speakers were similar to the division of protolanguages from Latin; as with Romance languages, some modern Njila languages have a closer "genetic" relationship than others. Over roughly eight hundred years, speakers of Njila languages made a series of divergences as their languages spread over the savanna of present-day Angola.[26] The first was between Northern Njila and Southern Njila speakers. Northern Njila speakers who diverged between the Kwilu River valley—not far from the homeland of Proto-Njila speakers—and the Kwanza River valley respectively became Kwilu and Kwanza speakers. Speakers of these languages and their descendants stayed roughly in the vicinity of these river valleys up to the present. More than any other Njila speakers, Kwilu and Kwanza speakers were the closest to the KLC speakers who inhabited the lands around and just south of the Congo River.[27] Over the centuries these neighbors and distantly related "cousins" had extensive contact and mutual influence with each other, highlighting the importance of geographic relationships between speakers as well as "genetic" ones between languages.[28]

The descendants of Southern Njila speakers moved more frequently over a greater spread of land, diverging into more protolanguages than Njila speakers in the north. Soon after the divergence of Northern and Southern Njila, Southern Njila speakers diverged into Proto-Eastern Njila speakers, who lived near the headwaters and watersheds of the Kwango and Kasai Rivers, and Kunene speakers, who lived near the eponymous Kunene River in the more arid southwest. In the middle centuries of the first millennium, speakers of these protolanguages diverged further into Lunda Block and Moxico speakers in the east and Umbundo-Okavango and Cimbebasia speakers in the southwest. Finally, around 1000 CE, Moxico speakers diverged into Northern and Southern Moxico speakers.[29] With a few more recent subdivergences in between, the speakers of these subgroups—Kwilu, Kwanza, Lunda Block, Moxico, Umbundu-Okavango, and Cimbebasia—were the progenitors of the modern Njila languages spoken in the region today.[30]

It was beginning around 1000 CE that significant political transformations across these sub-branches of the Njila family tree shaped the key idioms that people used to discuss power, morality, and individuals with extraordinary abilities to heal or harm. The remainder of this chapter explores these major concepts along with a Western European counterpoint to set the stage for Atlantic interaction.

Key Concepts

Issues of power were at the core of both Western European and West Central African discourses about "poison," but in different ways. Over a period of roughly fifteen hundred years, Western Europeans elaborated on Latin speakers' gendered connections between poison and the usurpation of legitimate power. In West Central Africa, this history is at heart one of healing as both an institution for critiquing power and, crucially, as an institution of power that was critiqued. From circa 1000 to 1500 CE, people spoke and worried about the responsibilities of leaders to community health and their ability to threaten the same through an abuse of their powers.

For medieval Europeans, poison was the weapon of the weak, and the archetypal "weak" were women. As historian Franck Collard notes in his analysis of poison in this period, "An entire cultural heritage encouraged the male of the Middle Ages to attribute to women a proclivity for poisoning."[31] From classical Roman sources, to the Bible, to the literary trope of the princess as poisoner, to frequent real accusations against royal women, the idea of women using poison to usurp power that was not legitimately theirs was ubiquitous. The core concern was about poison being a means for people to illegitimately rise above their station and overturn the "natural" order of things.[32] Links between women and poison extended into medical theory and the work of physicians: venom (from *uenēnum*) permeated discussions of gender and the human body. These physicians described women's bodies as inverted, inferior, and even "poisonous" versions of men's bodies. The idea of women as literally physically poisonous dated back to Pliny, whose description of the negative effects of contact with menstruating women continued to reverberate in late medieval Europe.[33] A popular medical book from the late thirteenth or early fourteenth century described women as "so full of venom in their time of menstruation that they poison animals by their glance."[34] Celebrated twelfth-century Sephardic philosopher Maimonides cautioned men against the malicious activities of adulterous women, who could cause their husbands' limbs to fall off by mixing menstrual blood into their food.[35] The spiteful and malicious connotations expressed by "venom" were not incidental but central and gendered.

Europeans further elaborated their gendered discourse of poisonous women during the early modern witch hunts. A major development in late fifteenth-century theory on witchcraft shifted the nature of the alleged crime from causing physical harm to devil worship, making the explosion of witch trials possible: in the eyes of the law, witches were no longer merely felons but heretics.[36] European elites associated witchcraft with women based on the idea that the devil more often chose women as followers due to their weaker and more sinful nature.[37] However, there was a gap between popular and clerical concerns. The former considered witches as primarily causers of physical harm: vindictive and unnaturally powerful women, whose actions could possibly be combatted by other "cunning-men" and "wise-women." The latter considered witches as idolaters—women reaching back to Eve being more susceptible to satanic seduction—and any "counter-magic" used against them as also inherently demonic.[38]

In addition to and often in conjunction with witchcraft, Europeans gendered poison as a feminine crime—particularly disturbing as a subtle act that could by devious means upend the so-called natural authority of the strong.[39] Alleged acts of poison and witchcraft were linked in European thought. Witch-hunting manuals, including the notorious *Malleus Maleficarum* (1487), described witches learning how to make poisons through their pacts with the devil.[40] Fears of female witches—and their alleged skills in poisoning—were partially fears of the devil inverting the social order by giving women power.[41] Poison could be a powerful tool of inversion; medieval European law codes reaching back to the Theodosian Code singled out poison as a particularly horrible crime and primarily a form of treason fueled by "unmentionable and illegitimate ambitions."[42]

In contrast to this central focus on poison as a means for those who should not have power to usurp it, people in West Central Africa in the centuries before the Atlantic period worried about poison as an *abuse* of power by those who already had it. These concerns were central to conversations about leadership. Beginning around 1000 CE and continuing up to the arrival of the Europeans in the late fifteenth century, speakers of Njila languages and some of their KLC-speaking linguistic "cousins" implemented radical changes in governance. At the same time, they innovated, elaborated, and borrowed new words to discuss healing and affliction with each other. Institutions of healing *were* political institutions; people developed changes in leadership through the language of healing.[43] These transformations went hand in hand because for people in the West Central African savanna, healing had been and continued to be a collective enterprise. The maintenance and insurance of public health, as well as the punishment of threats to this health, were themselves acts of governance—even as the forms of governance and healing that people created took different forms in different regional contexts.

In the relatively densely populated fertile river valleys of western Angola, Kikongo speakers, Kimbundu speakers, Umbundu speakers, and other smaller groups around 1000 CE began innovating leadership roles that linked new titleholders with responsibilities for ensuring public health and prosperity. These leaders were accountable for maintaining good relationships among the living by arbitrating conflicts between villages, as well as between the living world and the spirit world.[44] People in western Angola continued to build on this connection between leadership and spirit powers as they formed powerful new kingdoms. In the late fourteenth century, Kikongo speakers in polities on the savanna just south of the Congo River came together to form the federated Kingdom of Kongo, whose king was powerful first and foremost as a spiritual leader.[45] Wyatt MacGaffey's anthropological work yields insights for historians on the nature of this durable—though not unchanging—connection between health and politics. MacGaffey highlights the role of leaders as "ritually qualified figures through whom occult powers of benefit to the community and their followers were controlled."[46] In this role, a leader was at once both a *nkisi* and a *nganga* as a container for power ("as much object as person") and an expert in wielding that power.[47] Discussions of *minkisi* used to bring about various ends—mainly to improve well-being in this world for individuals and wider communities—have also been conversations about legitimacy in governance and power.[48]

West Central Africans had long discussed the prosecution of "witches"—here meaning people who abused their powers for selfish ends rather than the European idea of a "witch"—as an essential aspect of leadership, but people in these central river valleys also began to describe these powerful new rulers themselves as a potential and particularly threatening source of misfortune. In other words, they worried that their kings could be self-serving witches. As discussed above, the connections between the power to afflict and the power to heal in the root *-dòg- were ancient; what was new was an intensification of the links between this morally ambiguous power and political leadership roles. Kings of Kongo held this power of *kindoki* (power to curse or protect, described by MacGaffey as "the exercise of power in social relations") that shared the same root as *ndoki* (witch)—both ideas deriving from *-dòg- (to bewitch, to curse).[49] People made connections between leadership and potential harm with other roots as well. For example, Kwanza speakers—or possibly their Kimbundu-speaking descendants—innovated and used a noun *kilemba* for "negative or harmful sorcery (malefício)," employing the same root they had used to elaborate the *ndembu* title of leadership.[50]

Layered alongside the powers of new political leaders after circa 1000 CE were older and continuing networks of extraordinary people who had their own connections to the spirit world: particularly blacksmiths, hunters, and diviners.[51] In some ways, titles and political institutions overlapped with the power of these occupations of authority. The emergence of blacksmiths as culture heroes and the metaphorical connection between blacksmiths and political power is very well known to historians and anthropologists of Central Africa.[52] In the objects of power or "charms of office"—often made of iron—that gave rulers legitimacy to perform their duties of maintaining public health and ensuring the fertility of the land, people made concrete connections between the powerful work of smiths, diviners, and kings. For example, people in the Kwanza basin innovated and quickly spread the word *ngola* for both iron objects of power and a title for the kings of Ndongo (this word is also the root for the name of the Portuguese colony and modern country of Angola). For some of the descendants of Proto-Njila speakers, the root of this word, identified by Jan Vansina as *-kód- (to be strong, be hard), also continued to carry the connotations "to be in good health" and the causative "to make strong."[53] By discussing the kings of Ndongo in this way, people in the Kwanza basin made semantic connections and expectations between strong leadership and good health.[54]

Speakers of Njila languages in both the growing western kingdoms and the decentralized societies in what is now eastern Angola elaborated their roots on healing to discuss governance and power—even as the forms of governance after circa 1000 CE took significantly different paths. From the end of the first millennium to circa 1600, the descendants of Kwilu and Proto-Eastern speakers gradually developed and elaborated networks of societies based on age and gender that cut across clusters of small villages. These sodalities organized initiations as important rites of passage into these societies. People further expanded these networks into hierarchical oligarchies of "big men" and elders in the northeast and small polities led by "big men" in the Kwilu basin.[55] Some of the words they used to discuss initiation and governance overlapped with *-kítì and *-gàng- roots connected to spirit power and healing.[56]

People in both the west and the east found the near homophonic roots *-dèmb- (to calm, pacify, sooth, tame) and *-dìmb- (to trap by birdlime) productive for discussing power and how it could be used.[57] The sticky substance used to make birdlime came from a shady species of ficus tree connected to ancestors; the word was so widely attested in both Njila and KLC languages that I suspect it was used by a common ancestor of speakers of both language families. This tree—more specifically a cutting from an older tree— was commonly planted at the center of every new village and was a powerful symbol of leadership across the western savannas.[58] Kwanza speakers likely used the near homophony to innovate the new title, ndembu, that was both a political title for "lord" and a noun for "remedy, medicine."[59] With the final suffix—u, indicating a noun of quality derived from an adjective and in turn derived from a verb—ndembu could have been understood as "calmed person/medicine."[60] With this connotation, they would have spoken of their leaders and their medicines as both powerful and potentially dangerous— someone or something that had been "calmed." Further north, Kwilu speakers developed several new nouns, including *-lèmbà (from *-dìmb-) for "ancestor, grandparent, elder" and *-lémbà for "maternal uncle, chief of a clan, notable, pl. ancestors" and the "condition of the chief of a clan, his power."[61] Vansina describes this new *-lémbà "lineage leader" as a powerful "big man," coming from the ideas of placating, making a gift, and paying bridewealth (a payment made from the prospective groom to the bride's family). A *-lémbà leader—usually a maternal uncle, specifically the oldest brother of the resident mother—had an important economic role as the person who negotiated bridewealth and managed the estate.[62]

Central to these changes in governance were arguments about the respon-sibilities of leadership—how the strong with access to extraordinary powers should use those powers for communitarian ends. For the people who inno-vated and began using the term *-lémbà in the region between the Kwango and Kwilu Rivers between approximately 1200 and 1500 CE, the importance of amassing wealth to distribute to followers and manage bridewealth was connected to prosperity from the flourishing trade routes with KLC speak-ers around the Congo River.[63] When Kwilu speakers used their *-dèmb- verb ("to beseech, ask for"), they directed their requests to these powerful people, living or dead. From the same root, Cokwe speakers later developed a pair of verbs lembwisa (to subject, tr.) and lembwa (to be subject), describing these new political relationships.[64] Furthermore, people in the east connected these new ideas of governance to healing through the maintenance of rela-tionships with spirits. Most directly, Lwena speakers began using a new *-dèmb- verb, -lembeka (to consecrate with lilembu medicine), and the noun lilembu for this medicine itself in connection to kula (ancestors of elders), specifically contained in a calabash bowl or worn as leaves on the head.[65] Furthermore, in addition to the sacred mulemba tree connected to ances-tors, Pende speakers innovated a new compound word from *-dèmb-, gilem-biangola, to describe a "sacred enclosure" and a specific plant, translated as "sacred fence of Ngola king of the Pende and Angola."[66]

Discussions on the proper use of power were also important in the south—present-day southern Angola, northern Namibia, and northwestern Botswana—even as it was in many ways a different world. As Cimbebasia speakers and their descendants moved farther and farther south, to the arid edges of the Kalahari Desert, they developed forms of governance centered on cattle and rainmaking, a contrast to other Njila-speaking agricultural-ists.[67] As the climate in the region became even drier in the thirteenth century, cattle herders developed new forms of governance centered on nomadic patri-archal management of the herds and a tight social hierarchy that revolved around owners and tenants of cattle.[68] In adapting to new environments and in their encounters with new non-Bantu-speaking neighbors to the far south, Cimbebasia speakers and their descendants also abandoned or significantly altered many of the roots relating to health and healing that their ancestors had used. Cimbebasia speakers dropped almost all *-kítì and *-dèmb- words, with only a handful of surviving attestations of each in Kwanyama.

Of the practitioner nouns, people did continue to use the durable *-gàngà, but dropped or radically altered the innovations their ancestors had made with words like *-bàndà; however, even here people made links between these ancient roots and powerful people. The following attestations from Herero are difficult to date: I have found the associated meanings only in a single language, preventing the comparative historical linguistic method. In other words, Herero speakers could have innovated them at any point between the likely divergence of the Herero sub-branch from their close linguistic relatives in approximately the fourteenth century and when these words were recorded in a nineteenth-century dictionary.[69] With this caution in mind, the ways that Herero speakers discussed *-bàndà are intriguing for how they amplified new exceptional qualities of power while dropping all explicit connections to healing and divining that their linguistic ancestors had used. Among the Herero, a new ombande ("hero") or ombanda ("conqueror, a brave, unflinching one") could be described as ombande ("bold, brave, heroic") or ombandi ("active, alert, ardent, cheerful, determined, dexterous, earnest, energetic, industrious, smart, a painstaking or quick worker"). They did their actions oty'ombande ("boldly"), and others could yerura kombanda ("exalt, praise") their ouvande ("bravery").[70] The figure of the brave conquering hero at first seems a significant departure from the prototypical meaning of a *-bàndà healer-diviner; however, this idea maintains the strong connection to social power. Herero speakers created unique layers of meaning to talk about ombanda, but they did so as part of a very long and fraught conversation on the use of power by powerful people.

From the pastoral patriarchies of the south to the village sodalities of the east to the expanding kingdoms of the western river valleys, West Central Africans developed discourses of healing as a province of power—power that could be abused. Ideas about poison, healing, and power were intertwined with political changes because they were themselves political.

If speakers of Western European and West Central African languages differed strongly in how they discussed relationships between poison and power—whether as a weapon of the weak or an abuse of power by the strong—their ideas on the emotional significance of "poison" converged in interesting ways. Malice and negative social interactions were deeply embedded in European discourse of poison. For example, thirteenth-century Portuguese speakers used peçonha for both a "venomous secretion of certain animals" and a figurative connection to "malice"—in other words, the same way that Old French speakers and their descendants used venin (venom).[71] Potentially fraught social relationships are at the center of the Germanic root for poison as a "gift," given transitively from one person to another like an iconic poisoned apple. Old High German, Old Dutch, and Old English speakers—living in approximately the seventh to the eleventh century—had a common ancestor of West Germanic, but they did not use their inherited poison/gift vocabulary in the same ways. Old English speakers used *gift* to refer specifically to "payment for a wife"; speakers of descendant languages used *gift* in the senses of "the action of giving" and "the thing given." They did not use *gift* words with any connotation of poison.[72] Old High German speakers had a verb *këpan/gëban* (to give) from which they derived a noun, *gift* (with a dual meaning of "gift/present" and "poison"); a more specific noun, *firgift* (poison); a verb, *farkepan* (to hand over, forgive, safeguard); and a verb, *fargiftjan* (to inflict poison). The prefix *ver-* (Proto-Germanic **far-*) had several uses, including indicating an action resulting from the stem (for example, from *këpan*, as in "to give," to *farkepan*, as in "to hand over, forgive, safeguard"). It could also be used to indicate a negative connotation: while *gift* could mean either a gift or a poison, *firgift* was exclusively negative. Middle High German speakers from the eleventh to the fifteenth century continued to use *gëben*, *gift*, *vergift*, *vergëben*, and *vergiften*. They also developed a new practitioner noun, *vergifter* (poisoner), and a new adjective, *vergiftic* (poisonous, poisoned), from which they later created another verb, *vergiftigen* (to poison).[73]

Intriguingly, when discussing "poison," Middle Dutch speakers generally chose to use a French loanword laden with connotations of malice rather than an inherited Germanic word: *venijn* (poison, malice). Middle Dutch speakers did use their inherited noun *gift*—but only with the connotation of "donation" rather than "poison"—and the verb *vergheven* (to give away, remit, give forgiveness). The earliest recorded use of *vergif* (poison) in Dutch was only at the end of the Middle Dutch period (attestation 1485). Middle Dutch speakers in the late fifteenth century derived *vergif* from *vergheven* with the focus on giving/administering something. Early Modern Dutch speakers in the early sixteenth century began using their existing vocabulary in new ways, including *gif* (poisonous substance)—which Middle Dutch speakers had not previously used to refer to poison. While Middle High German speakers had used a poison adjective, the first Dutch attestation of *vergiftig* (poisonous) was not until circa 1500.[74] The fact that Middle Dutch speakers did not develop or borrow a practitioner noun relating to poison, in contrast with Middle High German and Romance language speakers of the same period, perhaps suggests a lesser degree of concern with poisoners. However, the changes in the late fifteenth and early sixteenth centuries point to a moment of transition toward increased interest and concern about poison.

Greed, selfishness, and negative social emotions were also central to West Central African discourse on poison in the centuries before the Atlantic period. With the power to maintain public health associated with new forms of leadership came the responsibility to identify and punish threats to that health, particularly in the form of people who abused their power for selfish reasons—"witches." Ideas about witchcraft as a crime of greed and envy were both widespread and very old in West Central Africa.[75] In addition to words derived from *-dòg- (to bewitch), speakers of Njila and KLC languages made connections between judicial activities and other roots relating to healing, harming, and leadership. For example, Kikongo speakers used the following verb and compound from *-gàng- (to tie up): kànga (to tie up, to harden, to imprison) and kànga nsatu (to have a voracious hunger).[76] The ideas of "voracious hunger" and "tying up" also connected to ideas about witches as the exploitative and powerful people who ate the souls of the living for personal gain; the fact that these specific words came from the same root as *-gàngà (expert, healer-diviner) points to an ambivalence regarding the extraordinary powers possessed by these specialists and the ways they could use or misuse them.[77]

Western Europeans and West Central Africans also developed similar idioms through the conceptual metaphor of power as tying/untying. A quick glance at some derivatives in English from the Latin root ligare (to bind, tie) highlight aspects of this metaphor of binding power—ligature, oblige, liaison, liable, reliability, religion. The idea of being bound to or by something resonates strongly in the context of social obligations (another derivative), with power embedded in these relationships. In West Central Africa—and indeed across much of the Bantu-speaking regions of the continent, as people from the equatorial rainforests to the east coast to the southern savannas inherited and continued to use *-gàng- (to tie up) and its derivative *-gàngà (expert, healer-diviner)—"tying up" was a durable way to talk about power and affliction.

The material aspects of the metaphor—the act of physically binding something together—also resonated through the material culture of power objects that proliferated in both pre-Atlantic Europe and Africa. Indeed, the main root that Ibero-Romance-speaking ancestors of Portuguese speakers used to describe both "poison/sorcery" and power objects used to prevent or treat it focused on this bound materiality. Instead of using words from pōtiō to form a verb and practitioner noun for the act of poisoning the way Old French and Anglo-Norman speakers did, Portuguese speakers elaborated on their inherited Latin root *factīcius* (manufactured, prepared, artificial) to create *feitiço* (spell, charm, something used to seduce) and *feitiçaria* (sorcery). From the root verb *facīo*, whose dozens of meanings included "to make, build, construct, cause, achieve," a *factīcius* thing was the product of a deliberate act of creation.[78] Portuguese speakers first recorded their use of *feitiço* and *feitiçaria* in a legal context, as part of antisorcery legislation from 1385 and 1403.[79] As anthropologist Roger Sansi has explored, these terms carry within them both ambiguity over what is real and what has been falsely constructed, as well as an idea of "sorcery" as an act of seduction—a way of swaying others to one's creative will. In the late Middle Ages, Portuguese speakers crafted *feitiço* amulets from powerful objects, like broken mirrors and pieces of hangman's rope, to protect themselves from potential danger and to influence their relationships with other people.[80]

Ideas about bound-up power objects in the Iberian Peninsula—and, more indirectly, across the rest of Europe—were significantly influenced by the Muslim presence in the region from 711 to the 1492 conquest of Granada.[81] Iberia in the Middle Ages—al-Andalus in Arabic—was a place of cohabitation not only for people of many faiths but also of many geographic origins. The eighth-century Muslim founders of al-Andalus were themselves a diverse combination of Arabs, Berbers, and sub-Saharan Africans; the Moroccan-based, eleventh-century Almorovid Islamic revival movement also had roots in the West African empire of Wagadou (also known as Ghana). Muslim practitioners from North and West Africa made popular talismans containing paper with Arabic writing tied up in pouches and tied to the body of the client.[82] Links between Moors and occult power had a long resonance in the folkways of the Iberian Peninsula. In the Kingdom of Portugal from the reconquest in the thirteenth century through the eighteenth century, common people told stories of *mouras encantadas*—Moors, especially women, who were reputed to have vast stores of occult powers for healing and locating legendary buried treasure allegedly left behind by the retreating Muslims.[83] This existing folk association between people of African descent and secret knowledge would have significant implications for healing practices in Portugal during the centuries of the Atlantic period and the ideas of the Portuguese at home and abroad in the Atlantic world.

In West Central Africa, binding together objects and networks of extraordinary people were ways to enact power that were central to the philosophy of good leadership.[84] If power in concept was morally fraught, then so was power in action through tying/binding. Europeans were primarily concerned with the *source* of power and who should or should not have it; West Central Africans worried about the *intentions* of the powerful and why they tied or untied with it. As Kathryn de Luna succinctly notes, "In the context of a moral philosophy whereby every affliction had a divinable cause and every personal gain came at the expense of others, the morality of tying was determined by intent: healing versus personal gain (witchcraft)."[85]

While they differed significantly in their views on the relationship between poison and power, both Western Europeans and West Central Africans in the centuries before the Atlantic period developed forums for creating narratives about poison, including rituals and institutions. In Europe in the Middle Ages and Renaissance, scholarly treatises were one such forum where elites debated occult virtues, demonic and natural properties, and what constituted "superstition."[86] As part of these debates, these scholars sought to create a definitive understanding on the nature and prevention of poison. For example, Maimonides wrote prolifically on a wide range of subjects, including his *Book on Poisons and the Protection Against Lethal Drugs* (1198). One of his eleven titles on medicine, this treatise combined knowledge of both Greco-Roman and Islamic medical theory, as well as practical advice based on his personal experience as a court physician in Cairo.[87] Maimonides's work on poisons became well-known and influential among scholars in Western Europe; in the century after his death three separate Latin translations of *On Poisons* were made and circulated.[88] French physicians in the fourteenth century used Maimonides's work as the basis for their own medical treatises and commentaries on poisons. Many of his specific remedies—such as the rapid consumption of oil or milk to both induce vomiting and to "coat" the poison, or the topical application of a *bezoar* (a stone taken from the stomach of a goat)—were included in the later boom of poison treatises of the eighteenth and early nineteenth centuries.[89]

Poison trials had a long history in medieval and early modern Europe, even as the focus and form of those trials changed over time. In several instances in the Middle Ages, practitioners who believed a person to have been poisoned conducted tests of the substances suspected to be "poisonous" on animals to see if they could have been the cause of death. Such tests reached back to the works of Galen testing poisons on roosters. These tests helped build narratives of specific cases: was a substance "poison," and did it cause the death in question? Poison also sometimes appeared as one of a range of ordeals, including trial by combat, that could be undertaken to try to determine guilt or innocence—ordeals that Pope Innocent III outlawed in 1215.

By the Renaissance, court physicians began testing proposed antidotes on condemned criminals while their nemeses—empirical street practitioners—demonstrated powerful cures to poison on their own bodies through public performances.[90] Such demonstrations also constructed narratives about the efficacy of various potions and other powerful substances, with both poisons and counterpoisons as things consumed or applied. From the sixteenth century onward, a wider world of exotic drugs greatly expanded the repertoire of such experimentation.

Rituals used to identify "poisoners" appear frequently in descriptions of West Africa and West Central Africa from the Atlantic period; word histories suggest that forms of such trials may have had a longer history. For example, speakers of several KLC languages used words from the ancient root *-kác- (to dry up, coagulate, be hard) to talk about poison ordeals—ritual judicial proceedings involving the swearing of an oath and a test of innocence through the consumption of a draught made from the bark of the tree *Erythrophleum suaveolens* (called *nkasa* by later Kikongo speakers).[91] It is plausible that the regional spread of this term for this ordeal—wielding a powerful "poison" for communitarian ends—had a relationship with the rise of the Kingdom of Kongo. With the elaboration of extensive trade networks in the region from circa 1200 to 1500 and the emergence of the Kingdom of Kongo as a regional power in the late fourteenth century, people living beyond the kingdom itself began adopting Kikongo words and prestigious Kongolese institutions.[92] The later presence of a powerful officer in charge of administering poison ordeals and advising the king in sixteenth-century Loango north of the Congo River is suggestive of both the widespread use of such poison ordeals and the connections between them and political power.[93]

*   *   *

The story these words from Western European and West Central African languages tell is one of power, who held it, and how they wielded it. For Europeans, poisoning was an illegitimate usurpation of power, a tool for the weak—especially women—to access power that did not rightfully belong to them. In West Central Africa, speakers of KLC and Njila family languages conducted a centuries-long conversation on the fraught relationship between healing and power with a focus on how extraordinary people used their abilities—for communal or selfish ends. The forms and metaphors of power through social relationships and acts of binding created possibilities for later convergences, and both Europeans and Africans developed ways to identify and create narratives about poisoning events. Understanding this story of power and its manifestations is necessary for understanding the subsequent interactions between Europeans, Africans, and their descendants in Atlantic spaces.

The distinguished historian of late antiquity Peter Brown once spoke of varieties in intellectual and cultural conversations over time as a "braided river."[94] Western European and West Central African discourses on poison flowed through significant changes over time on their separate courses before extensive cross-cultural contact, each with their own tributaries and meandering divergences. With the emergence of the Atlantic world in the late fifteenth century, the rivers of poisoning cultures began to intertwine.

CHAPTER 2

Cross-Cultural Exchanges and Poison

Francisco de Buitrago believed he had made a discovery of great significance: a new tool to combat demons.[1] He was a knight of the Order of Christ—a highly prestigious order that had included Henry the Navigator and Vasco da Gama—and a cavalry officer stationed in Angola from 1692 to 1718. In 1731 he drafted a manuscript on the uses of what he dubbed the "tree of life" in an effort to enter the realm of European intellectuals interested in bioprospecting and *materia medica*—materials that could be used to fight afflictions, including those believed to be caused by demonic agency.[2] He claimed to have spent a significant amount of time observing the work of health practitioners in Angola and the Kingdom of Kongo and asking them questions. It was through these connections, and through enslaved informants in Angola, that he learned about the "greatly esteemed" *cassa* tree, "the most singular counterpoison that there is in the whole world."[3] Buitrago saw healers use this small yellow tree with thick bark like a pine to cure a man who was greatly swollen from "malifícios" [sic] (evil spells) and noted the bark's efficacy against "feitiços" and "veneno."[4] Furthermore, Buitrago reported that people used this bark preventively, possibly in amulets or charms, to keep *feitiços* from reaching their target. Based on the bark's powerful and proven efficacy in the work of these healers—which Buitrago interpreted as casting out demons— he enthusiastically promoted its adoption in exorcisms.[5] Unfortunately, it appears that inquisitorial censors may have been less enthusiastic as Buitrago's work was never published; the Inquisition generally frowned on amateur exorcists.[6]

Buitrago's account of the "tree of life" is fascinating, but it is only part of the story. Based on his description and the term "cassa," he was very likely referring to the tree *Erythrophleum suaveolens*—called *nkasa* by Kikongo speakers in the nineteenth and twentieth centuries. Kikongo speakers used this tree and associated words from the same root to discuss ordeal draughts—beverages made to test the innocence of those accused of a crime—as well as the toxic bark used both for these ordeals and as a fishing poison.[7] The history of the ancient root of this word, *-kác- (to dry up, coagulate, be hard), among the linguistic ancestors of Kikongo speakers and their "cousins" in the Njila language family farther south reveals a long and fraught discussion of poison, affliction, acts of binding, and power.[8] Furthermore, very likely this same tree and its use in similar poison ordeals appeared in European descriptions of practices in seventeenth- and eighteenth-century West Africa. Buitrago's story is an illustrative window into the relationships between poison, healing, and power and how they changed over time in Atlantic Africa and Europe.

Cross-cultural interaction was a crucial and defining aspect of the Atlantic period. These interactions between Africans and Europeans began in the half-century before Columbus's 1492 transatlantic voyage and continued through the nineteenth century. The ideas of early modern Europeans and Atlantic Africans impacted each other, extending beyond early encounters into transformative effects over time.[9] This analysis is more than a prelude for that of poison cases in the eighteenth-century Americas; it is not simply a story of antecedents in the east that then moved west. Nor is it a study of "Atlantic Creoles" as a body of Atlantic Africans inhabiting a culture of fusion; as Roquinaldo Ferreira has argued, this conceptual category is too rigid to reflect the ways that people circumstantially adopted, adapted, and tapped into a range of practices.[10] If the previous chapter argued that African and European ideas on poison, healing, and the morality of power were regionally dynamic in the centuries before extensive contact, this chapter points to the processes of transformation and borrowing defined by cross-cultural interaction in the Atlantic period and embedded in this deeper context of change and continuity. Atlantic Africans and Europeans incorporated and domesticated new ideas into durable yet flexible frameworks for thinking about poison.[11]

I am not currently able to sketch West Africans' changes to their ideas about poison through their words over a deep time scale as I did for Western Europe and West Central Africa. Without the numerous written sources that make European philology possible, or the extensive published historical linguistic records of Bantu languages that I have for West Central Africa, at this time I have the sources to speak primarily to changes in West Africa over the early modern period.[12] My research for West Africa draws from a combination of three kinds of sources: descriptions from early modern European observers, analyses of word roots from dictionaries compiled in the nineteenth and twentieth centuries, and twentieth-century ethnography. As with all historical sources, each has its own flaws. Recognizing their uses and limitations, I compare and triangulate between them. I am not using the recent anthropological work to fill in the past with an ethnographic present; rather, this ethnographic work is useful for corroborating evidence from other sources and for fleshing out dictionary definitions. I cannot guarantee that people used the same words in nineteenth- and twentieth-century dictionaries or ethnographic work as they did in the Atlantic period, nor can I—without comparative historical linguistics—pinpoint the antiquity of word innovations. However, the conceptual connections between the roots of recently attested words can suggest important insights into the ways past peoples of West Africa discussed poison. There are also several challenges to using European narratives, as these observers filtered what they saw through the lens of their own changing ideas. Furthermore, Europeans visiting Africa had often read earlier European accounts and set their expectations accordingly. To help mitigate these challenges, I am only using firsthand accounts.

Indeed, many of the exchanges of ideas at the center of this chapter were written by Europeans who were in Atlantic Africa like Buitrago; these moments of ethnographic observation were themselves sites of exchange and not merely neutral recordings of evidence.[13] Buitrago's manuscript on the "tree of life" is one of thousands of such spaces of encounter—encounters that refracted the ideas of multiple actors based on what they expected to see. Gaps in perspective opened spaces for misunderstanding as well as convergence, such that multiple parties could come to similar conclusions about alleged poisonings for different reasons. The term "poison" itself in European linguistic manifestations held such strong connotations of illegitimate usurpation of power and a moral distinction from "medicine" that Europeans struggled to understand how this (mis)translation failed to fully encompass Atlantic African categories and ideas on the morality of power. This chapter, then, is as much about cross-cultural misunderstanding as it is about engagement.

Exchanging and (Mis)Interpreting Ideas About "Poison"

Discussions of cross-cultural exchanges in the Atlantic must begin by recognizing the internal exchanges between West Africans, who were far from hermetically sealed off from each other in the centuries before European arrival.[14] With important environmental differences between narrow bands of ecological zones from the Sahel to the savannas to the coastal forests, the history of West Africa had long been one of vibrant cross-cultural connections and trade. Caravans run by Mande speakers centered on the large trading cities and empires of the Sahel intersected with riverine networks, exchanging desert salt for gold and kola seeds. In forging these trading relationships, people developed ways of accommodating and incorporating traveling merchants.[15] Furthermore, many people were multilingual and interacted frequently with other groups. Indeed, throughout the Middle Ages, the West African Sahel was the center of not only major regional but transregional trade, as merchants, scholars, pilgrims, and captives circulated through trans-Saharan networks as part of the wider Islamic world.[16] During the era of the transatlantic slave trade, violence from wars and raiding spurred new exchanges through the formation of refugee communities. Some, like the collection of peoples between the empires of Dahomey and Oyo in the early eighteenth century who began calling themselves Mahi, created new languages and practices in this shatter zone.[17] This interconnectedness of West Africa, despite regional differences, is important to understanding overlaps and shared ideas about health, healing, and affliction.

While there were dozens of languages spoken between Senegambia and the Bight of Biafra in the early modern period, the main languages of interest for West African peoples connected to the Atlantic world fell into four related subgroups of the Niger-Congo language family: Atlantic (for example, Wolof, Fula, Limba), Mande (for example, Bambara, Malinke), Kwa (for example, Akan—with recent language divergences into Fante and Twi, and Gbe—with recent language divergences into Ewe, Fon, Aja, and Mahi), and Western Benue-Congo (for example, Yoruba, Igbo).[18] Geographically, in the early modern period, speakers of languages in the Atlantic family lived in the Senegambia and the Sierra Leone coastal regions—with Fula-speaking nomadic pastoral communities extending along the Niger River valley; speakers of Mande languages lived along the Sahel in the West African interior; speakers of Kwa languages lived along the Gold Coast and Bight of Benin; and speakers of languages from the West-Benue-Congo family lived in the Bight of Biafra and the interior of what is now Nigeria.[19]

Words and the ways past people used them to articulate their hopes, fears, and concerns are essential to understanding a long history of regional exchanges in ideas about health and affliction. In the words they developed to

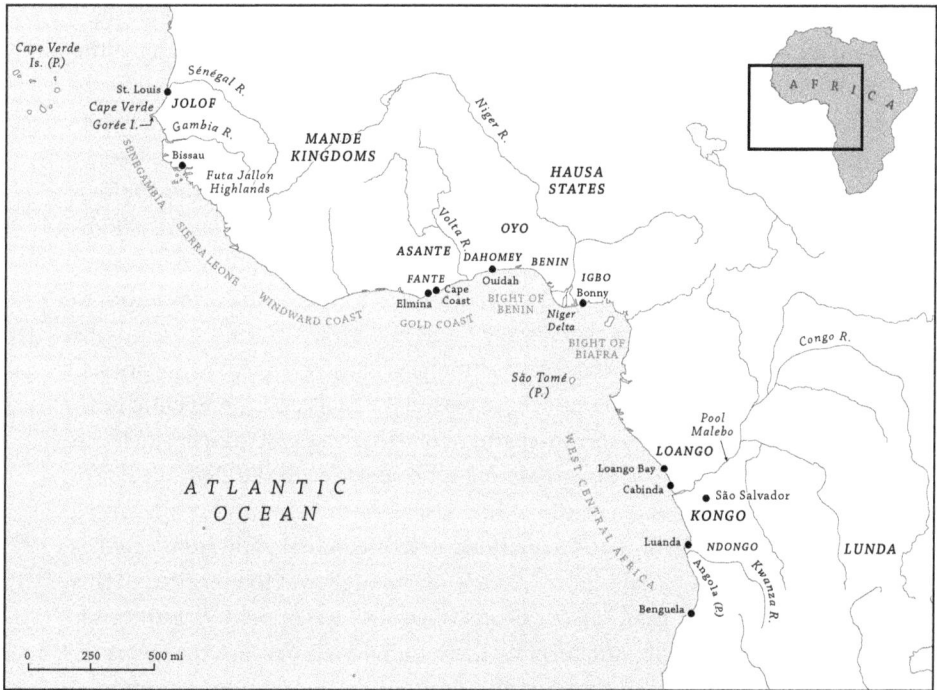

Figure 2. Map of Atlantic Africa, c. 1700. Erin Greb Cartography.

discuss harm caused by malevolent manipulation of power and efforts to prevent or treat it, West Africans made strong links between poisoning and
emotions. Like Europe and West Central Africa, West Africa was part of
and transformed by the expansion of connections to the Atlantic world;
people in West Africa became increasingly concerned with abuses of power
during the Atlantic period in connection with the violence of the transatlantic slave trade.[20]

Many of the rituals observed by Europeans in the late seventeenth and
eighteenth centuries centered on the maintenance of public health, often
in relation to seasonal events or in response to crises such as disease or war. In
the days before the rice harvest in Rio Sestro in the early 1680s, French slave
trader Jean Barbot observed a public ritual of sacrificing and feeding hens to
"their fetiche," a small shrine with a thick, human-shaped statue.[21] Likewise,
Willem Bosman, a Dutch West India Company merchant living on the Gold
Coast from 1688 to 1702, described divinatory rituals and sacrifices conducted

by practitioners before important public decisions on wars or major travel.[22] Perhaps the most well-known public healing cults surrounded Dangbe the snake in pre-Dahomean Ouidah. Dangbe was one of many *vodun*—frequently interpreted by these European observers as a "god" or "devil"—but more accurately described as a spirit force or power capable of impacting the lives of the living.[23] In times of fevers, people in late seventeenth-century Ouidah also made offerings to specific powerful *vodun* trees to restore health.[24] Public sacrifices of animals to "feed" benevolent spirits and soothe malevolent ones, predominantly conducted and performed by men, were also central to practices among Igbo speakers in the Bight of Biafra.[25]

Across West Africa, specialist practitioners, usually referred to as "priests" by Europeans, performed both these seasonal rituals and therapeutic healings. At least in late seventeenth-century Ouidah, these practitioners included both men and women, though among Igbo speakers in the Bight of Biafra they were usually men.[26] While in Rio Sestro, Barbot met and spoke with a local practitioner, who was "acquainted with medicinal plants and acted as a doctor to all his parishioners." People only sought out the services of this "greatly respected" man "on occasions when they felt in peril."[27] Europeans and locals alike sought out cures by these individuals because they were often effective.[28] Bosman begrudgingly admitted as much in his description of practitioners' successful use of the Gold Coast pharmacopoeia in ways that seemed counterintuitive to Galenic medicine: "How contradictory and improper soever these Med'cines may seem . . . I have seen several of our Country Men cured by them, when our own Physicians were at a loss what to do."[29] These practitioners on the Gold Coast charged some form of payment for their services, usually paid by the relatives of the patient and proportional to their means.[30]

West Africans discussed these practitioners as people particularly gifted in communications with the spirit world, as divination to determine causes and cures were a central part of healing.[31] The connection between healing and divination was embedded in the words people used to discuss these practitioners. Bosman referred to a "Feticheer" or "Priest" he observed on the Gold Coast as "confoe"—*o-kòmfó* in late nineteenth-century Twi. Twi speakers very likely derived this term from their verb *kom* (to be possessed with a "fetish" or to perform the practice of a "fetish man") along with related words for the state of being possessed, a revelation, and a child born through the help of a "fetish."[32] Twentieth-century Fon speakers similarly discussed *bokɔnɔ* practitioners as diviners, healers, and interpreters of *fa* (spirit and art of divination).[33] In the Bight of Biafra, Igbo speakers used the term *diaba* to describe specialists with a strong connection to spirits and expertise in both herbal knowledge and divination.[34] These practitioners were generally described as people of morally neutral power, who could choose to use it for communal or selfish ends.

European observers in West Africa described several common healing practices similar to their own; however, close attention to such spaces of convergence point to distinctly different ideas on what such practices meant and how they worked. Mary Hicks's work on bloodletting (phlebotomy) highlights this phenomenon. Phlebotomy on the Iberian Peninsula had deep roots in European medical traditions, centered on the Hippocratic-Galenic idea of restoring humoral balance. In contrast, multiple West African practices emphasized the "empowered word" in tandem with bloodletting: Yoruba speakers, for example, made incantations and used iron knives in both gathering healing plants and making incisions to invoke the *orixa* Ogun. In other words, the healing power of this practice was conditionally efficacious and rooted in speech: "Without '*Ohùn*' ('speech,' 'voice,' or 'the performed word') neither *Èpe* (the malevolent component of life-force), nor *Àse* (the largely beneficent component of life-force)—two sides of the same coin—can fulfill its mission."[35] Bloodletting was also common practice in West Central Africa, and the resemblances between Atlantic African and Portuguese practices facilitated exchanges.[36] However, while the practices themselves were similar, the underlying theories of *why* bloodletting gave relief were significantly different between Europeans and Atlantic Africans.[37]

Speakers of different West African languages innovated and used the same roots within their respective languages to discuss what Europeans separated into "medicine" and "poison"—often connecting them through a discussion of form, such as powders. For Fon and Ewe speakers, the very ancient root *-ti-* (tree) plays a prominent role. The root *-ti-* was not only widespread in West Africa; it is also a major root inherited into the Bantu language family—a sub-branch of the Niger-Congo tree.[38] In Fon, the noun *àtí* was used with modifications to discuss all trees and was also specifically used to discuss "medicinal powder made with plants" and "poison."[39] Speakers of both languages used words from this same root to discuss health practitioners and the charms they made with *-ti-* medicine in them.[40] When Twi speakers used *aduru* to discuss both medicines and poisons, the connection was in the noun's primary meaning of "powder." In other words, medicines and poisons were essentially both powdered things. Igbo speakers used the noun *juju*—from the verb *a-juju* ("to ask") and represented as *ọgwù* in modern Igbo—as an umbrella term for things with power, from shrines to medicines to poisons (treated separately in English).[41] In modern Igbo, this word is part of the compound verbs -*gwọ ọgwù* ("to prepare medicine"), -*kọ ọgwù* ("to practice sorcery against"), and -*rụ ọgwù* ("to neutralize effect of poison"). A compound noun from modern Igbo suggests the kinds of afflictions that might have required such treatment: *ọgwū ūde* ("native medicine prepared and stored in a bottle with palm kernel oil, used for curing convulsions, poisoning"). Igbo speakers also linked "poison" with "sorcery," with the noun *nsi* ("poison, sorcery"—also connected to *osisi* "tree") and associated verbs -*gwo nsi* ("work sickness or death by means of magic or poison"), and -*ku nsi* ("to poison, to practice sorcery against").[42] The distinction between "medicine" and "poison" embedded in European languages and idioms map poorly onto West African discussions of empowered powders or trees.

Another site of cross-cultural exchange, convergence, and (mis)understanding was in the material culture of power objects. These objects were created and ritually consecrated by specialists to achieve or prevent specific ends.[43] According to European observers from the late seventeenth and eighteenth centuries on their conversations with local informants, people commissioned objects ranging from pouches tied to the body to small statues. Bosman described people on the Gold Coast in the 1680s and 1690s wearing objects that were "consecrated or conjured" by "priests" and placing such objects in the rooms of the sick to help them recover. The fact that some Europeans on the coast considered this remedy efficacious and adopted these practices shocked Bosman.[44] Several decades later, British Royal Navy surgeon John Atkins described different "fetishes" or "Gregries" from Sierra Leone to the Gold Coast, querying his local informants on their composition and uses. In Sierra Leone, people told him that they wore and kept amulets tied to their houses and boats to defend from miscarriages and other misfortunes, while Atkins's friend and business partner at Cape Coast Castle explained to him that the multiple "fetish" that he wore and paid for from a "Fetish-man" were "to protect from Dangers, or recover from Sickness."[45] According to John Matthews, a Royal Navy lieutenant in Sierra Leone in the 1780s, people there wore several charms at once, each targeted toward protecting against a specific misfortune: "One is to preserve him from shot, one from poison, another from fire, others from being drowned."[46]

The power objects themselves reveal a long history of cross-cultural interaction. In Senegambia, Muslims and non-Muslims alike sought out *mar-*

abouts for pieces of Arabic writing—especially Qur'an verses—as powerful elements of protective amulets that the Portuguese called *bolsas de mandinga*.[47] Words in modern Wolof derived from Arabic for "feiticheur" and "fetichisme" (*jibar b-*), as well as a specific term for "talisman made with Koranic writings" (*téere*), point toward this history.[48] In the 1780s, Matthews noted similar "griggories" containing powders and pieces of Arabic writing in use farther south in Sierra Leone.[49] At the time of Mungo Park's 1793–94 expedition along the Niger River, he reported Mande speakers' use of similar amulets of animal horns filled with *saphoes*—paper with passages from the Qur'an.[50]

The act of composition itself is crucial for understanding the ways West Africans thought about health, healing, and misfortune, and for understanding how this cross-cultural synthesis was made. European accounts frequently commented on these compositions in pouches, horns, tubes, and mixed-media statues and on how specialists consecrated these powerful objects through their assemblage. While often disparaging in tone—from "nasty and dirty little trifles" to "trash"—these observations are important for their emphasis on the assembly and binding together of diverse objects.[51] In her work on objects of power (*bo*) among speakers of Gbe languages, particularly human-shaped statues or *bociɔ* (literally, "empowered cadaver"), art historian Suzanne Blier explains the reasoning and significance behind the main elements in creating these statues that caused such revulsion for early modern Europeans. Saliva "glued" ritual speech to an object; fire, metaphorically represented through the heat of powdered peppers, red palm oil, or alcohol, brought the power to heal and to harm; knots and twisted cords of raffia with hair, feathers, or fur bound or "fixed" the power of the composition together; and finally a patina of blood smeared over the surface acted as both a sacrificial transference of life-force to the object and an offering to higher powers, whether specific *vodun* or ancestors.[52] Historians working with more recent ethnographic evidence like Blier's work must always exercise caution to avoid simple upstreaming. However, when paired with texts from the Atlantic period, this evidence offers suggestive insight into the power of composition in West African thought on healing and "poison."

The act of binding or tying up, for example, benefits from this kind of source triangulation. Across Atlantic Africa, "tying up" was both the action of empowering these compositions and a key metaphor for understanding power and affliction. Speakers of Gbe languages interviewed by Blier in the 1980s associated cords and binding with the dead, describing illnesses caused by angered ancestors as the dead binding the living. At the same time, cords could signify life, with life itself understood as a cord (*kan*) and descendants attached through such cords to the lives of their ancestors. Furthermore, bound empowerment objects could be used to cause suffering—the fundamental act of selfish abuse of power conceived of as an act of tying up—at the same time that ritual bondage of the sick was part of healing.[53] Based on European descriptions, early modern West Africans likely understood similar ritual bindings as powerful actions of afflicting or healing. For example, Bosman described an act of binding with power objects through a ritual conducted by a specialist following a birth on the Gold Coast: "The Child is no sooner born than the Priest (here called *Feticheer* or *Confoe*) is sent for, who binds a parcel of Ropes and Coral, and other Trash about the Head, Body, Arms and Legs of the Infant: After which he Exorcises, according to their accustomed manner; by which they believe it is armed against all Sickness and ill Accidents."[54] Twentieth-century Ewe speakers referred to ritual practitioners as *dzosalá* (one who ties or wears charms) and their action of *dzosasa* (tying charms) using the same root *dzo* (fire, heat, light) they used to describe good fortune, misfortune, and empowerment objects.[55] Likewise, the Fon speakers Blier interviewed described a sick person as *bla u* (literally, "bound body") and used the word *kannumon* (literally, "thing belonging in cords") for "enslaved person."[56] Farther west, nineteenth-century Twi speakers described the action of a tightly bound charm driven into the ground of a house or town as "[catching]" or "[binding]" a "wizard," while they used their verb *tō* for a range of meanings, including "to twist, to entangle, to poison."[57] Convergences between Atlantic African, Indigenous American, and European ideas about "tying up" cropped up early in sixteenth-century accusations of women who "tied" men in New Spain.[58] Africans and their descendants in the eighteenth- and early nineteenth-century Americas, believing themselves to be afflicted by a selfish manipulation of power, also sometimes described themselves through this idiom of being "tied up."

Speakers of Fon, Ewe, and Twi—languages sharing descent from Proto-Kwa—used the root *-bo-* not only to discuss empowerment objects, but a whole suite of power and spirit words evident in dictionaries from the late nineteenth and early twentieth centuries. For example, in addition to *bo* (charm, empowerment object) and *bociɔ* (human-shaped statuette), both Ewe and Fon speakers used *-bo-* words to discuss healer-diviners (respectively *bokó* and *bokɔ́nō*).[59] Twi speakers used this root to form the words *o-bonsám* ("wizard, sorcerer, witch"), *abonsám-kürów* ("the abode of evil spirits"), and *bow* ("charm [fetish] hidden in the ground").[60] I can connect some of these ideas to the late seventeenth century, as Twi speakers in that period used *bossom* both to describe spirits generally and for what Bosman described as a "fetiche" used to injure others.[61] Having obtained the *bossom* from a specialist, a person could place it "in some place which their Enemy is accustomed to pass" to cause their death.[62] With his own ideas of poison centered on an ingested or otherwise internally applied substance, Bosman ridiculed the idea of a "poison" being efficacious by stepping over it.[63] The fact that Twi speakers innovated a specific word to describe a hidden charm that could cause an affliction when stepped over—and that they connected this word to spirits and practitioners—suggests considerable concern with this very particular kind of "poisoning."

West African specialists with access to powers and the ability to create empowerment objects were generally respected, feared, and morally ambivalent figures, as they could use their expertise selfishly or communally.[64] Among Fon speakers interviewed by Blier, ritual practitioners were powerful people, and concerns about them—often within a community or family—were fundamentally concerns about the abuse of power.[65] People sought out these specialists to make and activate *bo* empowerment objects for a wide range of purposes. Blier describes her lists of purposes for commissioning *bo* as a catalog of "individual longings, fears, hopes, and concerns," including desires to attract others, to cure illnesses, to cause an illness, to protect against the malevolence of another, and to poison someone at a distance.[66] However, it is just as important to see the ways in which benevolent manipulation of power commissioned by one person could be understood or felt as harmful to another. A defensive *bo* worked aggressively; to protect one from malevolent powers or to bring about one's desires, the *bo* could harm the source or negate the desires of someone else. Likewise, a malevolent or aggressive *bo* brought positive benefit to the interests of the person who used it.[67] If fortune is seen as a zero-sum game, then efforts to improve one's life and fortune could be harmful to others—and the line between a communal or selfish use of power depended significantly on perspective.[68]

*   *   *

From the arrival of Europeans on the Atlantic African coast in the fifteenth century to the start of the colonial period in the nineteenth century, new objects, ideas, and people posed new challenges and invited new ways of discussing health, healing, and misfortune. Much like West Africa, West Central Africa was a place of extensive cross-cultural interaction and trade long before Europeans arrived; speakers of Njila family languages and the Kikongo Language Cluster (KLC) had long borrowed, adapted, and elaborated on ideas connecting health, healing, and leadership. While engagement with European ideas and practices were therefore neither a foreign concept nor a rupture from some static past, the Atlantic period was a time of great change heavily marked by the transatlantic slave trade.

West Central Africans incorporated goods and ideas from Europe and the Americas into their existing practices and discussions of power. Robust research has been done on how Kikongo-speaking Catholics "domesticated" Catholicism by absorbing it into their ideas about relationships between the living and the dead.[69] For example, Kikongo speakers used *ukisi* (holy)—the abstract form of *nkisi* (spirit)—along with *nganga* (expert, healer-diviner) to talk about Christian priests as *nganga a ukisi*, which Linda Heywood and John Thornton translate as "religious specialist with the characteristics of idols."[70] Catholicism also played a crucial role in fifteenth- and sixteenth-century diplomacy and discourses of sovereignty and rights between Atlantic African and early modern European polities.[71]

As part of the Columbian Exchange, health practitioners in West Central Africa also began experimenting with and adapting plants and products from the Americas into their existing practices.[72] Atlantic African practitioners, just as early modern European ones, were keenly interested in experimenting with and using *materia medica* from around the Atlantic to "[craft] economic, social, and political power."[73] Tobacco, far more potent in the early modern period than today, took on a particular significance. Portuguese living in Angola described *ganga* practitioners incorporating tobacco smoking into existing healing practices where they had previously been using cannabis.[74] Mbui speakers in the upper Kwanza valley even innovated two new nouns for tobacco, *kambandu* and *mbandu*, from the same *-bánd-* root they used for *kimbanda* ("doctor, healer"), *imbanda* ("remedy"), and *umbanda* ("medical science").[75] The final suffix *-u* suggests that these new words derived from a verb of quality, while their respective noun class prefixes suggest respective indications of "tools" and "modes of action."[76] In other words, Mbui speakers may have described tobacco as a tool or action taken by someone—probably a *kimbanda*—for healing. While conducted in the early twentieth century, ethnographic work from José de Oliveira Ferreira Diniz on Hungu speakers, also inhabitants of the Kwanza watershed, noted that they used Brazilian ipecacuanha, an important emetic in the Atlantic pharmacopoeia, in their poison ordeals—ordeals where vomiting was key to the outcome.[77]

The Portuguese colony of Angola—territory around the capital of Luanda that the Portuguese, with allies from the Kingdom of Kongo, had conquered from the Kingdom of Ndongo in the last quarter of the sixteenth century—was a site of intense cross-cultural interaction between the Portuguese, local Kimbundu speakers, and speakers of a variety of Njila languages from the interior who were enslaved in the city or forcibly marched to the waiting holds of slave ships in the harbor.[78] Inquisition records in particular reveal interactions centered on religion, healing, and affliction—as well as fraught social tensions. The colony was ostensibly Catholic, and not just for the resident Europeans; many West Central Africans in Luanda converted and were active participants in churches and lay brotherhoods. However, much like Kongolese Catholics, people domesticated Christian practices into existing frameworks that added to rather than replaced the significance of *nganga* and other ritual practitioners, while Portuguese colonial officials also relied on *nganga* and syncretic practices for healing.[79] For the *sobas* (noblemen) outside of the colony, baptism offered both a chance to cement alliances with Portugal and an opportunity to tap into a new source of public healing power with new spirits; healing was political and a cornerstone of leadership.[80]

The content of the fifteen *feitiçaria* denunciations involving thirty-six people in the colony of Angola recorded in the *cadernos do promotor* of the Lisbon Inquisition from 1698 to 1724 illuminates this cross-cultural interaction in practice. Given this small sample size, any quantitative interpretations should be taken with caution. However, what is immediately striking is that while the clients included a cross-section of Angolan society—African, European, free, enslaved, wealthy, and poor—the practitioners identified in these cases were exclusively African; to the dismay of the Portuguese administration, people suffering from afflictions primarily went to *nganga* for their expertise.[81] These practitioners, evenly split between men and women, were well known in the colony for their cures, and the ceremonies they performed, while usually in private houses, involved communal participation from the afflicted and their relatives. These ceremonies involved divination, usually with spirit possession and sometimes animal sacrifice, to identify the source of illness, followed by therapeutic treatment and the removal of objects from afflicted bodies. When he became sick on a business trip to the Province of Libolo, free *preto* ("black man") Alexandre went to a *nganga*

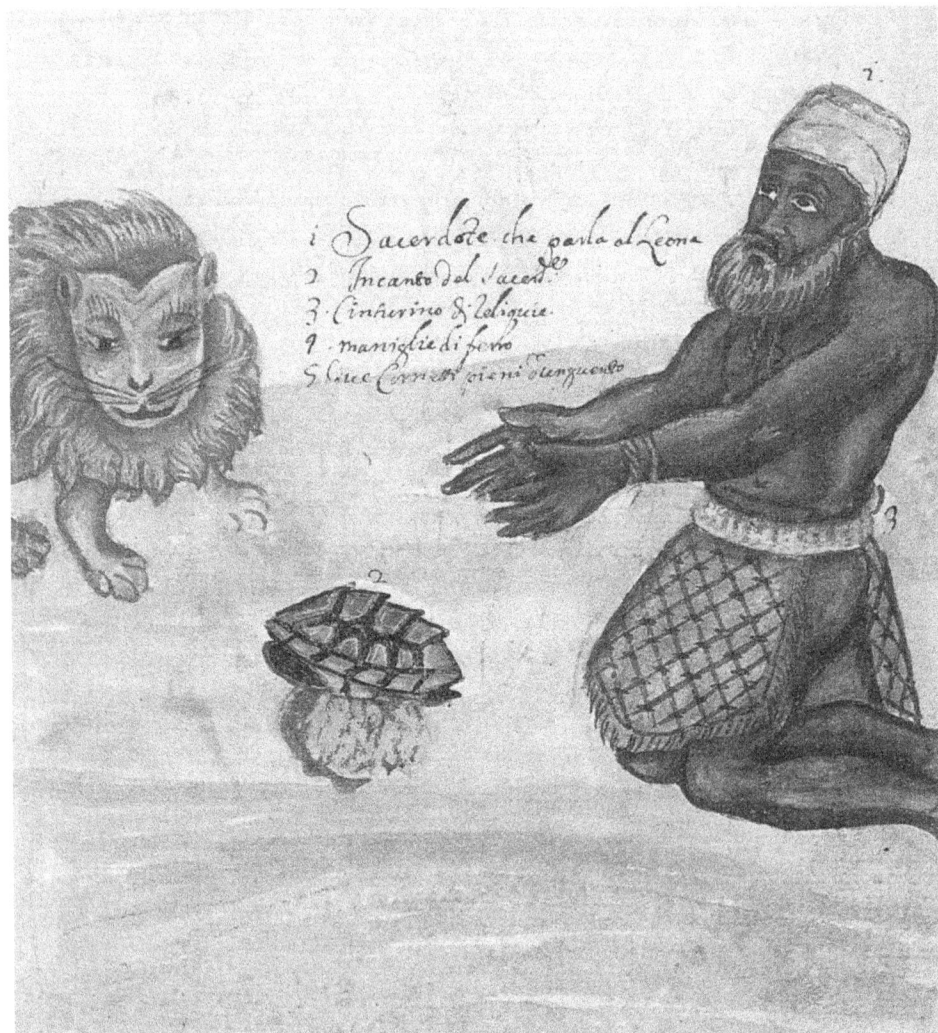

Figure 3. Capuchin missionary Giovanni Antonio Cavazzi wrote extensively—
and negatively—on religious practices in Angola during the mid-seventeenth
century. The text in the image reads, "1. Priest speaks to the lion; 2. Spell of the
priest; 3. Little belt of relics; 4. Handles of iron; 5. Two little horns full of oint-
ment." John K. Thornton writes extensively on Cavazzi and the context for this
watercolor. "Untitled Image (A Spiritual Practitioner and His Paraphernalia),"
*Slavery Images: A Visual Record of the African Slave Trade and Slave Life in the
Early African Diaspora*, accessed August 11, 2023, http://www.slaveryimages.org.

Domingos, who sacrificed a baby goat, fed Alexandre some of the meat, then pulled several "venomous animals" from his body.[82] In a Luandan "house of feitiçaria," two enslaved women—an unnamed expert and her "disciple," Guiomar—treated an afflicted Portuguese officer through a consultation with "demons" and the removal of *feitiços* that included a lion claw, human hair, and unspecified herbs.[83] Treatment involved a community of the living and the dead, through spirit possession and the participation of family and friends—such as the three cavalry officers who accompanied their sick friend to the house of Guiomar or the free *preta* Catherina Borges who went with her two daughters to a ceremony to treat her afflicted niece.[84] Finally, details in the denunciations in the *cadernos do promotor* highlighted the geographic mobility and fame of these practitioners.[85]

Another communal aspect of the activities of *nganga* and other practitioners was the swearing of the *bulungo* oath: a judicial ordeal involving the consumption of a substance to prove one's innocence or guilt. Three cases in the *cadernos* mentioned the *bulungo* oath, all in 1716 and 1717.[86] In one, Portuguese man Francisco da Silva Nevis denounced nine African residents of the city of Carinda for *feitiçaria*, and two of them—Pedro Quibuca Quiangolla and Fernão Lungariambamba—specifically for performing *bulungo* oaths. He also denounced a "fugitive" named Domingos Aganga who was widely believed to have injured people with *maleficios* and had taken the *bulungo* oath four or five times to try and prove his innocence before fleeing the city.[87] The names of the accused—particularly the use of some form of *nganga* in four of the nine names—are suggestive of the roles of the denounced as expert ritual practitioners in the Carinda community.

Not every action attributed to powerful practitioners involved communal healing practices. Both European and African witnesses denounced individuals in three cases for killing others with *feitiços* and *veneno* for selfish personal reasons.[88] The ways private conflicts could involve objects created by expert practitioners are highlighted by a 1720 case in Bengo Province. All of the individuals involved, including the four men who spoke with Capuchin missionary Padre Vicente Borges about the case, were identified as "black," and all but one were free. Returning home from business travel, João Baines de Souza was approached by an enslaved woman named Josepha, who had found a *feitiço* in the house. This composition included chicken feathers, other bird feathers, conch shells, roots, herbs, and a piece of bread. Baines de Souza publicly denounced Manoel da Costa; multiple denouncers informed the commissioner that it was "public" knowledge that da Costa made *feitiços*. Many people came to Baines de Souza's house to take a look at the *feitiço*; three of these individuals—notably not Baines de Souza himself—told the missionary that Baines de Souza's wife (unnamed in the document) had been having an affair with da Costa, and the purpose of the *feitiço* was to keep Baines de Souza from discovering them. The entire story, from the contents of the *feitiço* to the details of the affair, were stated to be public knowledge by the time of the denunciation.[89] João Baines de Souza had a clear motive for denouncing Manoel da Costa—and it is notable that he was the only person interviewed by the missionary to accuse his rival of killing with *feitiços*—but what is most striking about this case, even in Manoel da Costa's alleged use of power for personal rather than communal ends, is the emphasis on public knowledge and reputation associated with the practitioner.

How did European witnesses and participants in these rituals interpret them? Their statements in the *cadernos* offer clues. While still valuable, the full *processos* of the Inquisition as tried in Lisbon were predominantly shaped by the concerns of Lisbon inquisitors, in both their decision on whether to try the case and the questions they asked. Instead, the *cadernos* focused on the concerns of the people making the denunciation, who were often neighbors of the accused and sometimes had different priorities from inquisitors.[90] For example, while in full trials inquisitors relentlessly focused on pacts with demons believed to have been necessary to grant practitioners their healing powers, in only five of the fifteen *cadernos* cases did denouncers mention demons. However, close examination of *how* demons came up in these cases suggests ways in which Europeans interpreted practices involving spirit possession through existing demonological frameworks. Only European denouncers brought up demons, and they mainly did so to describe ritual possession as part of healing practices.[91] Heitor Cardozo in 1720 specifically accused an enslaved woman named Catherina of "copulating with a demon," a quintessential European idea of the gendered relationship between witches and demons and between demonic seduction and an unnatural female usurpation of power.[92] In contrast, when an enslaved man named Gregorio Pascoal denounced Victoria, a "master in divining," for holding large assemblies of about thirty people to divine and treat illnesses, he described the ceremony as a spirit entering Victoria's head and insisted to the priest taking his confession, when asked, that his participation did not constitute making a pact with a demon or leaving the holy Catholic faith.[93]

Western Europe was just as much a part of the new Atlantic world as Angola, embedded in the expanding web of connections following Columbus's voyage and transformed by these connections. While in a different context from the Americas or Africa, cross-cultural exchanges in Europe had an important impact on the way Europeans interpreted poison and medicine.

The impact of African ideas and practices on Europeans was most visible in Portugal and especially Lisbon—a city with an African population of 10,000 (10 percent of the total) by the mid-sixteenth century.[94] While precise census figures for the seventeenth and eighteenth centuries are lacking, an estimate from the 1770s noted about 15,000 African-descended people living in Lisbon.[95] The *Slave Voyages* database estimates that approximately 7,600 enslaved Africans disembarked in Europe during the years of the transatlantic slave trade, 3,887 of whom landed in Portugal.[96] These numbers represent a very small fraction of the approximately 12.5 million people forced from African shores. However, there were several other avenues for the African presence in Lisbon. Significant culturally but not demographically were diplomatic missions sent by the Kingdom of Kongo, a sovereign ally of the Kingdom of Portugal since 1485, as well as later missions from Dahomey and other Atlantic African states.[97]

As the central hub of the overseas empire, Lisbon was also the seat of inquisitorial trials from around the empire; after an initial investigation, individuals whose cases went to full trial were sent to Lisbon, and many of them served out their punishment in Portugal. Out of 569 people tried by the Lisbon Inquisition for crimes of *feitiçaria* or "magical" healing practices across the empire from 1536 to 1821, 77 (14 percent) were identified in the records as being African or of African descent. This number becomes more significant when considering that cases focused on magical crimes only accounted for 4 percent of the total full *processos* from the sixteenth to early nineteenth century.[98] For some—like the painter António Correira de Aguiar, born in the Kingdom of Kongo and enslaved in Minas Gerais, Brazil, at the time of his arrest in 1757, or freed man Sebastião arrested for *feitiçaria* in the Azores in 1691—their sentence was a period of convict labor in southern Portugal ranging from two to five years.[99] Others were sentenced to labor in the galleys, banished to other parts of the Portuguese empire, or released after the completion of a public shaming in the form of an *auto-da-fé*. None of the 77 were executed: indeed, executions for *feitiçaria*-related crimes were rare.[100] Many of the Africans and people of African descent brought to Lisbon by the Inquisition, whether they had been free or enslaved on entry, were released after an excruciating and often years-long process of torture and interrogation. From James Sweet's microhistorical analysis of one such individual, some of those who had ritually practiced continued to do so after release.[101]

Africans in Portugal had an outsized cultural impact on Portuguese ideas and practices regarding *feitiçaria* and healing. In terms of numbers, African descendants living in Lisbon and Portugal more broadly were accused of *feitiçaria* or related crimes only slightly disproportionately to their population. Of the 831 people in Lisbon accused but not tried in a full *processo* from 1671 to 1802, 98 (12 percent) were of African descent, a significant majority of whom were free.[102] However, popular folk ideas viewed Africans in Portugal with mystique, as keepers of secret exotic knowledge including healing practices.[103]

The name alone of popular charms of protection in early modern Portugal and the wider Portuguese Atlantic—*bolsas de mandinga* (literally, mandinga bags, "mandinga" being an ethnonym for Mande speakers in West Africa)—emphasizes this link to Africanness.[104] However, the origin of these charms is more complex. Portuguese speakers had been using small pouches as protective talismans since the Middle Ages, as part of an earlier cross-cultural exchange with Muslim North Africans in the context of Muslim rule over much of the Iberian Peninsula. Of the sixty-seven people accused of making or using *bolsas de mandinga* in the *cadernos* for Lisbon from 1671 to 1802, nineteen (28 percent) were identified as being African or of African descent, disproportionate from the population in the city.[105] By the eighteenth century, Portuguese folk practices of magical protection from misfortunes and malevolent affliction were intertwined both with African practitioners and ideas about African expertise.

Exposure to new ideas, peoples, and goods around the world had an impact on the work and ideas of European healing practitioners—a broad umbrella including licensed physicians, surgeons, household healers, barbers, and a range of "wise" or "cunning" women and men. Portuguese commoners associated Africans with secret knowledge and expertise and incorporated African health practitioners and their practices into their understanding of *curandeiros*—folk healers defined by Timothy Walker as "purveyors of a socially approved body of magical beliefs."[106] At the same time, physicians in the empire like Garcia da Orta in sixteenth-century Goa creatively fused empiricism with textual authority with a practical eye toward the health needs of people on the ground.[107]

The emergence of a robust global drug trade beginning in the sixteenth century was key to the shaping of early modern European medical practice and ideas about poison. Drugs and associated knowledge of their use also circulated in the Atlantic world and beyond. Spanish and Portuguese works on natural history cataloguing and narrating experiences with these drugs were profoundly influential, as was seventeenth-century Dutch commerce.[108] Bioprospectors sought new drugs to adopt into the European *materia medica*, "drug" being widely defined in the early modern period to include not only plant-based but also mineral, animal, and chemical substances—from tobacco to bezoar stones to quinoa.[109] New drugs and information on how to use them appeared not only in botanical treatises but also in manuscript medical recipes and the popular genre of household medical books. For example, in the dozens of manuscripts of medical charms and recipes collected by Hans Sloane, two from the early seventeenth century began including plantains—used by Africans on both sides of the Atlantic—for treating venomous bites and stings.[110] Early modern English gentlewomen were also collectors and cataloguers of colonial plants alongside local ones in their gardens and medicinal recipe books.[111] Among elites, new publications from the Royal Society and physicians across Europe drew upon polycentric knowledge from Africans, Native Americans, and European creoles living in the wider Atlantic world.[112]

Cross-cultural interactions—along with imperial ambitions and global networks of trade—shaped ideas about healing knowledge and practices expressed in early modern European pharmacopoeias.[113] These texts show how the act of classification was an attempt by their makers at asserting professional control; however, they relied heavily on African and Indigenous American knowledge—not as raw material for study but as *knowledge* produced by healing experts.[114] In the early eighteenth century, several Portuguese apothecaries and chemists connected to networks of knowledge across the Atlantic and Indian Oceans produced large vernacular pharmacopoeias cataloging drugs in manuals for practical use.[115] While the idea of a pharmacopoeia was certainly not new—quite a few had been published in Latin in the seventeenth century and earlier—the shift to the vernacular by these writers in the early eighteenth century unleashed a wave of widely read and reprinted works.[116] Influential pharmacopoeia authors João Curvo Semedo (1707) and João Vigier (1716) wrote about *bezoars*—stones taken from the stomach of a goat that authors claimed could cure any poison—and snakestones from the East Indies that allegedly had the power, when applied to the bite of a venomous snake, to suck out the poison.[117] In addition to bezoars and snakestones, these Portuguese writers included specific drugs from the Americas.

Semedo had entries in his catalog for the Virginian snakeroot as a treatment for rattlesnake bites, and the "Tambuape" and "Jamvarandim" roots used by Indigenous peoples in Bahia to treat poisons. Likewise, Vigier described the powdered beak of the horned screamer as "highly esteemed" by unnamed health practitioners in the Amazon against poison and compared the usefulness of powdered bison horn for treating poisons to that of the unicorn.[118] Semedo and Vigier also respectively discussed reports of people in Angola and Brazil eating the flesh of venomous snakes to protect against venom from future bites; both discussed people incorporating pieces of the Angolan snake or, in the case of Brazil, a venomous spider called *nhamdui*, in *bolsas de mandinga* worn around the neck for protection against illnesses.[119]

While never simple or straightforward, the ways that European physicians and naturalists interpreted and made use of cross-cultural healing knowledge and practices underwent significant changes in the eighteenth and nineteenth centuries. Historians have spilled much ink on the professionalization of medicine—with roots reaching back to the sixteenth century—as a major development.[120] Physicians increasingly framed other kinds of practitioners as dangerous usurpers of proper medical authority—even as they increasingly rejected their efficacy. Elite European institutions from universities to inquisitorial tribunals made a concerted effort to replace the existing "mosaic of practitioners" with professional, licensed physicians.[121] Like eighteenth-century cunning-folk in England or unwitching specialists in the Netherlands, *curandeiros* were commonplace in Portuguese society, despite efforts by licensed physicians to discredit and eradicate them; their cures aligned more closely with community interpretations of affliction than elite medical theories.[122] Still, by the end of the eighteenth century, the ground on medical authority in Europe was shifting.

Tracking references in eighteenth- and nineteenth-century poison treatises highlights how Europeans shifted their ideas about medical authority away from cross-cultural sources. In the early eighteenth century, it was well-established practice for authors of vernacular poison treatises to weave together anecdotes of poisons and cures from Africa and the Americas—along with references to recent scientific works and ancient authorities. Richard Mead, a Royal Society fellow and personal physician to King George II who did not himself venture beyond Europe, was unusually conscientious for his time in providing citations across the 1702, 1729, and 1747 editions of *A Mechanical Account of Poisons*, revealing a multistranded braid of authority on poison and medicine in the early to mid-eighteenth century. While, unsurprisingly, Mead cited Galen and Hippocrates about a dozen times each in every edition, he increasingly cited authorities with direct experience in Africa or the Americas: for example, Spanish physician Francisco Hernández's 1615 treatise on the Mexican tarantula (all editions); New England alchemist George Starkey on his "Pacific Pill" cure (1729, 1747); Portuguese merchant Duarte Lopes's *Report of the Kingdom of Congo* on the Kongolese eating vipers to cure diseases (1729, 1747); and Dutch naturalist Peter Kolb's 1719 work on the use of poison arrows near Cape Town (1747). Mead also cited several "personal communications" between himself and anonymous surgeons living in Guinea (a generic term for the West African coast) and Virginia—the latter reporting knowledge of how to suck poison out of a rattlesnake bite learned from unnamed Indigenous peoples—as well as a surgeon living in London on his own experiences with rattlesnakes.[123] Knowledge about rattlesnakes, poisoned arrows, and nature in Africa and the Americas for European authors like Mead had a polycentric creation, as knowledge from Africans, Native Americans, and European creoles on the natural world influenced and helped create European knowledge and ways of knowing about the world.[124]

While early eighteenth-century authors like Mead had made claims to credibility through references to African or Indigenous American informants—though rarely by name—by the end of the century these authors were far more likely to be dismissive of their practices—if they acknowledged them at all.[125] In the Portuguese empire, Enlightenment-influenced physicians in Angola and Brazil increasingly called in racialized language for crackdowns on the work of African healers as "superstitious," backward, and unscientific.[126] In poison treatises, European authors gave greater primacy to knowledge created in European labs through experimentation. It was not that experimentation itself was new but rather that knowledge from Africa and the Americas had much less authority for these authors than they had had for earlier eighteenth-century authors.[127] Felice Fontana's 1781 treatise was a collection of over six thousand experiments he had personally conducted, focused primarily on viper venom.[128] Instead of relying on reports from others, as Mead had—reports often rooted in the practices of unnamed Indigenous practitioners—Fontana incorporated his own experiments with poisonous plants of the Americas into his research. Fontana specifically conducted experiments on poison ivy (*Toxicodendron radicans*) from North America and *ticunas*—a plant-based arrow poison used by Yameo speakers in Amazonian Peru. Ignoring the knowledge and reports of others had risks of its own. Apparently, the rashes Fontana experienced when handling the poison ivy were so bad that he abandoned his experiments with it in defeat: "Thus have I dearly paid for my skepticism and want of precaution, in becoming, myself, the subject of my experiments."[129]

The story behind *ticunas* is particularly illustrative of changing European discourse on medical authority. Having read Charles Marie de la Condamine's 1745 report on *ticunas* from his travels along the Amazon, Fontana had the opportunity in London to conduct experiments with "American arrows well preserved, and well covered with poison," supplied by a friend and Royal Society member.[130] He saw these experiments as necessary, as he trusted neither Condamine's observations nor "the doubtful relation of some native of that country."[131] For many European intellectuals like Fontana, by the mid- to late eighteenth century the personal experiences of European travelers and creoles in the Americas and their Native American or African interlocutors counted for far less than experiments conducted by European professionals in a laboratory. This attitude stood in stark contrast with how European creoles in the Americas saw themselves as unique contributors to knowledge—often obtained without acknowledgment of African and Indigenous American informants—to scientific discourse in Europe.[132]

These cross-cultural exchanges from the late fifteenth century on were part of an explosion of Atlantic and global circulation—of goods, ideas, and people. They did not take place in a vacuum. Context matters for understanding exchanges and interpretations of healing practices and ideas about poison.

Poison and the Slave Trade in Atlantic Africa

For Atlantic Africa, the transatlantic slave trade was a key context. An area where the impact of the slave trade was most visible was in the expansion and transformation of judicial practices—many used to identify and punish "poisoners" and which themselves involved ritual access to spiritual power—and their escalating role in generating captives sold to Europeans and the plantations of the Americas.

The era of the transatlantic slave trade was one of increased anxiety for many people in Atlantic Africa; historians of the region have suggested that during this period people became increasingly concerned about the effects of abuses of power. People in the Bight of Benin had used *bo* empowerment objects to manage anxiety before the slave trade, but these objects became particularly important during this period as a means and strategy of response to increasing misfortune.[133] Farther east, the role of *diaba* specialists in villages of Igbo speakers also changed and intensified over the eighteenth and nineteenth centuries, as people increasingly sought the consultation of oracles, made more petitions and sacrifices, and commissioned more empowered objects for their protection.[134]

A combination of increased anxiety and the skyrocketing prices Europeans offered for enslaved people on the coast led elites in many West African societies to alter their judicial systems, selling many into slavery at tribunals for crimes that may have previously been punished with fines or possibly death.[135] European accounts of Sierra Leone over the course of the early modern period reveal changes in an emphasis on divination and "witchcraft" over time and their relationship to systems of justice.[136] In other parts of West Africa, rulers sometimes arrested and sold individuals identified as possessing powers into the transatlantic slave trade as a way of neutralizing a political threat. Such was the case of priests of the *vodun* Sakpata in the vicinity of Dahomey, as they became rival sources of political power for the many refugees of the Dahomey expansion.[137]

Trading enslaved people for luxury goods upended the social relationships embedded in West Central African governance.[138] West Central and Central African elites had participated in a robust trading network with each other for over a millennium and had reasons internal to their societies for wanting to participate in exchanges for imported trade goods.[139] Leaders faced a political paradox, as their ability to acquire and distribute highly desired Indian textiles and other imported goods to followers and dependents was made possible by selling some of these dependents to the Europeans on the coast.[140] Waves of civil wars and conflicts between polities, though arising from political struggles and not necessarily with the primary purpose of generating captives to be enslaved, nevertheless did so. As recent scholarship in the Angolan archives has explored, in addition to violence and war, people of West Central Africa were also vulnerable to kidnapping, seizure for debt, and tribunals reconfigured by *sobas* (noblemen) to punish crimes from adultery to theft to witchcraft with sale to the web of itinerant traders in the hinterlands of Luanda and Benguela.[141] Farther north, the decades-long civil war in the Kingdom of Kongo from the mid-seventeenth to the early eighteenth century opened the floodgates for rival factions to sell prisoners of war and civilians caught in the middle both to the Portuguese at Luanda and to the Vili merchants working north of the Congo River—business partners from the mid-seventeenth century with the English, French, and Dutch.[142] In this period of chronic instability and violence from the transatlantic slave trade, people in West Central Africa began discussing health and affliction in new ways.

Those who were involved most extensively and directly in the slave trade and with Europeans developed new institutions of healing in the seventeenth century. These institutions should be understood as political institutions, as West Central Africans innovated these new healing cults to manage the political paradox described above. Speakers of Civili and other KLC languages north of the Congo River heavily involved in slaving formed a new institution called *Lemba* that was both a form of governance, organizing and controlling the markets and trade routes from Malebo Pool to the coastal ports like Loango and Cabinda, and a form of public healing to manage the negative spiritual effects of accumulating wealth from the slave trade. *Lemba* became a form of arbitration and institutionalized justice through ceremonial exchanges.[143] Members of *Lemba* were predominantly elite healers, merchants, and leaders connected to the transatlantic slave trade who had suffered an affliction believed to have been caused by angered spirits. These spirits needed to be pacified for healing to take place.[144] Kikongo and Civili speakers specifically discussed the appeasement of angry *nkisi* with words from the same transitive verb *-dèmb-* (to calm, to pacify, to soothe, to tame) that speakers of Njila languages had inherited. Because of the flexibility of Bantu languages, it is easy for any individual to change a verb into a noun. From the main verb *lémba* (to calm, to speak, to appease; to turn away the anger of a *nkisi*; to invoke or conjure a *nkisi* so that it will be obliged to turn away its anger), they elaborated a verb "to neuter, to tame"; words for "appeasement" and "person who appeases"; and a noun for a specific *nkisi* capable of causing pain in the chest.[145] Because of the ease of change, these developments from verb to noun—from "to appease" to "appeaser"—were not necessarily themselves significant unless used as a title; what is more significant was the use of new nouns from the root to refer to objects ritually used by *Lemba* practitioners. As part of their initiation, future members participated in a public therapeutic purification and paid the *Lemba* society in goods such as palm wine and manioc, or cassava, root—an American plant that had become a staple food crop in the region. Kikongo and Civili speakers had termed the leaves of this new therapeutic plant *lembe*.[146] For *Lemba* devotees, public healing that incorporated new substances into an existing repertoire of powerful plants was a way of addressing concerns about the abuse of power relating to the same Atlantic networks of trade that brought manioc to African shores.

In some moments and places, mass movements of public healing became explicit institutions of political critique. For example, in its critique of the Kongolese civil war, the slave trade, and the actions of the current king of Kongo, the Antonian movement of Kongolese Catholics from 1704 to 1706—led by a young woman named Dona Beatriz Kimpa Vita who claimed to be possessed by the spirit of Saint Anthony—attempted to heal the country by redirecting the *kindoki* (power, from the root *-dòg-*, to bewitch, to curse) that they believed had been misused.[147] There is also evidence that some speakers of Njila languages elaborated on the connections they had made between leaders and their powerful relationships to spirits in new and more negative ways in this period. Cokwe speakers, who had fled into the wooded highlands to escape slave raiding and became middlemen in the transatlantic slave trade in the 1750s, innovated a noun *chikola* (brute, bully) and verb *kolema* (to rebel) from the same root, *-kód-* (to become strong, hard) that people throughout the Kwanza basin had previously innovated for iron objects of power and as a title for the king of Ndongo.[148] In the Kwanza basin itself, Kimbundu speakers began using the same root in the intransitive verb *kukóléla* (to do bad) and an adjective *úkola* (terrible, evil).[149]

Institutions of public healing and powerful practitioners were not only institutions of political critique; they were also political institutions that could *be* critiqued. This moral ambivalence of power—as the power to heal was also the power to harm, and the same action could do both depending on one's perspective—was not new in West Central Africa. However, evidence from the Atlantic period suggests an intensification of concerns about power and the individuals who wielded it. For example, words used by agropastoralist Nyaneka-Nkhumbi speakers changed the way they talked about *-bánd-* people and *onganga*.[150] While they had inherited a noun *-bàndà* (healer-diviner) and continued to use it in the form *otyimbanda* ("curandeiro," "feitiçeiro"), they innovated a new noun *ekongo-mbanda* ("malfeitor").[151] This was very different and new way of discussing a *-bánd-* person, as a criminal and a threat. While Nyaneka-Nkhumbi speakers still used their inherited word *onganga*, they also used several proverbs that emphasized the moral ambiguity of the position: most evocatively, *Tukatapela-pi, kuhen'ombingale? Tukatungila-pi, kuhen'ononganga?* ("Where will we have to go to water without there being muddied water? Where will we have to build a house without there being *nganga*?").[152] The people who created, shared, and used this troubled proverb expressed anxiety over abuses of power by the powerful, as well as an inability to escape their presence. Words and proverbs taken from single languages in modern dictionaries rather than reconstructed in deeper time through the comparative method of historical linguistics should be treated as suggestive rather than definitive evidence of change; there is a distinct possibility that mid-twentieth-century negative connotations in attested words for ritual practitioners could also reflect intensified Christian influence from colonialism. However, an increase in distrust of institutions and practitioners like *nganga* in the era of the transatlantic slave trade is a plausible interpretation given their links with power and judicial ordeals.

In their words about the slave trade, West Central Africans discussed it as an affliction and an act of violence. They did so primarily through metaphor, using the same roots their ancestors had elaborated on to discuss health and healing. Southern Moxico speakers took their inherited *-kód-* verb (to be strong, solid, hard) and layered on additional meaning with *nakolo*, the state of being "swollen" and "captured by illness."[153] This second meaning suggests overlap between the semantic domains of this verb and its homophone *-kód-* (to take, touch, with derivative *-kódè* captive, booty), while the former provides insight into the kind of affliction described. The idea of being "captured" by an illness is particularly evocative, linking the state of being ill with the state of captivity, and perhaps enslavement. Umbundu speakers innovated two new nouns, *ochimbandanga* (affliction of the legs, paralysis) and *okambanda* (young slave).[154] As they used *ochimbanda* for "diviner, witch, healer"; *owanga* for "charm"; and a noun class prefix *-ki* that included semantic domains of "outstanding people" and "diseases," this new condition could be translated as "extraordinary power affliction."[155] Likewise, to form the word for a "young slave," Umbundu speakers added the diminutive prefix ka- to the root *mbanda*—the same root for *ochimbanda*.[156] As a young enslaved person, perhaps a young adult highly sought on the transatlantic market, an *okambanda* would have been someone who had been split from their people and almost certainly bound. A 1738 inventory of a march of captives in this region from Caconda to Benguela vividly illustrates the frequency of leg afflictions, with nearly one in ten of the individuals on the march identified as having a leg injury of some kind.[157] However, the term could have also been metaphorically resonant for Umbundu speakers, as slavery could have been seen as a form of social paralysis.

Some attestations among Njila and KLC speakers suggest that they made a metaphorical connection between being tied up, malevolent affliction, and the marching of coffles. Dcrirku speakers in the Okavango Delta innovated a suite of new words from *-gàng- (to tie up): the generic term "disease," mukânga; "health," ukângure; "healthy person," mukângure; and "state of health," likânguko.[158] Dcrirku speakers used the *-kàng- variant of *-gàng- for these new words, indicating that they did not derive them from the same path of the ancient word ngangá that they continued to use for "medicine-man, doctor." Instead, they derived these roots from a verb that had either been innovated by Southern Njila speakers or had recently spread between the geographically contiguous Lwena, Southern Moxico, and Dcrirku speakers: an intransitive verb -kanguka-, "to be healed, become well."[159] At the same time, Southern Moxico speakers also innovated the term likanga livu (a line of people)—likely people who were "tied up."[160] A set of *-kàng- words innovated by Kikongo speakers also suggests a connection between tying up, affliction, and a marching line of people. While the primary meanings of their verb kànga (to tie up, to knot, to tighten) were the durable descendants of *-gàng- (to tie up), Kikongo speakers layered on very specific and unique meanings, "to imprison, to march." They further elaborated a reversive verb kàngula with a primary meaning "to undo, untie" and further meanings "to liberate, to defend, to acquit or declare not guilty" and a noun kàngulwa, "rope, cord."[161] In using these words, Kikongo speakers not only linked binding with enslavement but also with legal conviction or acquittal at tribunals—a mechanism of enslavement that ensnared so many in the era of the transatlantic slave trade.[162]

*   *   *

Francisco Buitrago's observations of the uses and virtues of the nkasa tree in the early eighteenth century did not end in West Central Africa. Before completing his circuit to Lisbon and sitting down to write his never-to-be-published manuscript, he sailed on the western currents in 1718 to Bahia in northeastern Brazil. He had received permission from his superiors to travel to Salvador for his health, apparently a fairly common reason for leave for Portuguese officers stationed in Angola.[163] While visiting a relative in Salvador, he discovered that there were many people there, free and enslaved, who were "sick of feitiços" and seemed "incurable" with drawn-out illnesses lasting for three or four years. An enslaved woman on the plantation was dying, with a swollen body and sluggish pulse. Other enslaved people said she was afflicted with "malificios" [sic]. Armed with some *nkasa* bark he had brought with him from Angola, Buitrago performed his first exorcism. He was considered successful enough that others went to him for treatment; Buitrago reported selling some of his bark to eager buyers and performing at least ten more exorcisms with it while in Bahia.[164]

Buitrago saw his cure as efficacious because the hidden virtues of the bark helped remove *feitiços* that had been diabolically "lodged" in the sufferers' afflicted bodies, but it is equally important that the enslaved people in Salvador also thought his treatment worked. In the decade leading up to Buitrago's first exorcism, more than seventy thousand Africans disembarked in Bahia, about 13 percent of whom came from West Central Africa; ledgers from Bahian plantations a decade later also suggest that African-born individuals made up about 75 percent of the enslaved population at this time.[165] There are thus reasonable odds that among the enslaved Africans Buitrago treated and encountered in Bahia, some may have recognized the bark and the Kikongo name he used for it, as well as the techniques he had explicitly learned from *nganga* in Angola and the Kingdom of Kongo. Though I imagine it would have been difficult to identify the tree from the well-traveled bark alone, it is significant that people from West Africa also had experience with *E. suaveolens* and could have possibly recognized it in Buitrago's work and particularly his preparation of the bark into an infusion of red water.[166] What we have in the moment of Buitrago's healing appears to have been a "dialogue of the deaf," where multiple parties agreed on a solution to an affliction caused by "poison" while maintaining very different ideas as to where the affliction came from and how and why this solution was efficacious.[167] As I turn now to eighteenth-century poison accusations and trials in the western Atlantic, I will explore these often violent moments as sites of contested ideas, productive misunderstandings, and creative formations of new ideas between people of African and European descent.

CHAPTER 3

Contested Idioms

In January 1746, smoke filled the air in Orange County, Virginia, as an enslaved woman named Eve burned at the stake. A panel of prominent local gentlemen in the county court had tried and condemned her for the murder of her enslaver, Peter Montague. "Induced by the Instigation of the Devil," Eve had allegedly "feloniously and traitorously" mixed "poison" into Montague's milk, causing him to languish for four months before dying.[1] The case of Eve is well known; the grassy hill where she was executed is locally called "Eve's Wail." Less well known is the case of Tom two years earlier and two counties away. Three enslaved men—Warrick, Mingo, and Roben—from three different plantations testified as witnesses before the Caroline County Court that Tom had prepared and given "Several Poysonous Powders Roots Herbs and Simples" to an enslaved man named Joe. Joe, trusting Tom, drank the concoction and died after "grievously Languish[ing]" for over two weeks. The court found Tom not guilty of murder; the act outlawing the preparation and distribution of "poisonous medicines" by people of African descent, regardless of harm or intent, did not pass until 1748.[2] However, since Tom was known to have "given powder to other negros," the court decided the safest course would be to forcibly transport him out of the colony as a potential threat.[3]

Eve's case exemplified European ideas about poison as a usurpation of power. The court saw her actions as a form of treason against her enslaver as the rightful holder of power; as an enslaved woman—someone who was doubly "beneath" Montague—her alleged poisoning of him upended the "natural" order. People of European descent in the colonies incorporated enslaved people into older gendered ideas about poison and weakness, racializing their alleged propensity for poison—for both men and women of African descent—by the nineteenth century. However, Tom's case reveals that this idea of poison as the weapon of the weak was not the only idiom at play. The enslaved witnesses who accused Tom in the courthouse highlighted how Joe had trusted him and how Tom was known to give powders to others, likely as a healing practitioner. Though the details are fragmentary, this case instead suggests an alternative view from the enslaved of poison as an abuse of power by the strong.

The very existence of records of these cases—not to mention their outcomes, even for those who were not convicted like Tom—recorded in colonial courts by the hands of Europeans and their descendants highlight very real disparities of power in the shaping of discussions about poison in these slave societies. The power of definition was key to making law and holding trials and any attempt to understand the waves of poison cases in the eighteenth and nineteenth centuries cannot dismiss the weight of this European conception of "poison." It was influential not only for shaping the development and outcomes of these trials but also in how poison appeared in abolitionist discourse. When antislavery philosopher the Abbé Raynal warned of enslaved "unfortunates" resorting to poisoning livestock and their fellows in a "spirit of vengeance" against their oppressors, for example, he drew upon this core idea of poison as a weapon of the weak, here used in acts of resistance.[4]

Existing studies of poison cases by historians have primarily discussed alleged poisonings by the enslaved as acts of resistance taken against enslavers—poison being a weapon of the weak and a tool of revenge.[5] This scholarship has done important work in identifying the significance of poison cases to slaveholder discourses on slavery and connections between poison and fears of rebellion. In these works, accusations of poison, obeah, feitiçaria, and so forth with enslaved targets have sometimes been framed as "anomalous behavior"—a deflection of aggression away from slaveholders.[6] However, frameworks of resistance obscure the fact that a significant portion—in some places the majority—of poison cases from Suriname, Bahia, Martinique, and Virginia in the mid-eighteenth century involved enslaved targets. Fraught relationships, not only between enslaved people and their enslavers but also within enslaved communities are important to understanding these poison cases.[7]

"Poison" was a slippery and unstable concept. Even individuals interpreting the same event as a "poisoning" and working to identify a "poisoner" often differed on what they meant by those terms. Examining any individual poison case reveals a kaleidoscope of possible meanings and interpretations. The line between what Africans and Europeans in these slave societies termed "poison" and "healing" was situational and relational. Supporting this fluidity in specifics was continuity in the baseline ideas of "poison" as an abuse of power by the strong or as a usurpation of power by the weak. When historians adopt the dominant European framework of "poison" as the weapon of the weak—or if we uncritically accept a singular definition of what "poison" meant to the range of people involved in these cases over time—we can miss the parallel conversations and definitions used by enslaved Africans and people of African descent that drew upon Atlantic African ideas on political morality.

Uses and Abuses of Power by the Strong

Europeans and their descendants had replaced gendered associations with weakness with racialized ideas of weakness in the context of slavery, with particular concern over African and African-descended healers as wielders of usurped power. From an African perspective, these same healers were powerful people within enslaved communities who could potentially abuse that power for selfish ends—and who could therefore be accused of "poisoning." Both perspectives focused on the powerful work of healing practitioners as possible sources of poison. With the exception of five people in Bahia, all the 190 healing practitioners accused in poisoning cases across these four locations for the entire 170-year period were African or of African descent.[8]

A demographic survey of surviving records of poison trials shows that the people accused of poisoning were generally enslaved, African-descended men, with relatively fewer women—even when accounting for demographic imbalances—and almost no white people.

I want to stress that this analysis reflects only the surviving records of those who were accused and not necessarily of those who practiced. There were also some nuances between the four locations on who was accused in poisoning cases; women and free people of African descent, for example, were accused much more frequently in Bahia than elsewhere. While the differences are not insignificant, what stands out are the similarities between regions and consistency over the peak decades of the eighteenth century. Healing practitioners were particularly prominent.

From the perspective of Atlantic African discourse on politics and power, these healers were not the "weak" as usurpers of power but rather the "strong"

Table 1. Demographics in Peak Decades of Poison Cases, 1740–1785

	Bahia[a]	Suriname[b]	Marti-nique[b]	Virginia: Cumber-land & Brunswick[c]
	(1740–1769)	(1740–1779)	(1742–1769)	(1750–1785)
Total people	105	151	117	32
Men	54	121	91	24
Women	51	30	26	8
African descent	81	151	116	32
Enslaved	40	144	101	32
Free Black	41	7	15	—
White	24	0	1	—
Indigenous	0	0	0	—
Healing practitioner	23	42	26	20

SOURCE: Inquisição de Lisbo, Procesos de Fé and Cadernos do Promotor; Oud Archief Suriname: Raad van Politie, Processtukken betreffende criminele zaken (1705–1828), vol. 793–836; Annales du Conseil souverain de la Martinique (1726–1778), Collection Moreau de Saint-Méry, vol. 244–246, ANOM; Brunswick County Court Order Books, vol. 3–14, Cumberland County Court Order Books, vol. 1752–58 to 1784–86, LVA.

[a] I am including all *feitiçaria* cases as an umbrella that included *calundús, bolsas de mandinga*, love magic, superstition, divination, and *maleficio*.

[b] Suriname volumes for 1747–1748 are fragments, missing data for the years 1746, 1749, 1751, 1755–1760. Martinique data missing for the years 1749 and 1760 to 1764.

[c] Virginia County Court Records only included criminal cases with enslaved defendants. While I used the numbers from Stuart Schwarz for total trial data in the Introduction, for detailed demographic information that Schwarz did not have (such as whether individuals were identified as healing practitioners), I focused on the two counties with the largest numbers of cases (Cumberland and Brunswick). Schwarz identified 179 total individuals tried for poisoning across the colony from 1740 to 1785; I identified 32 of them from these two counties in these same decades.

capable of wielding or potentially abusing their power; this central idea continued to resonate across the Atlantic even in the wider context of slave society power dynamics. There is evidence on how free and enslaved healing practitioners of African descent framed and talked about themselves: as powerful experts worthy of a reputation and respect. They were professionals: they learned their trade, acquired expertise, and were paid for their services. From Virginia to Bahia, slaveholders often relied on these practitioners, as white physicians were generally expensive, scarce, and ineffective. Furthermore, enslaved people specifically sought them out to treat illnesses and solve problems.[9] Their healing knowledge and expertise made them fixtures in colonial medical marketplaces, even when their practices were specifically outlawed.

The connection between power and knowledge for practitioners of African descent was apparent in the words they and their clients used to refer to themselves. In some cases, specific words from Atlantic African languages referring to professional healer-diviners traveled. Such was the case for Branca, an enslaved practitioner from Angola living in Bahia, who called herself a *ganga* and spoke when possessed with the voice of her dead son.[10] The root *-gàngà (expert, healer-diviner) had specific associations with communications with the dead as the ultimate source of knowledge and power.[11] With the root verb also centered on tying and untying, such a practitioner could bind powers into protective objects and unknot afflictions suffered by their clients. The fact that Branca and others who called themselves *gangas* both used the word and conducted practices as spirit mediums connected to contemporaneous uses and practices in West Central Africa indicates the movement, at least in part, of key ideas about who health practitioners were and how they operated in the Americas.[12]

More often, African-descended practitioners staked claim to their expertise through European vernacular terms. While called *empoisonneurs* (poisoners) and, less frequently, *sorciers* (sorcerers) by the courts and their accusers, in Martinique, healers of African descent called themselves *savant*: people of "great erudition."[13] As with the use of *ganga*, which in early modern West Central Africa was often combined with other terms to indicate the area of specialist skill, *savant* emphasized proficiency and command. In his journal, colonial prefect Pierre-Clément de Laussat noted that "savant is the name that they [slaves] give among themselves to these black poisoners. *I am not a Savant*, they say to indicate that they are not poisoners."[14] In Virginia, practitioners often referred to themselves as "doctor." For example, two advertisements from the county jails of Charles City and Isle of Wight County printed in the *Virginia Gazette* in 1774 and 1777 specifically noted that the captured runaway practitioners respectively called themselves "Doctor Dick" and simply "Doctor."[15] While the term "doctor" has connotations specific to emergent professional western biomedicine—leading many historians, including myself, to more frequently use "healer" to speak on a wider range of practitioners—it is important to recognize that to these practitioners it was the English term they chose to describe themselves and to communicate who they were and what they did. Terminology was complicated in Suriname:

wissiman, possibly derived from Dutch *wijs* for "wise" (that is, "wise-man") almost always had a negative connotation but referred to specialists with knowledge of plants and poisons.[16] Diviners more often referred to themselves as *lukumen* (or *locomen*—spelling in sources varied), a Sranan creole word glossed as "Wiessager" (seer) and "Zauberer" (magician, conjuror) by German missionaries in 1783.[17] The 1763 trial of Kwamina, well known to enslaved communities in the area as a "Doctor & Lukkeman," focused on his secret knowledge of herbs used to treat an enslaved man who had come to him from a different plantation.[18] Gramman Quassi, perhaps the most famous and successful health practitioner of African descent in the Atlantic world, also chose to go by the term *lockoman*—translated by John Gabriel Stedman as "sorcerer" and "sibyl."[19] In the words they chose to describe themselves, healers of African descent emphasized their knowledge and acquired expertise.

As part of their professional status, whether free or enslaved, healers generally received some sort of payment for goods and services rendered.[20] Such payment was part of the respect owed for their expertise. This was true both for slaveholders in the Americas who hired them to treat mysterious afflictions—though in cases where the practitioners were enslaved, payment would often be split or go primarily to their enslaver—and for the enslaved people who sought out their wide variety of services. For example, in late eighteenth-century Virginia, prominent slaveholders Robert Carter and Thomas Jefferson each hired healers of African descent and paid them, in consultation with their enslavers, in coin.[21] In Suriname, an enslaved practitioner named Scaramouche sold substances termed "poison" by the courts to five enslaved people on another plantation to guard against sicknesses.[22] While coins of some sort were the most frequently noted form of payment, if the form was noted at all, others included bananas, cows, and, in two Suriname cases, strings of "papa gelt"—possibly cowrie shells.[23] Free and freed healers generally had greater control over their services and charges than those who were enslaved.

Free status could also give practitioners greater flexibility as to where they conducted their work, although this was not without risk. While enslaved practitioners often had to face the chance of discovery by conducting healing rituals in their living quarters or in the spaces between plantations, free(d) practitioners were sometimes able to set up a private workspace. For example, Paulo Gomes and Ignacia, free and freed practitioners in 1740s Bahia, conducted *calundús* at a farm Gomes had purchased on the outskirts of the city of Salvador.[24] *Calundús* were ceremonial dances conducted to determine the causes of and solutions to illnesses for clients, organized and run by health practitioners. While the term *calundú* would gradually refer to a range of practices adapted from Atlantic Africa, in seventeenth- and early eighteenth-century Brazil the dance usually involved spirit possession with specific links to West Central African practices; the word itself originated from a Kimbundu word for a spirit capable of possession.[25] However, the relative privacy of a house did not guarantee safety. A large 1766 poison case in Martinique centered on meetings and activities held in the home of a free man of color named Jacques Pain, who allegedly orchestrated a series of poisonings.[26] Several decades later, another well-known case in the Bahian Recôncavo consisted of a police raid on a house of free Africans on a tip that they danced *calundús*.[27] While offering something of a private refuge, practices in homes or on farms could also attract suspicion; a frequently repeated sentiment in denunciations and trials was that everyone in a neighborhood knew where people went for illegal ritual practices. Free(d) practitioners of African descent may have had more opportunities and flexibility to conduct their healing work than their enslaved peers, but fixed locations could increase both success and risk.

The details about Ignacia, Paulo Gomes, and their work on their farm were embedded in a denunciation to the Inquisition, a denunciation from multiple neighbors—of African and European descent—focused on their work treating and allegedly causing illnesses with *malefícios* (malevolent spells). The idea that the same health practitioner could be accused of treating and causing malevolent afflictions makes sense in the context of an ambivalent conception of power; the power to cure was also the power to harm and those with power could abuse it for selfish purposes.[28] Furthermore, the separation between what constituted healing and harming could be relative: some practices performed to promote public health could be seen as malevolent to individuals believed to be harmful to that health. For example, an enslaved client might purchase an object to "tame" or pacify his or her enslaver—an act promoting personal and public welfare from the client's perspective, but invariably seen as dangerous and often "poisonous" from the perspective of the enslaver if discovered. Health practitioners of African descent who increased their visibility as powerful individuals also increased their risk of being accused of causing illnesses. The precarity of their position within a community hinged on public perception of how they used—or abused—their power.

Healers were highly valued in enslaved communities: people saw their work as efficacious and often took significant risks to avail themselves of their services. Enslaved people on plantations from Virginia to Brazil pushed against the varying limitations of their circumstances to take charge of their own health care. They frequently took the risk of punishment and potential execution to seek treatment from practitioners outside of slaveholder sanction and, frequently, beyond the borders of their plantations. Such was the case of an enslaved porter, Jan, who at his trial for running away in 1762 gave the explanation that he was sick and had run to the Maroons for treatment.[29] Several Suriname trials of health practitioners, including Kwamina in 1763 and Scaramouche in 1765, included accusations from enslavers of their healing of enslaved people who came to them from other plantations.[30] In the case of the latter, the practitioner was convicted of selling *vergift* (poison) and "superstitions" to an entire group of people on another plantation for protection against illnesses.[31] From the 1740s onward, Virginia, Suriname, Martinique, and Bahia each had laws and local ordinances forbidding or severely restricting healing by people of African descent; the fact that enslaved people continued to seek their services speaks volumes to their view of these practitioners.

With the imbalance of power in the plantation world between enslavers and the enslaved, afflicted individuals who desired the services of practitioners of African descent often found it less risky to negotiate care, when possible, within the system of slaveholder sanction. In Virginia, this system was codified: after 1748, it was only legal for an enslaved person to practice medicine if all enslavers involved gave their knowledge and consent.[32] When Robert Carter wrote to nearby slaveholders requesting the services of their enslaved practitioners, he identified these requests to cure fits and unusual ailments as specifically coming from the afflicted or from other people in enslaved communities on their behalf.[33] A remarkable pass R. Carter wrote for a man named Sampson in 1788 both framed the illness as an unsolved mystery and emphasized Sampson's request to seek medical care: "To any Person whom it may concern, The Bearer Sampson the Property of the subscriber has for some time been declining, but the subscriber does not undertake to Assign any cause for Sampson's decline. The subscriber doth at the request of Sampson, permit him to make enquiry for some Person who has skill in the Practice of Medicine and put himself under his care to perform a Cure— Whoevere may engage therin the subscriber expects that said Person will advise him of the Terms."[34] Sampson managed to secure an unusually flexible arrangement, but he shared the basic strategy of negotiation with many enslaved people in the Americas who wished to see healers without risking punishment. To obtain a degree of protection, some enslaved people conducted communal rituals of healing with the knowledge, consent, and sometimes the monetary profit of enslavers. For example, those who participated in the *calundús* on the Bahian plantation of Pedro de Sesqueira Barbosa could do so at a reduced risk—accusations, when they came, were not from the slaveholders sanctioning these practices but from scandalized neighbors.[35]

While they took risks or negotiated with enslavers to see these health practitioners with their extraordinary powers, people in enslaved communities often had ambivalent attitudes toward those they deemed powerful precisely *because* they were powerful. It was not an issue of "usurped" power as many slaveholders feared—that is, a question of *who* should or should not have power—but a moral judgment on *how* these individuals used or abused the power that they had. To deal with healing practitioners who had allegedly abused their power, enslaved people sometimes made use of the infrastructure of colonial courts.

These colonial courts were designed for the control of, not use by, enslaved people, and there are important variations on the functioning and record-keeping of these courts that should invite readers' caution. In Virginia, Martinique, and Suriname, enslaved people could not directly bring a case to court; when they brought their investigations to their enslavers, it was a slaveholder or overseer who initiated court proceedings. Natalie Zemon Davis's work on systems of justice on Suriname plantations suggests that enslaved communities often handled affairs internally—conducting ordeals, adjudicating outcomes, and enforcing punishments—for minor crimes like theft or adultery, often resulting in some form of compensation. However, they were much more likely to go to enslavers with accusations of "poisoning" as something far more serious.[36] Thirty cases in my dataset, mostly from 1730 to 1790, explicitly stated that enslaved people instigated the poison investigation in question and then deliberately brought it to the attention of slaveholders. None of the Virginia records I examined had enough detail to say with whom the case originated, and the disproportionately high number of these cases from Suriname—accounting for twenty-four of the total—does not necessarily reflect a difference in the geographic rate of investigations led by enslaved communities as it does the degree of recorded detail. It is reasonable to suspect that there were more cases that enslaved people brought to enslavers than ended up in courts, and even more cases that they handled internally—cases that were not recorded because they were never brought to the attention of slaveholders or the colonial judicial system.[37] However, by looking closely at the cases for which I do have information, I have identified some common patterns.

Enslaved people in these cases did not launch investigations on behalf of alleged wrongs done to slaveholders, but to the enslaved community on the plantation or in the neighborhood more broadly. Twenty-three involved enslaved targets, mostly from the same plantation, while the remaining seven had no stated target: they accused individuals only of having a reputation for being a harmful poisoner or for going about with poison. In the 1688 case of Simão, eleven of the enslaved people working on the same plantation as Simão and more from the surrounding neighborhood had died over the course of a year from "unknown illnesses," prompting people on Andre Gomes de Medina's plantation to search Simão's cabin.[38] Likewise, in 1773 the enslaved people on Plantagie Peperpot denounced Mars to the overseer for killing fifteen of their number with *wiriwiri* that he had hidden in corners around the plantation—instigating his trial.[39] The people on Inquisitorial Commissioner Manoel Anselmo de Almada's tobacco plantation in the Bahian Recôncavo were so concerned about the freed practitioner Thereza that they "clamored" for action, informing him on a visit that she was responsible for "causing them illnesses unknown to the art of medicine."[40] All but one of the healing practitioners of African descent accused by enslaved people in my dataset were explicitly accused of causing the illness or death of an enslaved person through "poison."

A case from 1732 Suriname illustrates how enslaved people accused healing practitioners based on how they used or abused their power within the community. Two enslaved men—Mainbij, a driver (an enslaved manager responsible for labor and punishment), and La Lande—were accused of causing the deaths of nine people and illness of five others across the living quarters of the enslaved in a neighborhood of plantations, using herbs "to poison" that caused stomach pains, swelling, and weakness. It was La Lande himself who led a crowd to investigate Mainbij's cabin while he was out, producing evidence including bottles of liquid and a boiling pot with dead animals in it. A woman named Beluche from a nearby plantation, whose daughter was among the afflicted, said that she knew well the healing practices of both Mainbij and La Lande, which involved baths with certain leaves, preservative treatments for children, and rituals involving placing dead birds on afflicted bodies and then burying them. Because she believed the men had caused the death of her daughter, she said she "did not want to hide" them. The enslaved people in the neighborhood saw Mainbij and La Lande as practitioners with access to power and the deaths they allegedly caused as an abuse of that power. Following the deaths, even La Lande's own mother-in-law, Venus, joined in the accusation.[41] This trial record is a fragment; while it contains an initial letter from the overseer, the court's interrogation of the accused, and information from several enslaved witnesses, I was unable to find the conclusion. For many of these cases tried in colonial courts, the results were gruesome executions designed as a demonstration and reassertion of power by its "proper" wielders. While enslavers and colonial courts recorded fragmentary glimpses of enslaved communities' alternative discourse on the morality of how power was used, their dominant frame for understanding poisoning cases was instead centered on who had the proper use of power.

Healers as Usurpers of Power and Controlling the "Weapon of the Weak"

If the colonial courts and enslavers in the Americas talked about poison as primarily a usurpation of power, then a key concern was to assert control over possible threats to that power—namely, African-descended health practitioners. Slaveholders from the Chesapeake to Brazil had a fraught relationship with these healers and their practices more generally: they frequently hired and depended on them for the medical care of enslaved people—and, occasionally, themselves—but they did not entirely trust them. There was a tension between what enslavers saw as the secret knowledge of these practitioners and their anxiety over the potential application of that knowledge outside of their own control.[42] This anxiety was reflected in a series of poisoning laws of the 1740s that built on accusations against healers in earlier cases to criminalize healing work by practitioners of African descent.[43]

One of the ways in which this unease over the dependence of plantations on practitioners' knowledge manifested itself was through attempts to draw lines on which kinds of healing practices were acceptable and which were not: this strategy was particularly common in the Catholic church. As early as 1682, Jesuit R. P. Mongin, on Saint-Christophe, set out a list of classifications and recommendations for action on what he described as types of magic practiced by enslaved people. Mongin allowed tolerance for healers who used herbal remedies but called for the suppression of any enslaved people who combined herbs with spells as these were connected to demons.[44] The Lisbon Inquisition was also concerned with cures deriving from the power of demons and with policing the boundaries of what constituted legitimate practice. Their concern extended to priests incorporating some of the practices of African-descended healers into their exorcisms, like the Dominican missionary Alberto de Santo Tomás whom the Inquisition interrogated in 1713.[45]

Enslavers in Virginia, Martinique, Suriname, and Bahia also hired health practitioners of African descent, especially but not exclusively to treat unusual afflictions.[46] Even on plantations with hospitals based on European design and heavy involvement from slaveholders as professional or amateur healers—such as that of Virginian Landon Carter in the mid-eighteenth century—much of the actual work of care was done by enslaved practitioners.[47] In Virginia, enslavers like Robert Carter in the 1780s and Thomas Jefferson in the 1790s and early 1800s explicitly hired enslaved practitioners to treat strange declines and "fits" among the enslaved population that they could not explain.[48] French colonists in the Caribbean often turned to both enslaved and European healers, the latter of whom were often undercertified, poorly paid, and a constant source of concern for medical reformers due to widespread malpractice.[49] In Suriname, while overseers were responsible for maintaining the health of enslaved people on a plantation, they often outsourced healing work to enslaved practitioners.[50] In Bahia, slaveholders frequently sought the services of free and enslaved healers of African descent to treat malevolent afflictions among themselves and the enslaved. For example, Jacome Rodrigues put himself under the care of a well-known "black *feitiçeiro*" Pedro Nunes, who used divination to identify a woman enslaved by Rodrigues, Philipa, as the source of his illness.[51] Even the Jesuits at Sergipe de Conde, when overwhelmed by an outbreak of fevers in 1745, decided to experiment by sending one of the afflicted priests to stay with an "angola" near the coast for treatment.[52]

Another way enslavers sought to manage the potentially subversive powers held by African-descended practitioners was to insert themselves into rituals of public healing and investigations held within enslaved communities to identify poisoners. The descriptions I found of slaveholders turning to enslaved practitioners for help—especially for conducting rituals to identify poisoners—were predominantly from Bahia and Martinique. While instances of enslavers hiring ritual health practitioners certainly appeared in cases from Virginia and the Dutch Guianas, I did not find evidence of enslavers' direct participatory role in curing rituals. In Bahia, several slave-holders were denounced to the Inquisition for not only allowing practi-tioners to perform *calundús* but in some cases taking a participatory and profiteering role. Secret denunciations to the Inquisitorial commissioner named enslavers Pedro Coelho Pimentel in 1686, Pedro de Sesquira Barbosa in 1701, and Manoel Lopes in 1743 for their roles in such practices.[53] In the denunciation of Pimentel, he and his wife, Maria Pereira, were well known to have purchased the enslaved practitioners in question specifically for the purpose of making money off their reputation as healer-diviners. Barbosa likewise made a tidy profit from the *calundús* run by his enslaved diviner, Branca. Like other enslavers, Lopes hired out one of his enslaved healers in the city of Salvador to perform *calundús* and cure afflictions caused by *feitiços.*[54] Although these three cases did not go anywhere beyond the de-nunciations, they are intriguing for the glimpses they offer of the ways slaveholders attempted to control both health practitioners and their en-slaved clients. Granting permission for ritual healing practice was one way to try to assert control over them.

In Martinique, several cases involved enslavers taking a more physical role in divinatory rituals run by enslaved communities. French doctor Raymond de Laborde, who resided at the time in Cayenne but had spent years in both Saint-Domingue and Martinique, reported disdainfully in 1775 on slavehold-ers' "superstitious" methods. Such methods included digging up the heart of an individual believed to be poisoned and damaging it with quicklime or a firebrand to make the "author of the poisons" fall into convulsions, as well as to line up suspects and tap them gently with the branch of a certain tree with similar results.[55] While I did not find instances of the former in the Con-seil Supérieur trials—perhaps Laborde was referencing a passage from Père Jean-Baptiste Labat on poisoning—the ritual with the branch appeared in at least two cases. In the case of an unnamed enslaved man from 1755, the en-slaver, suspecting one man of poisoning another, tapped him with a small branch of the *medecineir* tree (*Jatropha curcas*), with the expectation from commonly held opinion that doing so would cause the poisoner and "dis-tributer of spells and *malefices*" agony. Tapped by the branch, the man col-lapsed into convulsions and confessed to poisoning.[56] The incident in a 1767 case offers more intriguing details, as the enslaver Lahuassaÿe Due Cipre had a three-year-old enslaved girl place the branch of the *medecinier* tree on the man Jacques, whom he suspected of poisoning.[57] Known in English as the "physic nut," "Barbados nut," and "poison nut" tree, *Jatropha curcas* has oily seeds that have been used as a purgative; physical contact with the branch or leaves alone would not explain a physical reaction like the convulsions and agonized cries described in these cases.[58] Apparently, this practice, including the role of the child, was still prevalent enough in the early nineteenth century that Pierre-Clément de Laussat noted its continued use in a journal entry from 1807.[59] In both cases, enslavers had a central role in using the ritual—with the wider participation of the enslaved communities on each plantation—to try and identify culprits allegedly responsible for the afflictions and deaths of enslaved people.

By inserting themselves into healing rituals and offering limited sanction of the actions of healers, these slaveholders sought to prevent a usurpation of power—in ways that could come into conflict with other forms of authority. Clergymen in Martinique and Bahia, for example, were dismayed at enslavers relying on the enslaved for ritual aid. Even before official poison trials existed, Labat described slaveholders he met in 1698 "going over" to enslaved people by using occult means to identify malefactors on their plantations.[60] A friend of Labat on a sugar plantation on Martinique, believing several enslaved people there to have been murdered, cut open one of the bodies, removed the heart, and buried it "with certain ceremonies" in quicklime with the intention of thus killing the "sorcerer." Embarrassed by the scandal, Labat went to his friend and delicately reproached him for not providing a good Christian example to the enslaved. Labat's interference was unwelcome: "He said that although I [Labat] was his Curé, I should not enter into his domestic affairs. . . . He warned me once and for all not to trouble myself with his conscience, nor that of his slaves; but only to make the evil spells of the slaves on our plantation stop."[61]

Labat described an encounter with an enslaved practitioner on a Martinique plantation that highlights both his battles against what he saw as demonic sorcery and an emerging concern with unsanctioned healing by enslaved people in the late seventeenth century. After the local surgeons had given up on an enslaved woman, who had been mysteriously ill for some time, she was taken (presumably by her enslaver) to the quarters, where enslaved people often got "involved in treating these sorts of ills" as slaveholders expected them to "know the composition, & sometimes the remedy" for poisons.[62] Suspicious of interference, Labat prevented the enslaved community from giving the woman any medicine and tried to bring back the surgeon. Later that night he heard the woman crying, broke into her hut, and discovered a crowd of enslaved people from multiple plantations with a ritual practitioner, incense, a small sack with various ingredients, and a figurine. A voice had apparently spoken through the figurine to inform the crowd that the woman would die in four days. Labat then severely punished the practitioner, destroyed the ritual objects in front of the horrified onlookers, and informed the slaveholder of his proceedings. Specifically, by his own published account, Labat tied the man up, gave him three hundred lashes with a whip, placed the figurine in front of him, and told the crying man to ask the devil to deliver him. When the gathered crowd "tremble[d]" at his disrespect toward the figurine and said that it would kill him, Labat burned it along with the rest of the ritual objects and threw the ashes into the river. He then had the practitioner put in irons and his wounds rubbed with a common combination of hot pepper and lemon juice (both extremely painful and supposedly a method for preventing gangrene). Labat brought the man to his enslaver, who promised to pay Labat for his trouble and whipped him again "in good manner." Labat later remarked that the enslaved woman did indeed die on the fourth day, in his analysis due to the effect on her imagination, but as he was able to hear her last confession he "had the consolation to see her die a good Christian."[63]

Several key details stand out from this grim account. First, Labat claimed enslavers frequently relied on enslaved healers when surgeons trained in European medicine were ineffective. Second, these slaveholders connected the expertise of enslaved people particularly with knowledge of poisons. Third, the practices that accompanied healing for a suspected poisoning involved a ritual specialist and a network of people across plantations gathering to consult a spirit via a figurine and other ritual objects, interpreted by Labat as idolatry. And fourth, Labat was convinced that demons were the source of the voice and any of the enslaved practitioners' powers, meaning that they were illegitimate usurpations. This incident from the 1680s, preceding Martinique's laws on medical practice, highlights both a religious concern and the emergence of enslavers' concern with unsanctioned and potentially dangerous ritual practices of the enslaved. Labat's interpretation of what he saw also encapsulates European thought on poison as a usurpation of power and weapon of the weak.

Slaveholders and colonial officials who feared a usurpation of their power sought to control healing activities—even when there were no suspicions of death or even physical harm. The work of practitioners of African descent was always potentially subversive to people of European descent precisely because it involved "the weak" wielding power. Enslavers employed a range of legal tools to try and contain this potential. While he did not explicitly link a wave of illnesses in Salvador to alleged poisoning, in the early 1740s the Conde das Galveas, viceroy of Brazil, issued new ordinances that made any suspected administration of "poison," even if it did not cause death, worthy of close investigation.[64] In the following decades, denunciations to the Inquisition of causing illnesses through poison/*feitiçaria*, or for the unsanctioned treatment of such afflictions, rose rapidly. If the denunciations in the *cadernos* entries from Bahia serve as some measure for public concern, then they indicated great if not greater alarm regarding illicit healing methods to treat poisons/*feitiços* than the infliction of harm. From 1740 to 1769, *feitiçaria* accusations involving cures—some but not all of which were explicitly conducted through *calundús*—consistently outnumbered those involving some sort of specific harm.[65] The relative degree of concern with practices over instances of harm is also evident in the alleged targets referenced by the *cadernos* cases. In thirty-two of the forty-six *feitiçaria* cases in the *cadernos* in these decades, there was no specific target of harm.[66] However, details from cases indicate that despite enslavers' fears about the "weapon of the weak," people of both African and European descent made frequent use of these practitioners' services in Bahia.[67]

Members of the Suriname Court of Policy and Criminal Justice considered health practitioners and their "poisons" to be a serious threat, even if they did not always believe their practices to be efficacious. Taming services—sold to enslaved clients to "soften" or "cool" their enslavers and by doing so make the lives of the enslaved easier, appeared in several Suriname poison cases.[68] One case in 1749 gave the court an opportunity to discuss the implications of these taming practices. The court tried an enslaved healer, Bettie, for "poisoning" her enslaver: on examination, the court decided that the suspected substance she had given him was not technically *vergift* (poison) with a physical effect but something that enslaved people used to put their owners "in a good humor." The court determined that this and other such "superstitions" were still "evil and dangerous" and that their use, whether to "poison their owner or slaves," should be punished.[69] While the court described taming as a superstitious practice, in other cases they took African-descended healers' knowledge of "poisons" very seriously. In fact, another woman also named Bettie in 1766 was able to at least delay her execution by agreeing to work with a Dr. Moedner to conduct experiments on the *vergiften* (poisons) and *tegengiften* (antidotes, literally, "against/contra poisons") that she knew.[70] Slaveholders and the colonial court both recognized and feared the powers of practitioners as they scrambled to control them.

A 1748 Virginia law made healing by "any negroe, or other slave" a felony crime, regardless of whether any harm had occurred—justified by the idea that many people of African descent "under pretence of practising physic, have prepared and exhibited poisonous medicines."[71] Of the twenty-seven Brunswick and Cumberland County cases in the mid-eighteenth century, just over half involved healing practitioners accused under this law of preparing, exhibiting, distributing, and sometimes administering "poisonous medicines."[72] After 1748, the number of cases for "poisonous medicines" increased significantly and in tandem with cases with no target. This phrase, which did not appear in cases or law before 1748, now appeared in a majority of cases up to the end of the century.[73] Courts in Virginia associated healers of African descent so firmly with poison that an enslaved person seeking the services of such a practitioner was considered inherently suspicious. In 1771, Sharper's enslaver had him arrested for "Endeavouring to Procur[e] Poison from a Negroe Doctor or Conjurer as they are Call'd but for what Purpose unknown"; his purpose was later referred to as "his Intended Villiany [sic]."[74]

Slaveholders' concerns with alleged poisoners of African descent also began to shape colonial policy in Martinique. While earlier cases had identified enslaved Africans generally as suspected poisoners, by 1741 the Conseil Supérieur specifically attributed deaths to African healing knowledge, creating "poisonous" powders and drugs from plants and distributing them under the guise of remedies within enslaved communities. While enslaved people and livestock were the primary targets of this alleged practice, the council raised the specter of these enslaved healers turning their skills toward "recrimination" against their enslavers or against whites who "trespass on their debauches." Furthermore, they argued that it would be impossible to distinguish healing from poisoning, as practitioners carefully guarded knowledge of their compositions and other enslaved people would not denounce them for fear of becoming their victims. As with Virginia, the council concluded that enslaved people should be banned from giving "any remedies, powders, or drugs for any malady."[75]

The enslaved practitioner threatening the established social order with usurped power emerged as a central figure in Martinique poison cases. The content of these cases frequently linked "poison" with both secret knowledge of "drogues" and invocations of *malefice*—evil spells.[76] In mid-eighteenth-century trials, the expression *"poison et malefice"* appeared in just under half of the forty-six poison cases from 1740 to 1769. "Drogues," sometimes

specified as being made from herbs and roots and often in the form of powders, appeared in over a third as a possible threat grounded in secret knowledge.[77] Simply the possession of unknown substances could be cause for
alarm, as was the case in 1753, when an enslaved man was branded and
whipped for carrying "suspicious and unknown drugs," the use of which
"could be nothing but very prejudicial."[78] Suspicion of free and enslaved
healers in this colony became enough to try individuals as potential "poisoners," even when there was no specific accusation of causing affliction.[79]

Several of these new laws that enslavers created went beyond existing legal
treatment of poison as extreme measures taken to try and control this weapon
of the weak. Two examples—of new forms of punishment in Suriname and
in alterations to the definition of "poison" in Virginia—highlight the ways
that colonial officials perceived poisoning as a unique threat. In 1740s Suriname, the governor and court first struggled to control the supposed poisoning crisis—"one of the greatest troubles today of this land"—through an
escalation of public and terrifying executions intended as a deterrent.[80] This is
not to say that executions were not gruesome before; several cases in the 1730s
ended with beheadings, burning at the stake, and bodies broken on the wheel.
The increasingly favored punishment in the 1740s involved branding and
pinching with hot tongs until dead, then displaying the head on a spike in
the Suriname River: this was the fate of Baron, Sambo, Abraham, and
Emanuiel in a chain of cases in 1742.[81] This waterfront display, visible to all
who moved in or out of the city, was part of what Marisa Fuentes describes
as "architectures of terror and control" in the urban spaces of eighteenth-
century slave societies.[82]

However, by 1745 the governor believed that these grisly executions were
ineffective, as "this rabble does not fear death" or even "the most wretched
torments."[83] The court decided it was necessary to try new tactics. While a
brief December 1745 ordinance addressing poison cases in Suriname did not
expand its definition or alter what constituted "poison" in the eyes of the law,
through the proposed changes to punishments it specifically targeted the un-
controllable networks of connections that had grown between enslaved
communities and African-descended healers. The Society of Suriname began by acknowledging that more and more enslaved people "[went] about
with poison," undeterred by execution because they allegedly believed they
would return to their homelands after death. As a new punishment, enslaved
people convicted of poisoning livestock or other enslaved people would have
their tongue removed and forehead branded and would be sent to work in

chains in Fort Nieuw Amsterdam. The ordinance emphasized the isolation of these convicts, "secluded and without communication and meeting," from other enslaved people, explicitly "so that they never have a community."[84] The violence of this ordinance was not only physical mutilation but a specific attempt to sever bonds of community and mourning among the enslaved.[85] The Society did not continue this practice for long, reverting instead to their terrifying public executions and displays of heads along the river bank: I have found no mention of such a punishment for poisoning used after the 1740s. However, this punishment was the fate of at least three men: Goliath, Philip, and Bossoe.[86] The Society tried to solve what they saw as a poisoning crisis by breaking webs of connection and communication among people of African descent.

Colonial leaders in Virginia forged new conceptions and associations with poison that deviated from contemporary English law, most visible through the exceptions carved out in the 1748 ordinance forbidding healing by African-descended practitioners. Two key provisions tempered the death sentence for such practice. First, if the court determined that the "poisonous medicine" was not made or given with "ill intent, nor attended with any bad consequences," the court had the option to choose a more lenient, though still violent and humiliating, punishment—in practice, a standard brand mark on the hand and thirty-nine lashes at the public whipping post. Second, this law would not apply to enslaved people "administering medicines" with the mutual knowledge and consent of all the enslavers involved.[87] The idea that "preparing, exhibiting, or administering" a medicine deemed "poisonous" could be done without "ill-intent" was in direct contrast with contemporary English law; there poisoning, "the most detestable of all" crimes, could not be tried as manslaughter, as "it carries with it an internal evidence of cool and deliberate malice."[88] In English law, the act of poisoning was inherently intended to harm. By eliminating the need for proof of harm or ill intent to try enslaved people for "poisonous medicines," the Virginia legislature gave county courts—which only had jurisdiction over criminal cases with enslaved defendants—the flexibility to punish those with the perceived potential to "poison." The second provision makes clear that this law was designed to police enslaved practitioners as much as it was to prevent alleged poisonings. By framing healers of African descent as a threat—their practice a possible front for nefarious deeds, the "medicines" they created "poisonous"—while leaving an opening for enslavers' controlled use of these practitioners, the law placed the power to sanction healing practices in the hands of enslavers. By creating a mechanism of slaveholder sanction, the law centered the key issue of avoiding a usurpation of power by enslaved practitioners.

The overlap between their roles as slaveholders and judges also encouraged enslavers in official positions to sometimes bend their own laws on jurisdiction and punishments. As an Inquisitorial commissioner in Bahia, Manoel Anselmo de Almada did not have the authority to make arrests without orders from the Lisbon office.[89] However, Anselmo was also a slaveholder, born and living in the city of Salvador, and owner of a tobacco plantation in São Felipe parish in the Recôncavo. His status was not uncommon; many of the Bahian ecclesiastics and Inquisitorial commissioners were locals: for example, João Calmon, one of the longest-serving commissioners from 1701 to 1737, came from a powerful Bahian family with a sugar plantation.[90] Anselmo appended a letter explaining his unorthodox actions to a 1778 case file denouncing free practitioners and alleged *feiticeiros* Thereza and Luis. While visiting his plantation away from the Salvador office, Anselmo claimed that enslaved people there and across the parish repeatedly came to him calling for action against this "preta Mina" Thereza, who had a bad reputation as a *feiticeira* and who had allegedly killed entire families with "infirmities unknown to the Art of Medicine." Claiming that he was so moved by these accusations, and not wanting Thereza to escape arrest, Anselmo took the initiative to capture her and conduct an investigation without waiting for the authority to do so. He expressed confidence that there was sufficient proof from the testimonies he gathered for her trial, an opinion that was not shared by the inquisitors in Lisbon when they received his case file.[91] Though the Lisbon office declined to take the case, it is illustrative of the ways enslavers involved in cases in an official capacity often had personal stakes in the investigation of poison trials and acted accordingly.

The marriage between slaveholder interests, laws, and courts was not always smooth; in their efforts to control "the weapon of the weak," enslavers sometimes took vigilante action. As Natalie Zemon Davis has noted, colonial Suriname was held in tension between multiple simultaneous systems of justice: that of slaveholders on their plantations, the local colonial government, imperial governance, and that within enslaved communities.[92] A similar tension existed in Martinique.[93] In his letter informing the Ministère de la Marine of the Conseil Supérieur's 1753 decision to suspend portions of French law in establishing the extraordinary commission for poisoning cases, Governor Maxim de Bompar expressed concern that, however valid their alarm at perceived poisoning and their desire to maintain order, it would be dangerous for the colonial enslavers on the council to think that they had the right to act unilaterally.[94] Bompar's unease was part of a jurisdictional tension that was a perpetual factor in poisoning cases.

Some enslavers and overseers chose to take matters into their own hands—torturing and executing suspected poisoners on their plantations—rather than work within the court system. In 1743, the same year as Bahia's ordinance on poison, the royal secretary of the judgment of crimes in Bahia reported numerous enslavers in the city, Recôncavo, and *sertão* practicing extrajudicial punishments of enslaved people for alleged crimes.[95] The situation was similar in Suriname, leading to one high-profile case of a white manager for torturing and beheading an enslaved woman he had accused of poisoning.[96] By choosing to interrogate, torture, or even execute suspected poisoners on their own, slaveholders and managers became a challenge to the legal judicial system and authority of the colonial government.[97] In Martinique, efforts to address poisonings by and of enslaved people highlighted tensions and compromises of judicial power between enslavers and colonial officials. In the earliest cases, Governor Vaucresson was as alarmed by slaveholders' usurpation of legal violence in extracting confessions from enslaved suspects as he was by the economic threat of poison. While the Code Noir set explicit limitations on enslavers' rights to violence toward enslaved people, Vaucresson deemed it necessary to remind them of their limits in a 1713 ordinance in the wake of these cases.[98]

When enslavers suspected poisoning, they sometimes attempted to extract confessions on plantations that conformed to their expectations of poison as a usurpation of power, targeting whites, and especially involving substances placed in food or drink. Case records from eighteenth-century Suriname are rife with such practices. In 1735, an enslaved man named Kees told the court that when the overseer suspected him of poisoning his water—due to a bad smell—his enslaver Jon Kramer tied him to a plank, beat him, and refused him food and water until he confessed and named accomplices. Kees renounced his confession to the court.[99] Similarly, in the 1742 case of Sambo, his enslaver and a group of neighboring slaveholders interrogated him harshly on the plantation until he confessed to being a *"vergeevanaer* [sic]" (poisoner).[100] Similar gangs of neighborhood slaveholders conducted interrogations of Jean Baptiste in 1766 and Jacques in 1767 in Martinique.[101] Enslavers arresting, interrogating, and torturing enslaved people they suspected of poisoning to extract a confession in 1770s Martinique was apparently both commonplace and accepted, however begrudgingly, by the Conseil Supérieur.[102]

The degree to which these actions outside the courtroom affected the outcome of cases varied; during peak periods of poison accusations, their questionable legality appeared to have mattered little if at all. While the court found Kees's claims to have been forced to confess under abuse troubling enough to result in an ambiguous outcome, the same court seven years later had no problem condemning Sambo to be branded, pinched with hot tongs, and beheaded.[103] In fact, when Sambo attempted to deny his earlier confession from the plantation, the court ordered him to be tortured at Fort Zelandia until he affirmed the confession.[104] Likewise, while the Trinité court mildly chastised Seigneur Lahoussaye Du Cipre for overstepping his bounds in interrogating and extracting a confession from Jacques on his own, they nevertheless accepted the confession as valid and proceeded to find Jacques guilty; the Conseil Supérieur confirmed their verdict on automatic appeal.[105]

Furthermore, in relatively rare instances when courts found enslaved defendants not guilty, or determined that they had insufficient evidence to convict, enslavers continued to pursue the matter on their own plantations. Enslaved people found not guilty in Virginia, Suriname, and Martinique were almost always discharged back to their enslavers, often the same people who had brought the case to trial. While colonial prefect Pierre-Clément de Laussat was greatly concerned with the threat of "poisoning" in Martinique and recorded his observations of a wave of cases in 1807 and 1808 in his diary, he was also deeply troubled when he discovered that the Dominicans at Saint-Jacques plantation—one of the largest in the colony—had established their own private jail and had locked up enslaved people who had been implicated but released in the recent Basse Pointe case. The conditions in these cells were so "horrible" as to upset Laussat greatly but apparently were not bad enough, in his view, to justify exposing them.[106] The courts themselves sometimes worked with enslavers to deal with enslaved people they did not convict. In the case of Tom that opened this chapter, the Caroline County court sentenced him to deportation in 1744 as a potential threat, even though they had determined that he was guilty only of giving out powders but not of killing: this case came four years before the Virginia legislature outlawed such activity.[107] Laussat also reported enslavers quietly working with the Saint Pierre jail to deport enslaved suspects they arrested for poisoning without a trial.[108]

Even as slaveholders sought to control "poisoners" and spoke emphatically of their threat, the idea of what "poison" was remained contested and slippery. This was true even within European languages. Europeans living contemporaneously on opposite sides of the Atlantic differed in their analyses of the relative threat of African-descended healers as "poisoners," and the details of what Europeans considered to be "poison" changed from the late seventeenth to early nineteenth century. Changes in dictionaries suggest shifts in how Europeans thought about "poison" as a physical substance. The *Dictionnaire de l'Académie française* is an excellent source for tracking such changes among French speakers between the first (1694), fourth (1762), and sixth (1835) editions. Between the 1694 and 1762 editions, the academy dropped tobacco as an example under "poison," while between the 1762 and 1835 editions, it changed the primary example for "contre-poison" from theriac to milk—used frequently by nineteenth-century physicians to induce vomiting as the first step of treatment in accidents.[109] Under the entry for the verb "empoisonner," the 1835 edition included a new example: "He poisons himself with arsenic."[110] While both the 1694 and 1762 dictionaries discussed "vénéfice"—a word loaded with implications of "sorcery" in contemporary usage—as a "crime of poisoning . . . only used in criminal procedures," by 1835 the academy had made a small but crucial change in saying that *vénéfice* "was only used in former criminal procedures."[111] Though small, each change contributed to a pattern where European elites increasingly discussed poison as chemical substances with a greater emphasis on criminal justice and forensics.

While European authors of poison treatises earlier in the eighteenth century had focused on trying to understand how poisons and venoms worked on the body—and by extension, how bodies worked—these later treatises had a practical focus on medical jurisprudence. Samuel Farr, a Bristol physician, and William Dease, an Irish surgeon, respectively published treatises as educational pieces to improve the accuracy of autopsies and correct firmly held popular ideas about poison that could lead to false accusations.[112] Mathieu Joseph Bonaventure Orfila's multivolume *Traité des poisons* was a significant turning point in that his work brought together the goals of medical jurisprudence with an effort to comprehensively catalog known poisons as the basis for a new field of "toxicology"—itself a newly coined word.[113] Orfila described this new field as the widest of all branches of medicine, of interest to many, including the "Practitioner"—always seeking ways to "quickly ruin [poisons'] deadly action"; the "Chemist"—"revolted by the crime of homicide" who seeks to help magistrates "punish the guilty"; and the "Gentleman"—who "[deplores] the fate of victims of negligence or scorn," sympathizes with suicides, and feels "horror at the idea of the heinous assassin" who attacks in silence.[114] First published in 1814, *Traité de poisons* was almost immediately translated into English, Italian, German, and Hungarian and went into three French editions in just over a decade. This work was so foundational to nineteenth-century toxicology that in the 1870s Émile Littré's massive *Dictionnaire de la langue français* cited Orfila and his work as the primary example for the word "toxicologie."[115] As with Farr and Dease, Orfila explicitly directed his work to the tasks of training physicians to be able to identify and properly treat poisons in living patients and to perform autopsies to identify causes of death. Like Farr, Dease, and other writers, Orfila was emphatically concerned with educating physicians who might be called to testify in criminal cases and with reinforcing and policing the boundaries of professional medicine.

What is striking about these works of medical jurisprudence is that they are each completely void of *any* discussion of the waves of eighteenth- and nineteenth-century poison trials across the Atlantic. As part of his comprehensive catalog, Orfila did discuss several plants and local treatments from the Americas, including the *guaco* plant, used by Indigenous peoples and people of African descent in New Granada to treat snakebites, and the arrow poisons *ticunas* and *curare* from the Amazon and Orinoco; in each of these cases he cited the reports and experiments of others—including Fontana—without conducting his own.[116] This treatment was in stark contrast with his extensive and personally conducted experiments on poisons of greater concern to him, especially mercury sublimate, arsenic, and antimony.[117] Orfila did not mention any of the cases of enslaved or free people of African descent accused of poisoning in contemporary Martinique, Suriname, or elsewhere, or the theorizing and practices conducted by enslavers intent on identifying "poisons" and "poisoners." The anecdotal cases Orfila cited to accompany his experiments were exclusively focused on European cases from Orfila's practice as a physician and frequently involved accidents and deaths by suicide.[118] While stating a concern with homicide, Orfila gave very few examples of it in his case studies; in fact, he appears to have been perhaps more concerned with doctors claiming to have found poison when there was none or running their experiments poorly. Bizarrely, in one passage Orfila railed against the crime of secretly introducing a poisonous substance into the rectum of a cadaver with the intent of skewing the autopsy and framing an innocent man: "of all the crimes committed today, there is none which inspires as much horror."[119] European authors of these late eighteenth- and early nineteenth-century poison treatises had their eyes fixed on Europe; the experiences of enslavers, enslaved people, and health practitioners of African descent in the ongoing poison trials of the Americas were apparently not considered relevant enough for inclusion. While the idea of the "weapon of the weak" endured with nineteenth-century tropes of arsenic-wielding female poisoners, and while Orfila presented his catalog of "poisons" as comprehensive, the definition of "poison" and who was a "poisoner" in the Atlantic world remained constructed, contingent, and intertwined with contested narratives of power.

*   *   *

Two durable idioms of talking about poison—a weapon of the weak versus an abuse of power by the strong—that Europeans and Africans had developed over centuries produced waves of eighteenth-century poison cases in the slave societies of the Americas with a shared focus on health practitioners of African descent. In both moments of contestation and convergence, the relationships of power between enslavers and the enslaved were dramatically uneven and are essential context for understanding how these moments played out. On plantations and through institutions of the state, enslavers interrogated, tortured, and executed hundreds of people of African descent as "poisoners"; violence and terror were defining pillars of eighteenth-century slave societies. However, despite this enormous power, enslavers did not have complete control over the way that everyone involved in poisoning events saw, interpreted, and discussed them. While slaveholders' fears about the usurpation of power formed the dominant discourse evident in the trials, theirs was not the only perspective. People in enslaved communities had their own concerns about the actions of extraordinary individuals in their midst and, most important, *how* they chose to use or abuse their powers. It is through close analysis of poison investigations and trials—from ideas about emotions, to the tying/untying work of "poison," to overlaps in narrative building—that we can catch glimpses of Atlantic African ideas, their transformation in the Americas, and the ways that European-descended enslavers (mis)understood them.[120]

CHAPTER 4

Poison and the Belly

Swart Jan was an enslaved driver at Plantagie Jagtlust, a large coffee plantation of two thousand acres almost directly across the Suriname River from the capital of Paramaribo.[1] The morning of June 18, 1744, he and his wife, a "Coromantee" named Griet, ran east into the woods.[2] Earlier that morning, an enslaved man named Quamina had led a group from the quarters to the main house to speak with Gerrit Versteegh, the manager and overseer of the plantation. They accused Swart Jan of being a "Wijsman"—*wissiman*—and he and his wife of "going about" with *vergift* (poison).[3] Their testimony, listed by name by Versteegh and later read before the Suriname Court of Policy and Criminal Justice, revealed that they suspected the pair as the cause of a series of illnesses and deaths in the neighborhood.

As evidence, they described their symptoms and linked them to moments of relationship conflict with Swart Jan. Among the specific accusations, one man named Leveilje claimed that Swart Jan had recently given him a bitter "soopje" (dram or broth), after which he had felt a heavy pain in his body, fallen to the ground, and was "touched" with swelling—interpreted as clear evidence of "poisoning." Primo claimed that Swart Jan had poisoned him in a dispute over Primo's cotton hammock. The crowd also told Versteegh that the recently deceased Quassiba, who was "also a doctress," had predicted her own death and the deaths of others by poisoning and claimed that Swart Jan would be the one responsible. One person claimed to have seen Swart Jan later taking dirt from Quassiba's grave, further evidence of his alleged abuses of power. Other accusations were not restricted to Jagtlust but came from enslaved people across the neighboring plantations of Peperpot, Meersorgh, and Mopentibo. Several people at Peperpot told their overseers that they had seen Swart Jan moving between the plantations, collecting *wiriwiri* (leaves from empowered plants) and threatening people.[4]

Relationships and the fraught emotions they engendered were key to this story—through evidence warranting suspicion within the enslaved community, through the fear and pain that suspicion could cause, and through the methods used by another practitioner to resolve the case. The crowd led by Quamina had searched Swart Jan's cabin, claiming a pot of what he protested was "medicine" was actually "poison"; they then beat Swart Jan and locked him in irons before bringing him to the overseer. Later that day, Griet helped her husband break free, and the couple ran. Three days later, a group from Jagtlust recaptured Swart Jan in a nearby meadow, wounded and with no sign of Griet. Brought again to the overseer Versteegh, Swart Jan told him that Griet had hanged herself in the woods and that he had struck himself with a knife, wanting to die.[5] When later asked by the court why they had run, Swart Jan replied that he had been afraid following the accusation of poisoning from the neighborhood. Before Versteegh took Swart Jan to the court in Paramaribo across the river, the enslaved community of Jagtlust, with Versteegh's knowledge, invited another enslaved man named Maskree to come to the plantation. Bearing a calabash and a sheep's horn, Maskree spoke with people in their living quarters and with Swart Jan. It is unclear from Versteegh's report exactly what happened next, but later that day Versteegh sent Swart Jan across the water to the cells of Fort Zelandia. Maskree and the others watched him leave.[6]

Swart Jan's case is significant in its own right as a microcosm of the tensions and fraught relationships between enslaved communities, enslavers, and practitioners of African descent; it is also illustrative of the ways these relationships were entangled with poison. The people who first investigated and locked up Swart Jan accused him of being a *wissiman*: of using empowered substances to "poison" rather than to cure. In conducting their investigation, they chose to involve both the white overseer and an enslaved healer from another plantation. I am not arguing that poison accusations were merely covers for "real" social conflicts involving negative relationships; instead, I want to explore the idea that negative relationships *were* "poison" and that people in the Americas drew upon Atlantic African ideas about selfishness, malice, swelling, and the belly in their understanding of what they described as poisoning events.

Borrowing from the history of emotions is not only useful for untangling the fraught relationships and motivations in poisoning events, but also for seeing connections between ideas about poison in Atlantic Africa and in the diaspora. Historians and anthropologists of Africa have long described widespread idioms linking aspects of "the exercise of power in social relations"—from discussions of *kindoki* to links between "witchcraft," cannibalism, and negative emotions like selfishness and greed—with physical and metaphorical ties to the belly as both the source of emotions and the physical place where extraordinary people could access powers.[7] Numerous works in African history over the past twenty years have embraced and contributed to many of the insights from the history of emotions, including reexamining oral traditions and the archive of words generated by historical linguistics for the language of affect.[8] As Tom McCaskie and others have explored with oral traditions, the ways that Atlantic Africans and their descendants spoke of and responded to affliction and alleged poisoning events in the Americas are useful not solely as sources of data but for the insights they can yield on the affective significance of these events to the actors involved.[9] Emotions shaped how individuals of African and European descent saw and interpreted poisoning events—including whether to even define an event as a "poisoning," what they meant by that definition, and which details were relevant for making these claims. The relative significance of details— the gender of the accused, the history of their interactions with their alleged target, the location of symptoms on the afflicted body—was embedded, expressed, and recorded through emotions and relationships. "Poison" was not solely an individual experience but a communal one.

Emotions and Tropes

Close attention to recorded symptoms claimed by people of African descent reveals an emphasis on seizures and sudden collapses, long declines, and swelling, especially in the belly: attention to Atlantic African ideas about poisoning gives us insights into the social and emotional significance of these symptoms. Unfortunately, I must begin with a caveat on what I mean by *recorded* symptoms. Of the 190 total poison cases with enslaved people as targets in my entire dataset from 1680 to 1850, only thirty-four (26 percent) described the symptoms of the afflicted in any kind of detail; the rest used general terms, mainly variations on "sick" and "ill." Documents from different courts contained differing degrees of detail, with cases from Suriname most likely to include details of symptoms and cases from Virginia the least. However, by combining information from these trials with more anecdotal evidence from plantation papers and correspondence from colonial officers, common symptoms among enslaved people claiming to have been afflicted with poison stand out. Often these symptoms were combined. For example, in the 1778 case of Thereza and Luis in the Bahian *sertão*, their alleged *"malefícios"* caused their free and enslaved victims to slowly lose their color, strength, and health before dying with identical swollen bellies.[10]

The most common symptom reported by those believing themselves to have been poisoned centered on the belly, opening up spaces of convergence between diverse European and African ideas focused on the abdominal region. Pain in the stomach could be sharp and sudden or involve long, drawn-out declines like that suffered by Samson in Suriname for three months before his death in 1732.[11] Belly pains were common enough in Martinique poisonings that enslavers there cited *mal d'estomac* as both a key symptom of poisoning and a scourge that almost exclusively affected people of African descent.[12] The effects of these stomach pains could be devastating: more than thirty enslaved people on M. Aurenae's plantation—the entire enslaved population but one—apparently died from such pains in less than a year.[13] In several cases before the eighteenth-century Suriname courts, afflicted individuals identified stomach pains with poisoning. For example, multiple people who gave their testimony against Swart Jan to the overseer Versteegh in 1744 described his causing "heavy pain in the belly."[14]

Enslaved people across the Americas referenced swelling—especially of the belly—more than any other specific symptom as a sign of "poisoning."[15] While various physical objects found in investigations were wielded as proof against the accused, suspicious swelling was often the first indication that poison was afoot and the spark of an investigation. The people who gave their testimony against Swart Jan cited swelling of the belly that in one instance caused a man to collapse as a powerful indication of poisoning.[16] In his 1739 testimony against Coffie, an enslaved man named Dosoe from the same Suriname plantation described how two people had swelled up before dying a few days later. In the ensuing investigation a jawbone was found—it is unclear from the testimony by whom—buried in the ground under the hut of the afflicted and linked to Coffie, evidence that led to his conviction and burning at the stake in Paramaribo.[17] The significance of swelling as a sign of poisoning appeared in even earlier cases, such as the alleged poisoning by Manoel Petécaba of three other enslaved people in 1699 Bahia, who suddenly began to swell all over, dying several months later.[18] Beyond the trial records, plantation papers from early nineteenth-century Virginia and Martinique noted strange swellings as a sign that something was seriously amiss. Such was the case with the "extraordinary swelling" of Agalé that preceded a poison investigation on Pierre Dessalles's plantation in 1822 and the swelling that began in Ursula's legs and spread to her whole body at Monticello in 1800.[19]

Stomach pains or vomiting overlapped with European conceptions of poison as primarily an ingested substance affecting the stomach. It is possible that these were not necessarily the primary symptoms reported by the enslaved but rather the ones considered to be most significant by the slaveholders and judges in these cases.[20] However, it is also possible that the convergence of ideas about poisoning symptoms could lead to enslaved people and their enslavers talking past each other. While early modern Europeans connected pains and problems associated with poison to the digestive tract, as their main idiom of poison centered on a consumed harmful substance, people in Atlantic Africa discussed similar symptoms as indications of poison but through the idiom of the belly as the source of emotions and poison as an abuse of extraordinary powers originating in negative emotions.[21] The shared focus on the belly—with symptoms of pains, cramps, vomiting, and diarrhea—opened up the possibility of people of European and African descent interpreting the same affliction as "poisoning" for very different reasons.

The act of vomiting and its connection to the belly could have resonated strongly with people of African descent due to its significance in Atlantic African practices. In Atlantic Africa, vomiting was often a central component to oath-drinking ordeals as a way of proving one's innocence. A common idiom in West Africa connected the stomach, vomiting, and illnesses of the stomach to antisocial emotions and malevolent afflictions. Suzanne Blier's work among Fon and Ewe speakers suggests that the consumption of a substance that made one vomit was key because it could clarify that the oath taker had nothing emotionally hidden in their stomach.[22] Fon speakers discussed the stomach as the "seat of human emotions" and used it metaphorically to express ideas like "peaceful" (fa xomɛ, literally "cool stomach"), "innocence" (xomɛ vo, literally "the stomach is empty"), "evil" (e gmlan xomɛ, literally "he has a bad stomach") and "to be in a bad way" (e gble xomɛ, literally "the stomach is spoiled").[23] Similarly, nineteenth-century Twi speakers used the same root for aya-ase (lower part of the belly), ayare-sá (the act or power of healing), o-yaresáfo (one that heals or cures a disease), and o-yàré (wickedness, illness, disease).[24] The stomach, afo, was also the "seat of the affectations" for Igbo speakers, who used this noun to identify particular stomach-based afflictions.[25] Ideas about the belly and the power of binding came together in *bociɔ* statues in the Bight of Benin, as people often tied cords around the bellies of those statues particularly associated with causing or preventing afflictions.[26] The act of binding was also one of "taming": to bind the belly was to tame or harness an emotion.[27] Blier had the insight that the physical symptoms Fon speakers cited when discussing afflictions caused by selfish abuses of power were very similar to those caused by extreme stress and anxiety and were primarily centered on the belly. These symptoms included "stomach cramps, vomiting, diarrhea (or constipation), weight loss, sleeplessness, and nighttime pain," as well as menstruation difficulties.[28] Stomach pains, vomiting, and other symptoms relating to the belly opened possibilities of convergence and (mis)understanding between European and African ideas about poisoning.[29]

Slaveholders in Suriname, Martinique, and Virginia focused on the belly and digestive tract because they claimed that enslaved people primarily poisoned their enslavers by knowingly placing something into food or drink consumed by the intended victim with intent to harm. In other words, enslavers brought enslaved people to court for alleged poisoning in ways that were consistent with durable European ideas about poison as an ingested substance—reaching back to the Latin root noun *pōtiō* (drink, potion)—and a usurpation of power through the underhanded method of attack. In 1769, Seba, Roselina, Quassiba, and Margo were tried for poisoning on suspicion of putting herbs in their mistress's soup in Suriname; likewise the Suriname court tried a group of enslaved people on Plantagie Paracabo three years earlier for attempting to poison their enslaver by placing an unknown substance in her milk.[30] In four trials from 1763 to 1798, the enslaved people in question were accused of poisoning their enslavers under the guise of administering them medicine. In one of the most famous Caribbean poisoning cases, a thirty-five-year-old enslaved woman named Émilie was burned at the stake in 1806 for allegedly putting crushed glass in the ragout of Madame La Pagerie—the mother of Empress Joséphine. La Pagerie had not been injured from the food, as she had been immediately suspicious of the texture. As she was well connected, she went directly to Captain General Louis Thomas Villaret de Joyeuse with her concerns; Villaret gave permission to his special tribunal to arrest and interrogate Émilie, burning her a day after convicting her of "forming a design to poison and kill" her enslaver.[31]

The case of Émilie also highlights how European descendants translated their ideas about gender, emotions, relationships, and poison to a plantation context. Villaret's letter summarizing the case described Émilie as having been born and lived her whole life in La Pagerie's house. She had been La Pagerie's chambermaid for twenty years, since she was fifteen. Both Villaret and Pierre-Clément de Laussat—a colonial prefect in Martinique at the time who wrote about this sensational case in his diary—described Émilie as having the trust and confidence of La Pagerie at the time of her alleged "poisoning."[32] This framing of "the most trusted" enslaved people as potential "poisoners" emphasized an idea of betrayal: enslavers who used it positioned the people they accused as not only dangerous but *ungrateful* and lacking what they saw as the appropriate emotional response to their alleged treatment. However, Laussat's diary entry from the week of Émilie's trial—copied out and rearranged as a draft for a future memoir—also contained a detail that he chose not to include in the published work: Madame La Pagerie had apparently caught her husband sexually exploiting Émilie before his death in 1790.[33] This detail highlights the extreme precarity of enslaved women in domestic labor and the sexual violence enslavers visited upon them; the warped history of this relationship also suggests why Madame La Pagerie's suspicion fell on Émilie so quickly. For Laussat, this story was evidence of Émilie's supposed "libertine" nature. Interrogated by unspecified means on the plantation, Émilie said that she got the idea to poison La Pagerie from an old woman known for her knowledge of poison. Laussat concludes that the women had worked together for years on "their vengeance."[34] The idea of a female poisoner, easily influenced, bent on malice, and driven by her passions drew directly on centuries of early modern European discourse about witches, gender, and poison.

Witch theorists at the height of the European witch hunts in the sixteenth and early seventeenth centuries associated witches with women because they believed women were inherently weaker and more emotional than men, and therefore more susceptible to demonic temptation in exchange for "unnatural" power.[35] Significantly, devil worship and the elaborate Sabbath rituals at which witches allegedly gathered were usually absent in initial depositions and accusations from neighbors, and only came up in interrogations and confessions extracted under torture.[36] For the magistrates conducting trials, poisoning was most significant as an indication of knowledge and power lent by the devil. For the common people who accused their neighbors, *maleficia* such as poison or crop destruction conducted by malicious members of the community were a primary concern. Both associated poison with witches and with women.

Overlapping with ideas about witchcraft, early modern European poison
accusations and discourses of poison in the public imagination centered on
the idea of spiteful women poisoning their husbands or romantic rivals.[37] The
idea of poison-wielding wives even appeared in new dictionary definitions.
Jean Nicot's *Thresor de la language françoyse* (1606), compiled from multiple
editions of sixteenth-century dictionaries, made such direct connections between poison and women. Under the verb *empoisonner* (to poison), Nicot
demonstrated the passive with the example "empoisonné par sa femme"
(poisoned by his wife).[38] Thomas Elyot included in his 1538 English-Latin
dictionary an entry "*Venenarię mulieres*," or "women that do sel [sic] poison."[39] In English law the murder of a husband by a wife through poison or
other means was a form of "petit treason," as the rule of a husband over the
household was a microcosm of the rule of the king over the kingdom.[40]
While not necessarily involving demonic power, these ideas framed wives as
the weak finding a way to "unnaturally" defeat their stronger husbands—
in English law a literally treasonous usurpation of power.

European gendering of negative emotions in relation to "witchcraft" per-
sisted long after they stopped putting witches on trial and beyond the major
areas of witch hunting.[41] The connection is strongly evident in the vernacular dictionaries of the late seventeenth and early eighteenth centuries. In the
first dictionary of the Portuguese language, a massive work of eight volumes
written over the 1710s and 1720s and published in 1728, Raphael Bluteau included not only definitions but also short essays and numerous citations with
many of the words. His entries for *feiticeira* (female sorcerer) and *feiticeiro*
(male sorcerer) and associated words are particularly illuminating. First, Bluteau firmly linked *feiticeiros/as*, *feitiçaria*, and *feitiços* with poison by trans-
lating them into Latin with his examples as *veneficus*, *veneficium*, and
venenum—words from the Latin root *uenēnum* that suggest "sorcerer-
poisoner" as a more accurate translation of *feiticeiro/a* for the early eighteenth century. In a lengthy definition, Bluteau pondered why there were
apparently so many more women sorcerer-poisoners than men. He theorized
that as women were "naturally more vengeful and envious" and so they "with
more curious malice study the means to satisfy these passions," rendering
them more easily taken by demons. In contrast, in the entry on *feiticeiros*,
Bluteau emphasized not interpersonal conflicts and passions but stories of
famous men using "Diabolical Arts"—making an implicit or explicit pact
with demons to exert power over nature. While the theory of demonic agency

necessary for going beyond the bounds of nature held, these differences in definition separated "sorcery" between feminine acts of women seeking vengeance and envy from a position of weakness and masculine acts of powerful men seeking greater power over nature.[42]

The European tropes of women as poisoners and poison as a usurpation of power also centered on fraught personal relationships. In 1707, João Curvo Semedo discussed "homens enfeytiçados" (bewitched men)—or more accurately, but very inelegantly, "ensorcelled-poisoned men"—affected by the love magic of women "fearful that they [the men] will leave them," as a common and serious medical problem. These women "secure[d]" their men and altered their behavior by putting various substances in their food and drink, most potently menstrual blood. Echoing physicians from the middle ages, Semedo went on to describe menstrual blood as a substance "so poisonous, and prejudicial" that it could cause "a thousand … pitiful symptoms" of madness, furies, fears, and tears.[43] In France, the "cultural script" of poison, to borrow Lynn Wood Mollenauer's term, in the late seventeenth century focused on women using poisons and potions, with ingredients like menstrual blood, to make men fall or stay in love with them—a form of female control over men that was considered deeply threatening to the social order.[44] Gendered ideas of poison and emotions continued in Victorian Britain; tales of vindictive wives poisoning their husbands was a staple of nineteenth-century British popular culture and novels with poisoning plots.[45]

European associations between treachery, cunning, and poison also appeared in a rather convoluted recurring trope whereby enslaved people allegedly hid powdered poison under a fingernail and stealthily dipped it into a drink while handing it to their intended target. In specific relation to Africans and people of African descent, this trope emerged in the late seventeenth century and had a robust longevity over the eighteenth century. To be clear, I am not here referring to fingernails used as an ingredient in "poisons" but of an alleged and particularly devious method of poisoning.[46] Yet in all of the 542 poison cases in my dataset, I found only one explicitly involving this fingernail method—the alleged act admitted during a forced confession on a plantation.[47] While this absence in trials and formal investigations does not necessarily mean a complete absence in practice, the gap between discussion of the method and the trials themselves is significant.

The history of the idea of the fingernail method and its emotional connotations had an interesting path in the Atlantic world that included a wide range of supposed poisoners—not all of whom were of African descent, but each of whom was stereotyped to different audiences as possessing malicious cunning. In exploring this idea, I found references to Africans, Native Americans, and Jesuits authoritatively identified by different European authors as supposed masters of the technique. In 1700 the Earl of Bellomont, governor of New York, reported a series of poisonings among the Onondaga involving an Indigenous woman from New France whom the Jesuits had "taught to poison as well as to pray." Bellomont identified the Jesuits as the origin of her technique. Allegedly, they "had furnished her with so subtill [sic] a poison and taught her a leger de main in using it, so that whoever she had a mind to poison, she would drink to em [sic] a cup of water and let drop the poison from under her nail, (which were always very long, for the Indians never pare 'em) into the cup."[48] Transatlantic English anti-Catholic sentiment—combined with the border tensions between the English, the French, and their respective Indigenous allies just three years following the close of King William's War and only two years before Queen Anne's War—undoubtedly influenced Bellomont's ascription of such an underhanded poisoning strategy to a Jesuit and his unnamed Indigenous apprentice.[49] The emphasized duplicitousness of the action—as the woman allegedly toasted her victims—had an emotional resonance.

References to this supposed method and the malice of those who used it abounded in published treatises discussing "poison" in the Caribbean. Labat described an incident on a plantation near Saint Jacques in Martinique, where an enslaved man confessed to hiding a poison made from plants gathered from the sea under a long fingernail and dipping it into the brandy of over thirty other enslaved people.[50] By the time Edward Long wrote his *History of Jamaica* in 1774, his description of the technique—in this instance apparently used by both Indigenous Americans and Africans—had changed to a rather elaborate description of placing powdered worms that had been bred from putrefying cassava juice under a thumbnail, grown long for the purpose, and skillfully dipped into a drink to "impregnate" it.[51] Anthony Blom, a former overseer turned plantation owner in Suriname who published a work on agriculture and plantation management in 1786, warned overseers to watch out for this technique of hiding powdered poison under a fingernail.[52] John Gabriel Stedman in two separate sections likewise credited the "Accawaw Indians" and *wissimen* of African descent for their skill and treachery in hiding poisons that caused slow lingering deaths under their fingernails to administer in beverages. Stedman further stated in a footnote that "after the most scrupulous enquiry, and even ocular demonstration, I can assert the above as literally true." [53] None of the ten poisoning cases tried during Stedman's time in Suriname, from 1773 to 1777, made reference to the fingernail trope, and the idea of him physically observing someone hide poison under their nails and kill someone is a bit absurd.[54] I think it far more likely that Stedman repeated this trope that slaveholders in Suriname and across the slave societies of the Americas had constructed on the dreaded fingernail method. In both 1775 and 1804, French colonial officials in Martinique reported on widespread belief among enslavers of enslaved people poisoning by means of hiding powders under their fingernails: Laussat added a new twist by describing "learned sorcerers" among the enslaved mixing the poisonous sap from the *manchineel* tree (*Hippomane mancinella*) with a gummy substance to more effectively hide it under their nails.[55]

Where did this idea of the cunning fingernail method come from? While frequently ascribed to Africans, it did not appear in the firsthand accounts of Bosman, Barbot, Atkins, or Matthews. Indeed, the earliest reference I have encountered had nothing to do with Africa; fourteenth-century chronicler Matthias of Nuremberg described hiding powdered poison under a fingernail to add to food or drink.[56] To the best of my knowledge, the earliest reference of the fingernail method in relation to *Africa* came from a 1686 work by Robert Boyle. Boyle shared an anecdote from a man who had traveled in Senegambia:

> A sober gentleman, who was governour of a colony in the torrid zone, and had sailed far up the river *Gambra* in *Africa*, assured me, that the blacks had a poison, slow and mortal, the dose whereof is so small, that they usually hide enough to kill a man under one of their nails; from whence they very dextrously [sic] convey it into any liquid aliment, for the person they design it. He added, that in another part of *Africa*, a famous knight, who commanded the *English* there, and lately died in his passage home, was in this manner poison'd by a young *Negro* woman of quality.[57]

Boyle's anecdote contained several key elements repeated in the eighteenth-century works: hiding the poison under fingernails, dipping these nails into a beverage, and a certain degree of admiration for the dexterity and skill involved. The second part, on an English knight poisoned in this manner by an African woman, connects these ideas to a European sense of both the gendered dynamics and political intrigue related to poison. The fingernail trope was interconnected with enslavers' ideas about both poison as a "weapon of the weak" and Africans as sneaky and cunning "poisoners."

Relationships and "Taming"

People in enslaved communities were embedded in webs of relationships with others; these relationships are essential to understanding the ideas surrounding poison and emotions. Friends and relatives of the afflicted were prominent advocates for their care and were often the parties who negotiated treatment with enslavers and health practitioners. In one of Virginia slaveholder Landon Carter's recurring confrontations in the 1770s with a middle-aged woman named Betty, he noted with frustration, "She has been her own doctor and now I have taken her in hand she will not do as I direct. . . . Indeed she has too much encouragement from within doors to be thus obstinate."[58] In the contemporary letters of Robert Carter, enslaved people trying to take an active role in the care of their relatives and friends were prominent. In the case of a woman named Suckey afflicted with fits, it was a man named Michael who suggested R. Carter seek out the services of "Black Hannah"; in the case of Katty, who was also afflicted with fits, it was Katty's mother who negotiated the assistance of "Negro David Doctr."[59] The relatives of those believed to have been afflicted with *feitiços* in Bahia likewise organized to pay healers to conduct *calundú* divinations and had an important participatory role in the dance.[60] In the 1704 denunciation of Mai Caterina, a well-known enslaved practitioner living in Salvador, her accuser described how free and enslaved people from all over the city brought their children to her for her to "bless" with protection and perform cures of afflictions.[61] While enslaved parents and relatives had drastically limited control over their kin, sources like these show some of the ways they did their best to negotiate and seek out both preventive care and therapeutic treatment for them.

Poisoning ranked highly among the health concerns of enslaved people suffering from affliction as well as their friends and relatives, and a significant number of alleged poisonings had enslaved targets. Between 10 percent and 60 percent of poisoning cases, varying by region, had enslaved targets; when reckoned as a proportion of cases with any target—given that there were many cases with no stated target at all—those numbers jump to 34 percent to 70 percent.[62] It is not that cases targeting white people were insignificant, especially considering that they were a small proportion of the total population

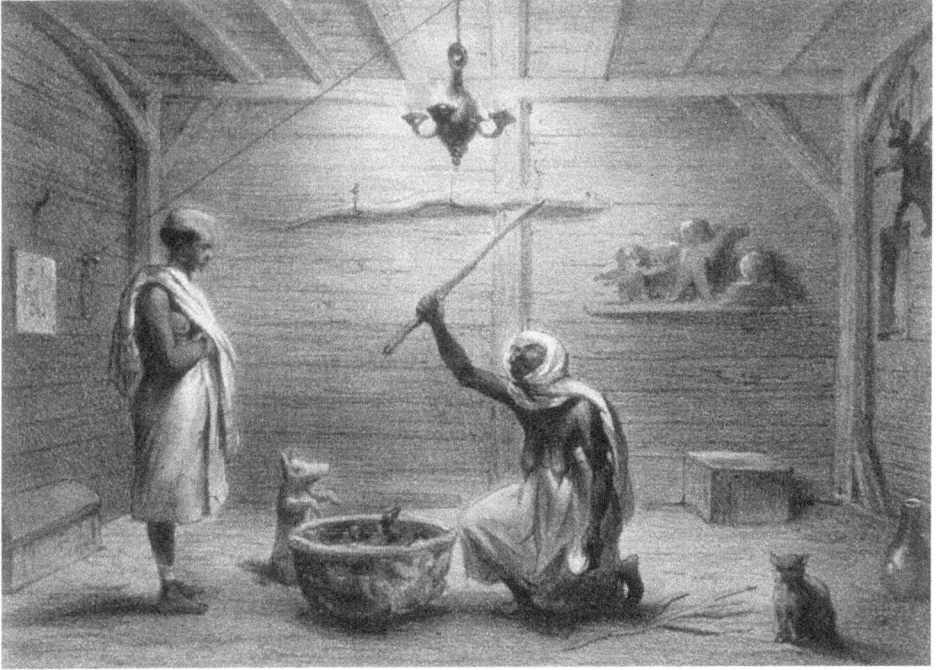

Figure 4. Artist Pierre Jacques Benoit made this lithograph to accompany his published account of his travels to Suriname in the 1830s. While other historians like Jerome Handler and Kenneth Bilby have closely analyzed the objects and actions of the practitioner, I want to point out from Benoit's accompanying text that the client—the woman on the left—was not a patient herself but a mother seeking help to cure her afflicted child. "La Meme-Snekie, ou Water-Mama, faisent ses conjurations," *Slavery Images: A Visual Record of the African Slave Trade and Slave Life in the Early African Diaspora*, accessed August 11, 2023, http://www.slaveryimages.org.

in Martinique, Bahia, and Suriname. However, the numbers of enslaved targets are significant considering both the context of trials where enslaved people could not—with the exception of Inquisitorial denunciations—bring cases to court themselves and the historiographical focus on poisonings of enslavers. Enslaved people were frequently represented in cases where a person was accused of poisoning a specific target. In cases where the words of enslaved people were recorded, fraught relationships were a key component of these cases.

On Jagtlust plantation, enslaved accusers pointed to damaged relationships followed by illnesses as damning evidence of Swart Jan's poisoning. Multiple people from the neighborhood claimed that Swart Jan used his knowledge of *wiriwiri* herbs to threaten people. A woman claimed that Swart Jan had wanted her for a second wife; when she refused him, he threatened to poison her and told her that she would die of disease. Since then, her menstrual period had stopped. The theme of a male health practitioner attacking a woman who rejected him was not uncommon, nor were alleged poisonings of romantic rivals. Allegations of both were especially prevalent in Martinique cases.[63] Other conflicts stemmed from relationships particular to the plantation context, such as that between drivers and other enslaved people, the former being in the fraught position as both leaders within enslaved communities and the individuals responsible for enforcing labor and meting out punishments.[64] Two men declared that, following a confrontation, Swart Jan, who was the Jagtlust driver, told them that they would "no more have a healthy hour."[65]

It is significant that when the practitioner Maskree came to Jagtlust, the first action he took was to interview Swart Jan and the wider enslaved community; establishing the "complex web[s] of social relationships" surrounding the afflicted was a crucial step for health practitioners in their diagnosis and treatment.[66] As Pablo Gómez argues on his work on African healers in the seventeenth-century Caribbean, to focus only on the biomedical properties of cures and not these social dimensions is to significantly misunderstand the actions and ideas of practitioners and their patients. Maskree's interviews were not separate from the work of healing but rather central to it. The relational vison of health and affliction with its emphasis on social networks and community context is a well-known and durable concept in the history of Atlantic Africa; manifestations appeared in African diasporic health practices, from the streets of mid-eighteenth-century Rio de Janeiro to the living quarters of the enslaved in Berbice to the conjure narratives from the nineteenth-century US South.[67] Healing—which included identifying threats to community health—was inherently about relationships.

As these cases were so deeply embedded in social relationships, poison accusations within enslaved communities could have a profound effect on the accused. Suspicion from enslaved communities was a powerful force, driving some accused of poisoning to flee. In Suriname in particular, several cases of enslaved people caught in *marronage* involved poison accusations as their stated motive for running away. This is a curious detail, and one that I have not found so directly stated elsewhere. One would imagine that drawing attention to accusations of poisoning—which were taken very seriously by eighteenth-century courts—would not be considered a useful strategy for reducing punishment for running away. And yet, I have found six cases from 1744 to 1776 of enslaved people telling the court that they ran away specifically because of accusations of poisoning levied against them by their fellows.[68] Swart Jan told the court that he ran "out of fear," that his wife's death by suicide and his own desperate attempt to cut himself stemmed from the accusation that they "went about with poison."[69] A poison accusation within an enslaved community could be a powerful force with devastating social and emotional consequences.

A subset of alleged poisonings hinged on the relationship between enslaved people and their enslavers: the idea of "taming the master"—altering the emotional state of slaveholders to produce better conditions for the one commissioning or performing the taming. In many of these cases the practices were explicitly not intended by the tamer to kill or cause physical harm—though enslavers were certainly horrified at the thought of being emotionally manipulated through occult means and interpreted this action as harm. In their position of extreme precarity in slave societies, many enslaved clients turned to taming practices as a way to try to manage and improve the conditions of life in this world. From the perspective of enslavers and overseers, the efforts by the enslaved to tame were also efforts to flip the "natural" power relationships of the slave society.[70] Slaveholders reacted to "taming" with great alarm, but the people who attempted to change their enslavers' behavior likely saw their actions very differently. For African-descended practitioners, taming practices were an important source of income as enslaved clients sought out their valuable services.

The use of empowered substances and rituals to manipulate the target's emotions was not exclusive to the context of the relationship between enslavers and the enslaved. Emotional manipulation through "poison" also had a history in early modern Europe, particularly through "love magic." In the court of Louis XIV, where proximity to the ruler translated to power, the infamous Affair of the Poisons in the 1680s centered on potions used by noblewomen to get close to the king.[71] Manipulation of powerful substances in matters of marriage, affairs, and sex was also an important part of the repertoire of folk healers in the early modern Iberian Atlantic, frequently appearing in eighteenth-century inquisition cases in Europe and in the colonies.

Several women in 1710s New Spain approached inquisitors to confess to using the services of Indigenous women to "tame" their husbands, while cases nearly a century earlier in Cartagena involved a network of Afro-Caribbean women and their free and enslaved female clients seeking to control the affections of the men in their lives.[72]

Nor were taming practices isolated to plantations; they were flexible and used by practitioners of African descent to try to create favorable outcomes in a range of contexts. One case in the Fort-Royal prison in Martinique highlights this effort as well as the risks involved. Two enslaved men, Jupiter and Gouan, were awaiting an appeal trial by the Martinique Conseil Supérieur in late spring 1754. Jupiter, captured in a state of *marronage*, had been originally tried and convicted in Fort Royal for carrying arms, a purse filled with unknown ingredients, and several *garde-corps* (charms). As capital crimes received an automatic appeal, he waited in the Fort-Royal prison for the Conseil Supérieur to meet.[73] At first, affairs seemed to be improving for him, as his sentence from the lower court of a hanging was commuted in exchange for giving information on others involved in the "distribution of secret drugs."[74] However, during his trial the council discovered that he had covertly continued to make and sell his "poisons and *maléfices*" in the prison itself, instructing new apprentices, including fellow prisoner Gouan, with his secrets. He showed them how to hide ingredients from their captors, how to put taming charms on the jailers and clerks to ensure their "benevolence," and how to make other substances that caused "close to sudden death with the extraordinary symptoms" of the "sickness of the blacks who have been poisoned."[75] The substances for taming were distinct to the substances allegedly used to cause death. The court sentenced Jupiter to be burned alive; for helping him distribute the drugs and charms, his assistant Gouan was hanged.

For African-descended health practitioners, taming practices were among a wide range of services offered to clients in diverse and highly competitive medical marketplaces. There were mundane economic aspects of taming in addition to the social-relational dimensions and slaveholders' conceptions of control. African-descended practitioners capable of composing substances or objects for use in taming practice competed with a diverse range of health specialists in the Americas, including each other.[76] This diversity and competition of healing practices were not exclusive to the Americas; historians of medicine have examined these issues more broadly in early modern Europe and in colonial settings from Atlantic African trading posts to the streets of sixteenth-century Portuguese Goa.[77] Historians focusing on the particular context of slave societies and working with Brazilian records from the Inquisition in the seventeenth and eighteenth centuries and police records from the nineteenth century have highlighted the long history of health practitioners who offered these taming services and the economic transactions involved.[78]

To study the taming services offered by practitioners of African descent—made in exchange for payment—is also to study the interests and ideas of their clients.[79] For the people who commissioned empowerment objects for the purposes of altering the emotional state of enslavers or overseers, taming could have been understood as a form of public healing. The general purpose of empowerment objects was to improve security and the conditions of life—to improve individual health either as part of community health or selfishly at the expense of others. Taming was one of a variety of ways to try to assert control over one's life and possibly to make things better for a wider community.[80] Empowerment objects could have a profound psychological impact as tools for people to manage anxiety as they navigated survival and relationships with others.[81] Slavery in the Americas was a state of extreme precarity, and enslavers and the system that supported them had enormous power over enslaved people's ability to maintain their health and relationships. In other words, while enslavers considered actions taken by the enslaved to bend others to their will as alarming and harmful, those working with taming powers could have seen the same actions as working toward a communal good and an act of healing.[82]

Enslaved people often used verbs like *soften, cool,* or *make gentle* when describing their taming efforts. The idea of coolness in the Bight of Benin is connected to language on the act of healing, often described as the application of "cooling" measures, soothing the fiery anger of a spirit, and a range of emotional states and characteristics, including the terms mentioned above: "peaceful" (*fa xome,* "cool stomach") and "friendliness" (*xome fifa,* "coolness of the stomach").[83] Cooling and soothing were also key to seventeenth-century healing practices relating to *Lemba* just north of the Congo River.[84] Several cases in the Americas included similar descriptions of taming actions. In 1789, a man enslaved by the archbishop of Bahia was caught attempting to place a small packet into the archbishop's chocolate drink. He confessed that it contained small pieces of *pedra de ara*—a "stone from the altar" in Catholic churches frequently noted in Bahian love magic—as a "remedy to soften his master" who had refused to free him.[85] Similarly, in a 1733 case in Suriname, a woman named Clarinda sought the services of Nero, an enslaved practitioner from another plantation, to "soften" the ill nature of the mistress who was "malicious" toward her.[86] An unnamed woman in Martinique was also convicted and sentenced to assist in the execution of the man from whom she purchased "drugs and ingredients" in order to "make her mistress agreeable and prevent the *Commandeur* (driver) from wanting to hurt her."[87] What is particularly significant here is that the action of the taming was specifically directed to the emotional states of the targets: not simply to avoid punishment but to make the person responsible for meting out punishment unwilling to do it.

In some cases, like that of the enslaved man and the archbishop's chocolate above, the act of taming was intended to result specifically in manumission—or at least claimed as such. For example, in 1754 two enslaved women named Roze and Sarra confessed that the powder a man on their plantation had given them to put in their mistress's water would "procure liberty."[88] In a much later case, Bahian police recorded a group of free "Nagô" (an ethnic label likely meaning Yoruba), who had been liberated from an illegal slaving ship and set to work at the Navy Arsenal, caught helping the enslaved laborers there achieve manumission through spells.[89]

Given that these sources are records of trials and investigations, it is possible that the defendants in these cases claimed to have had no intent to kill to try to save themselves. For example, in the case of Clarinda and Nero above, both repeatedly insisted that their actions were not intended to harm but to tame. Nero had sold Clarinda a concoction made from herbs gathered in the bush to put in her enslaver's water. Clarinda was alarmed when the woman then became ill and later died. According to Nero's interrogation, shortly before her arrest Clarinda came back to tell him what had happened, exclaiming that they were both going to die for what they had done.[90] It is possible that they each claimed to have been trying to "tame," not kill, in an ultimately unsuccessful effort to save themselves in the context of the trial.

However, recent work revisiting the famous Makandal poisoning case in Saint-Domingue suggests that many taming efforts were likely to have been genuine and not necessarily intended to kill. This massive case began after what appears to have been an uncoerced confession on the initiative of an enslaved man named Médor, who in 1757 told the court in Cap Français that he and many others had purchased powders—called "poisons" by his enslaver—to persuade slaveholders to grant manumissions. John Garrigus has linked the timing and spread of the deaths attributed to poison with an outbreak of anthrax among cattle and through the consumption of tainted meat, suggesting that Médor and others who confessed to using "*poison et malefice*" to tame slaveholders or treat afflictions may have believed, due to a coincidence of timing, that their actions had accidentally killed them. Enslavers were quick to latch on to the idea of a malicious "poisoning" conspiracy—despite an alternative epizootic explanation offered by contemporary European veterinarians.[91] The case culminated in the 1758 arrest and execution of Makandal, a healer and spiritual leader living in *marronage*.

For Makandal and the empowered objects he made—pouches containing small crucifixes that would thereafter bear his name in Saint-Domingue—the act of healing, the emotions involved, and their relationship to "poison" was quite complex. One of Makandal's followers, a woman named Brigitte, claimed that his packets could be used to identify "the poisoner"—the person or people responsible for the recent mass deaths of enslaved people. Indeed, as Kathryn de Luna argues in her recent linguistic analysis of the Makandal case, the speech used by Makandal in his healing practices as well as the wordplay embedded in his name (with the root stems *-kànd-*, a widespread root "relating to the semantic domain of pressing, often in the context of healing wounds," and *-kánd-* more narrowly distributed, "strike; punish") reveal efforts to "[hunt] the target responsible for causing the illness."[92] Furthermore, de Luna identifies the words he used in his invocations spoken while creating and activating these power objects with roots from the Kikongo Language Cluster, words that expressed a goal of punishing whoever was abusing their power and, in doing so, "soothing" the *mayangangue*: the "group repeatedly yelled at, tormented, pained, paid as a fine for injury or offense, refused, hated"—the enslaved.[93] The Makandal case was a tangle of fears, suspicion, and commentary on relationships of power in 1750s Saint-Domingue.

Beyond Saint-Domingue, enslavers across the Americas were horrified and offended by taming practices, which they saw as a usurpation of power and an inversion of the social order—similar in kind to the inversion performed by the devil in early modern European discourses of witchcraft.[94] For enslavers, the idea of taming was a special threat because of its implications for their power; enslaved people controlling the emotions of their enslavers would be a radical usurpation—a complete inversion—of the power hierarchies constructed and reinforced by slave societies.[95] Slaveholders did not need to believe that such methods were effective in order to see them as a threat. The Society of Suriname, after hearing about the case of Bettie—accused of having poisoned her enslaver by giving him something to put him "in a good humor"—passed a resolution in 1749 outlawing such "super-stitious, bad, and dangerous practices," regardless of any ill effect. They de-scribed the presumption of enslaved people believing in the efficacy of such practices and attempting to use them as exceedingly dangerous to the col-ony.[96] The Conseil Supérieur in Martinique had a similar discussion in the case of an unnamed enslaved man and woman in 1756, condemning practi-tioners of African descent who sold "pretended secrets" to enslaved people to make their enslavers agreeable and framing these practices, however "pre-tended," as a gateway to attempts to physically harm or kill slaveholders.[97]

The language of cooling and softening enslavers appeared even in loca-tions where I did not find explicit references to taming practices. Despite the fact that conjure packets and bundles were used in the nineteenth century for a wide range of purposes in Virginia, I did not find any specific references to "taming" practices targeting enslavers in the county court trials.[98] Yvonne Chireau's work notes enslaved peoples' use of conjure in the nineteenth-century US South to protect from violence and punish slaveholders but not exactly to modify their behavior by altering their internal emotional state.[99] However, there are some intriguing similarities between taming and the rhe-toric of evangelical sensibility in the late eighteenth century that called on enslavers in Virginia to "soften" their hearts toward the enslaved.[100] The pe-riod from 1785 to 1790 was one of intense conversion in the Chesapeake, as free and enslaved people of African descent embraced evangelical Baptist and Methodist movements and made them their own.[101] While Black evangeli-calism and conjure practices were complementary rather than mutually ex-clusive, it is possible that taming efforts by enslaved people after the late eighteenth century may have found greater or at least more visible expres-sion in the former than the latter.[102] As the eighteenth-century trials from Virginia are limited in detail, more work would need to be done scouring plantation papers to be sure of an absence of "taming"—or at least an absence of slaveholders' awareness of such practices. Here the limitations of the sources created by enslavers are starkly apparent: it is difficult to know if en-slaved people in eighteenth-century Virginia attempted to use taming prac-tices if their enslavers did not write about them.

*   *   *

Within enslaved communities, access to power in both its mundane and otherworldly dimensions was fraught with social and emotional peril. As

McCaskie notes on Asante ideas about power, "All people come into the world and eventually leave it, and between these two fixities trafficking in power can lift up and cast down in all kinds of ways that may appear arbitrary and opaque to understanding."[103] The efforts by an extraordinary individual with access to powers to "tame" enslavers or overseers by cooling or harnessing their emotions could reduce harm to the whole community; this same individual could quickly become a subject of community concern by abusing their power—"poisoning"—through broken relationships. While fragmentary, the voices of the enslaved that appear in poisoning cases repeatedly emphasized relationships and negative emotions as evidence against suspected individuals.

Swart Jan's case did not end well for him. During his three separate interrogations in Fort Zeelandia from late June to early September 1744, the court repeatedly challenged his denials of poisoning with statements from the enslaved people at Jagtlust and the overseer Versteegh. Finally, on December 10 the court brought the case to a close, declaring Swart Jan guilty of poisoning and running away. Five days later he was broken on the wheel in the plaza just outside of the fort, his head mounted on a pike in the Suriname River as a warning to others.[104] This case provides not only a vivid reminder of colonial violence and power over the lives of the enslaved but also insight into the importance of relationships in ideas about poisoning within enslaved communities. No other enslaved people from Jagtlust were physically present at the trial, but their testimony made up the bulk of the evidence; it was their investigation that prompted judicial proceedings. The entwined nature of public healing and community justice in the Jagtlust living quarters of the enslaved was laid bare in the last haunting image from Versteegh's account to the court: of Maskree and the people of the Jagtlust enslaved community standing together by the waterside, silently watching the boat take Swart Jan across the river.

CHAPTER 5

<hr>

Binding Power

By the time they opened their healing clinic on the outskirts of Salvador, Bahia, health practitioners Paulo Gomes and Ignacia were already well known in the sloping streets behind the city center.[1] Their neighbors, interviewed in 1749 by the city's Inquisitorial commissioner, had shared a street with Gomes for decades; their work performing cures with *calundús* was not a secret, nor were their efforts to continuously expand and improve their practice. Gomes, a free *pardo* (likely Brazilian-born) stonecutter, had purchased both the freedom of Ignacia, an African woman and master *calunduzeira* (dancer of *calundús*), and a farm where they could work together as partners. Ignacia led divinatory dances and prescribed and made cures for the afflicted who came to them. Gomes continuously sought out new streams of healing knowledge and advertised this knowledge to potential clients. One of Gomes's neighbors, a *pardo* stonecutter who worked side by side with Gomes for more than thirty years, said that Gomes confided in him many times that he wished to be successful and that he sought out "various black *feiticeiros*" to learn; another neighbor similarly noted that Gomes had traveled widely to visit other "*feiticeiros*." A middle-aged white widow, also a resident of Rua de Poeyra, told the commissioner how Gomes had offered her treatment, claiming that he could use his practice to bring her luck, wealth, "and everything she hopes for." Once, while hearing mass at Igreja de Nossa Senhora da Piedade, Gomes turned to another neighbor and pew mate, a white painter, and told him about a Castilian book he had acquired that taught both how to make *maleficios* and how to cure them. People across a wide social spectrum—free, enslaved, of African and European descent—went to Gomes and Ignacia for their knowledge and expertise. Their success as health practitioners rested on two forms of binding power: the compositions of their cures and their reputation built through networking.[2]

However, success went hand in hand with risk. As the reputation of Gomes and Ignacia grew, so did the suspicion that they were responsible for afflictions in the area. The same power that attracted clients also made these practitioners morally ambiguous in the eyes of their neighbors. Multiple witnesses said that Gomes was "notorious" for killing the white husband of a former lover with *feitiços*. One neighbor referenced this piece of public knowledge in her testimony to explain why suspicion in her household landed so quickly on Gomes. When several enslaved people had become sick and died in the months after the discovery of a *malefício* hidden in the house, "all attributed [it] to the *feitiçaria*" of Gomes. The reputation of Gomes and Ignacia, and attendant suspicions, extended well beyond their personal network as some of their neighbors sought outside help with their afflictions. When a white neighbor brought his afflicted wife to another African healer across town, part of the attempted cure involved divination to identify the person who had made the *malefício*. After spending some time in Gomes's neighborhood, the practitioner told the man that Gomes was responsible and a "bad neighbor."[3]

Two different competitors in Salvador's medical marketplace denounced Gomes and Ignacia in two different ways; both denunciations hinged on their powerful fame as healers. The unnamed *preto* (Black, likely African) practitioner consulted by the white neighbor and his wife did not instigate any sort of trial from the Inquisition or secular court, but he did identify Gomes as the source of affliction as part of the medical narrative he built with his clients. The formal denunciation that led to the documentation of this case came from Dr. José Xavier Tovar, a white surgeon and fellow parishioner, who had heard about Gomes and Ignacia's *calundús* after speaking with several of Gomes's neighbors. Climbing the hill to the office of the Inquisitorial commissioner in the center of the city, Tovar denounced the couple for superstitious practices and *feitiçaria*. In the ensuing investigation, the commissioner conducted further interviews with neighbors, and the details on the partners' practices came pouring out.[4]

The act of binding was essential to the work of African and African-descended practitioners such as Ignacia and Gomes. They bound together preventive and therapeutic cures for clients, and they could also "tie up" others. Tracking the actions and relationships of these healers through poison cases reveals not only complex webs of intimacies and relationships but also "networks of knowledge."[5] Practitioners like Ignacia and Gomes built their reputations over many years, establishing a wide clientele and incorporating multiple strands of medical authority. Their practices bound together multiple sources of power that they adapted and creatively expanded in new circumstances. Carefully cultivated networks of clients and knowledge formed the basis of prestige for healing practitioners, placing them in a powerful but precarious position. The same reputation, visibility, and expertise necessary to successfully attract clientele also made these practitioners vulnerable to denunciations.

These denunciations took place in the context of slavery and in the highly competitive colonial medical marketplace. Historians, especially those focused on Iberian colonies, in the past two decades have focused their attention on the circulation of medical knowledge and practices in the Atlantic world and the ways in which ideas on illness and health impacted each other and changed through their interaction.[6] In doing so, they have traced the ways healers constantly reconstructed, tested, and incorporated new practices through vast networks of knowledge. To adapt a phrase from historian Pablo Gómez, the Caribbean was a space of "medicinal promiscuity": practitioners continuously adopted and adapted diverse practices to serve a diverse clientele.[7] Though they coexisted and competed with a wide range of European health specialists and, in some local contexts, Indigenous practitioners, African and African-descended healers numerically dominated and did much of the healing work in these slave societies in the seventeenth and eighteenth centuries.[8] Several historians have focused specifically on examining the efforts of white physicians to try to assert their authority and to suppress the activities of these healers.[9] In the nineteenth century, as physicians of European descent increasingly asserted exclusive claim to effective practice through racialized language, the healing work of practitioners of African descent found greater expression in therapeutic rituals of new Afro-Caribbean religions.[10]

Bringing insights from African history into this ongoing conversation and taking a wide perspective on binding power across a range of slave societies enriches our understanding of the connections between the specific strategies these practitioners used to build their networks of knowledge and, crucially, the ways that these same strategies made practitioners vulnerable. In their highly influential 1995 article, Africanists Jane Guyer and S. M. Eno Belinga proposed a modification to the well-known "wealth in people" thesis as "wealth in knowledge": that the composition of knowledge through networks of practitioners—and through the soft boundaries between personhood and objects that allowed for storage of knowledge in things—was the key to wealth.[11] While their work focused on equatorial Africa, this insight has informed a wide range of historical, archaeological, and anthropological scholarship increasingly focused on knowledge, health, and healing and their relationship with morality and political culture in Africa.[12] While African and African-descended practitioners in Bahia, Martinique, Suriname, and Virginia did respond to local circumstances of the local medical marketplaces in these varied locations, their acts of composition *also* drew upon this idea of wealth and power through binding knowledge. In an irony, the very cultivation of networks of knowledge and clients that made these healers successful also put them at higher risk of being accused of being poisoners by enslavers, enslaved communities, and other practitioners.

Composition, Binding, and Power Objects

Free and enslaved healers of African descent were purveyors of a wide range of services for fees, including treating illnesses; making preventive, curative, and aggressive power objects; and identifying culprits suspected of "poisoning." For example, in 1755 the Martinique Conseil Supérieur convicted one unnamed enslaved healer, "famous in his neighborhood," for all three: composing and distributing "*drogues malefices*" (evil magical drugs) and "pretended remedies" for enslaved people who believed themselves poisoned; having "mysterious understandings" of dangerous plants; and discovering poison and poisoners on plantations.[13] At the farm of Paulo Gomes and Ignacia, clients received consultation and treatment through both divinatory practices and the application of herbs and objects. None of the seven witnesses from the neighborhood questioned by the commissioner admitted to attending a *calundú* at the farm, so details on the exact practices involved are scarce. One of Gomes's neighbors did claim to have once seen Gomes and Ignacia dancing, with her covered in ribbons and white powders—which they also sold at their farm. The white powder is suggestive of *pemba*, a white clay contemporaneously used in West Central Africa, as well as in two denunciations of Bahian *calunduzeiras* from 1701 and 1757, to symbolize and enhance contact with the dead.[14] In addition to their divinatory practices, Paulo Gomes and Ignacia also sold therapeutic herbal baths and, on at least one occasion, a small pot with unspecified contents for an enslaved client to leave at a crossroads to ensure the "obedience" of his enslaver—a form of taming.[15]

The services and rituals performed by practitioners of African descent often involved physical objects; close attention to the materiality of their practices helps illuminate what they did for people.[16] Practitioners made and sold protective amulets—called *bolsas da madinga, garde-corps,* or simply variations on "packet"—to prevent misfortune and help ensure success in life.[17] Health practitioners were also understood to be capable of causing afflictions—through *feitiços,* conjure objects, and so on—whether on behalf of clients or on their own account. For example, when the enslaved man Toiny sought means to kill Antoine in 1754 Martinique, allegedly out of jealousy, he went to an elderly enslaved woman who was apparently a well-known source of "poison" in the neighborhood.[18]

Bolsas physically bound together multiple sources of power—both the composition of individual components and the act of tying or binding itself were significant. The form of the *bolsa* varied—from bags to calabashes to animal horns. Horns appeared in several poisoning cases, both for their use in cupping—a widespread healing practice shared by Europeans and Africans in the Atlantic world—and as a way to contain and bind other power objects together.[19] In descriptions of these objects, certain materials came up repeatedly. Pablo Gómez's work on Black ritual specialists in the seventeenth-century Caribbean offers a useful framework for thinking about these bags not merely as containers for herbs and objects, but as both "[inventories] of healing and protective substances" and the "amalgamation of knowledge" from a practitioner's specific experiences.[20] Practitioners included specific objects of power and developed rituals to use them for specific purposes—to offer protection, for example, from injuries or the malevolent actions of others. In a long 1775 letter decrying the "superstition" of both enslavers and enslaved people in Martinique, Dr. Raymond de Laborde of French Guiana included a detailed, if disparaging, description of the collections of drugs he had seen used in Martinique by enslaved practitioners and their uses as explained to him:

> [Their drugs are] a mixture of twenty or thirty different drugs inside a box or little sack; each one has their different properties: there are some that otherwise combine in the little bottles, they are human fingernails, the claws of different animals, horsehair, different [illegible], feathers, seeds, roots, leaves, flowers of many trees or plants of the land, [illegible—possibly coral], red or of other nature. Each of these ingredients had their particular properties. That root is infallible for

the bite of such a serpent; the Requeim will touch no one who has been rubbed with such a leaf; this small piece of wood has the property to make such a girl fall in love with the one who carries it. This dirt infallibly cures this sickness. There are those who have talismans with figures, by means of which they become invisible . . . others for taking game in the woods, others so they are never discovered when they are maroons.[21]

While Laborde was clearly mocking his competitors, his inventory offers insights into how practitioners of African descent chose and shaped different material objects for specific actions—each with the goal of affecting outcomes in the material world. Both the goal-oriented use and the emphasis on composition resonate with practices involving power objects in Atlantic Africa.

While each practitioner developed a repertoire from personal experience, local sources, and local needs, several kinds of materials appeared frequently in both practices to heal and to cause harm. It is important to remember the limits of using poison trials and investigations here: the objects recorded were only those identified by the enslavers, courts, or enslaved communities as suspicious, and the records for court systems did not always include the kinds of ethnographic details that historians would like.[22] With that said, certain materials did come up repeatedly in trials and in anecdotal evidence.

Grave dirt was a way of connecting to the knowledge and power of the dead. Formerly enslaved people recalling practices in nineteenth-century Virginia described conjurors using grave dirt and other powerful powders to cause afflictions.[23] During the early nineteenth-century poison crises in Martinique, materials from graves and cemeteries played a particularly prominent and detailed role in accusations. One large case centered on an alleged underground network of grave robbers using the bodies of children from the cemetery to make "poisonous" powders from their bones.[24] While such elaborate accusations mainly came from the nineteenth century, earlier cases made connections to grave dirt, either through explicit mention or more implicit association. For example, in the 1742 case of Goliath in Suriname, witnesses claimed that he went to the place where enslaved people were buried in the bush to make his "poison."[25]

African and African-descended practitioners in Catholic colonies also sometimes incorporated Catholic power objects into their compositions. One element particularly prominent in the *bolsas* made in the Portuguese Atlantic was the *pedra d'ara*, a "stone from the altar" commonly used for love magic.

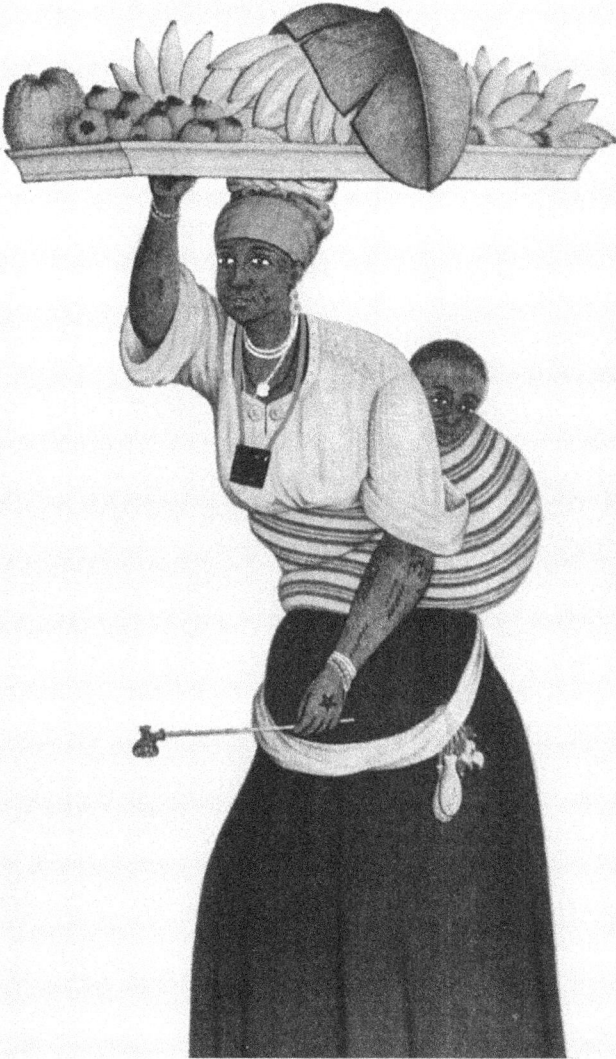

Figure 5. This detail from a watercolor by Carlos Julião highlights the objects worn by an enslaved food seller. While Silvia Hunold Lara cautions that Julião's images should not be taken uncritically at face value as ethnography, the wide array of *bolsas* around the woman's neck and waist are consistent with the idea of each composition having a unique material function. "Market Woman or Hawkers, Rio de Janeiro, Brazil, ca. 1770s," *Slavery Images: A Visual Record of the African Slave Trade and Slave Life in the Early African Diaspora*, accessed August 11, 2023, http://www.slaveryimages.org.

These special stones appeared in denunciations to the Inquisition originating in Bahia and in descriptions of *bolsas* from Angola to Lisbon to the Bahian Recôncavo with a range of healing and protective purposes.[26] In Bahia, pieces of consecrated host from the Eucharist, papers with the written names of saints, and small crosses were also sometimes used as power objects.[27] One of the most famous poison cases in the French Caribbean, that of Makandal in 1758 Saint-Domingue, centered on the charge of sacrilege for a tied-up power bundle that contained a crucifix.[28] The case of Maria Monjola is particularly interesting, as she allegedly caused afflictions with a pouch of power objects worn around her neck that included a cross and a *caboclo*—a figurine connected to Indigenous Tupí forest spirits.[29] Other common materials included feathers, animal parts, and herbs—usually, and frustratingly, unidentified in the records.

The act of tying up—often represented by tightly binding the *bolsa* in cords—as an idiom for causing or treating affliction is well known to historians of the African Atlantic and had deep linguistic roots in Atlantic Africa. Recall, for example, that the ancient, durable, and very widespread term for expert healing practitioners in Bantu languages, **-gàngà*—regularly used with either the noun class referring to people and proper titles or the noun class referring to people and tools—derived from the transitive verb **-gàng-* "to tie [something/someone] up."[30] These words and another derivative in the form an abstract noun **-gàngà* "medicine" appeared frequently in the Americas: from early eighteenth-century Inquisitorial denunciations from Bahia, to the "Congo" dictionary compiled by Louisiana slaveholder Louis-Narcisse Baudry de Lozières in 1803, to discussions of *wanga* in the late eighteenth and early nineteenth-century US South.[31] Archaeologists digging at the nineteenth-century Valongo Wharf in Rio de Janeiro found numerous tightly knotted, twisted, and bound objects made from indigenous Brazilian plant material and noted similar objects from contemporary Cuba, Haiti, and African American communities in the United States used to bind and hold spirits.[32]

Individual components of power objects had specific meanings, but they worked in bound compositions designed and crafted by health practitioners. For example, one case from the Bahian Recôncavo in 1754 involved an affliction caused by a branch of an unidentified tree knotted up with a piece of iron; in the case of April in Suriname, the object he purchased and allegedly used to harm others on his plantation was a little stick packed with herbs and tied up with "papa monies" (possibly cowrie shells).[33] It was the binding and composition of objects together and associated rituals that held power. In the earliest surviving poison case I have found from Suriname in 1731, the object in question was a calabash containing pieces of a red stone and a bird's beak: several enslaved people on the plantation also reported having seen the practitioner, Isaac, around the grave sites of others and using the calabash to pray to leaves behind his house. Isaac did not deny owning and using the calabash and its contents but insisted that it was for healing purposes and never used to cause harm.[34] While Isaac had chosen each of the materials in his calabash for specific purposes based on their properties, their power was in the composition—and in the words and gestures he used to activate them.

Bolsas bound and assembled multiple sources of power to achieve specific ends; each bolsa often had a unique composition and function. While the ingredients and composition of bolsas yield insights on the ideas and material knowledge of practitioners, the uses enslaved clients made of these pouches or charms offers an index of the concerns, hopes, and fears that they attempted to manage with them. Their contemporaries in West Africa shared some of these concerns, while others were more specific to the particular circumstances and violence of slave societies in these colonies. As with the bo power objects described by Blier's twentieth-century, Fon-speaking informants, the bolsas commissioned and used by enslaved people in the Americas had a common theme of trying to achieve security, to improve the conditions of life in this world.[35] While I did not find reference to specific empowerment objects in the Virginia county court records, Sharla Fett's work on Works Progress Administration narratives regarding nineteenth-century conjuring practices describes "conjure packets" used to cure, protect, or harm, as well as the common trope of the conjure doctor finding the packet when investigating the cause of malevolent illness.[36]

Like the minkisi in West Central Africa, the bolsas that appeared in trials in the Americas were bound to conflict and social tension, both between enslavers and the enslaved and within enslaved communities.[37] For their role as aids in crisis, bolsas or consecrated powders rubbed into the skin appeared frequently in descriptions of battles or uprisings. Maroons and fighters wore bolsas or obis to deflect bullets during Tacky's Revolt in Jamaica (1760), the Cottica River Maroon Uprising in Suriname (1770s), and the Muslim Uprising in Bahia (1835).[38] However, enslaved people used bolsas and other empowerment objects for a wide range of concerns. Archaeologists working with those materials found in the slave market at Valongo Wharf developed a theory on the layering of such objects—beads, cowries, crystals, teeth, horns, medallions, twisted rings of metal and plant fiber—with tattoos and scarification patterns to "weave the second skin" and protect against evil.[39] The following is a list of uses of empowerment objects I have found, in addition to protection in battle:[40]

To cause death by poison[41]
To protect against enemies[42]
To prevent snakebite[43]
To prevent poisoning[44]
To prevent various injuries[45]
To prevent a whipping[46]
To make someone fall in love[47]
To avoid or treat illness[48]
To catch game in the woods[49]
To make oneself invisible or avoid detection when running away[50]
To increase courage[51]
To "tame" or make someone kinder[52]
To procure manumission[53]

While some of these concerns (for example, attracting love) had broad applicability, others (for example, preventing a whipping) spoke directly to the challenges, anxieties, and violence of life in slavery. The reported frequency of instances of *bolsas* intended to cause death should be viewed with caution, as many of these sources were trials for alleged poisoning. It is entirely possible that there were uses of *bolsas* ignored, unreported, or misunderstood in these court cases as they were not connected to alleged harm. There is also the major issue of confessions extracted by torture, which could skew descriptions of what enslaved people intended to do with these packets. However, while deadly use may have been exaggerated, it was consistent with the uses of such objects described in seventeenth- and eighteenth-century Atlantic Africa.[54] Members of enslaved communities in the Americas took action to try and improve their health and well-being, which could involve identifying or targeting threats to their lives.

Binding was not only important for making power objects and harnessing the power of spirits but also as a way of understanding the actions causing affliction.[55] The way that enslaved people who claimed to have been poisoned talked *about* their symptoms was significant. In the cases of Marquis and Akkra in 1771 and Persenet and Abraham in 1798, their alleged targets described their symptoms not only as belly pains but specifically "belly pains and bonds/ties."[56] Suggestively, in an anecdote from a poison case in the *assises* court that Dr. Rufz de Lavison sat on during his time in Martinique in the late 1830s and early 1840s, a young enslaved woman testified with "passionate eloquence" against an older woman for "[tying] up" her child by passing her hand over his chest.[57] Speakers of Njila and KLC languages in West Central Africa made use of the idiom of "tying up" in relation to healing and affliction, and innovated and expanded these words during the era of the transatlantic slave trade to discuss marching coffles and the local tribunals that convicted and sold so many for crimes that included alleged "poisoning."[58] Ewe, Fon, and Twi speakers in West Africa also used the idiom of binding to discuss enslaved people, the ill, and verbs to "bind" practitioners and "to poison."[59] While the African *words* largely did not survive the crossing to the Americas, people of African descent continued to adapt and make use of these durable *idioms* to talk about the experience of being "poisoned," as well as their efforts to prevent it.

Networking: Strands of Knowledge and Power

Binding power also had a social dimension through personal networks and the ideas and practices connected through them. Knowledge and the accumulation of different kinds of expertise were the keys to healers' power and their ability to offer a wide range of services. One possible source of knowledge was previous experience in Atlantic Africa. In the case of Gomes and Ignacia, several of the witnesses referred to Ignacia as the "greater *feiticeira*" of the two—a "master" *calunduzeira* and "Queen"—and emphasized her connections to Africa as a "Mina."[60] The idea of African practitioners deriving secret knowledge from their countries of origin—having "learned in the land," as one accusation from a slaveholder in 1743 Suriname termed it—was not unique to Bahia.[61] In an essay on poison and *maléfice* attached to a 1756 case sent to the Minister of the Marine, the Martinique Conseil Supérieur pointed to the knowledge of simples for curing illnesses "used in their counties" as the source for enslaved Africans' poisoning expertise.[62] Some enslavers purchased or hired enslaved healers specifically for their connections to Africa and African knowledge.[63]

However, the use of specific African rituals was not restricted to the African-born, nor did African-born practitioners restrict themselves to practices from their region of origin.[64] Focusing only on direct personal links to Africa obscures the myriad ways in which healers of African descent made claims to knowledge. They appropriated, incorporated, and adapted sources of knowledge in specific local social and botanical environments to solve health problems, building their reputations and networks of clients on demonstrable successes.[65] As part of their efforts to bolster their practice and attract new clients, practitioners like Gomes worked constantly to build their networks of knowledge.[66]

One major strand in a health practitioner's network was the expertise of other practitioners. In the case of Gomes, one of his neighbors, a fellow *pardo* stonecutter who knew Gomes very well, claimed that he frequently attended the *calundús* of others before establishing his own. He described Gomes as constantly seeking out "various black *feiticeiros* to give him fortune." In the years before Gomes had saved enough money to purchase both the freedom of Ignacia and a farm where they could conduct their practices, he used to go to Rio Vermello and Itapagipe "to make *feitiçaria* and dance *calundús*" every Sunday and holy day. Not only did Gomes attend *calundús* organized around the outskirts of Salvador, but he also traveled as far as Pernambuco to visit the houses of other "*feitiçeiros*."[67] This detail of one practitioner specifically traveling to learn from others stands out among poison trials, but it was not uncommon for practitioners to know one another.

Practitioners of African descent also incorporated knowledge from European sources into their networks of knowledge. Convergences in ideas about the power of binding/tying and a long history of cross-cultural interaction in the Iberian Atlantic shaped the widespread use across social hierarchies of *bolsas* in colonial Brazil and in Lisbon.[68] Several practitioners in the Portuguese Atlantic also adopted European divination methods like the "scissor and sieve" technique into their practices.[69] Printed books were also sometimes taken into practice. João Roiz da Silva, the white painter who had been Paulo Gomes's neighbor and pew mate for ten years, told the inquisitorial commissioner that Gomes once described to him a Castilian book that taught how to make *malefícios* and their remedies. This was likely the same book that Antonia de Mattos, another of Gomes's neighbors, described as "um livro de curar, e matar" (a book to heal and to kill).[70] Books and other physical pieces of writing could be highly empowered objects and sources of authority in this period.[71] Significantly, Gomes not only sought out the Castilian book as a powerful source of knowledge, but he also advertised his possession of it to a potential client like Roiz da Silva.

For some practitioners of African descent, the healing practices and ideas of Indigenous peoples were also important sources of knowledge. Indigenous sources are not immediately apparent in poison cases from these colonies, as very few Indigenous Americans were accused or mentioned explicitly in the trials.[72] Unlike cases from the Mexico City Inquisition, where defendants of African descent frequently followed a strategy of identifying Indigenous sources of knowledge in accusations of "witchcraft"—sources who could not legally be brought before the Inquisition—defendants in the locations for this study generally did not follow suit.[73] This was even true for locations that did have relatively large Indigenous populations through the eighteenth century, such as Bahia and Suriname. However, there is evidence of exchanges of healing knowledge and interactions between Indigenous and African ideas about healing. In Virginia, enslaved healers learned the uses for many local plants—such as snakeroot, frequently used to treat poisons—from Native American interlocutors.[74] Reporting to the Royal Society from Barbados, English seaman Thomas Walduck described "the observation[s] of Dreams & omens" in conversations between Native Americans, European colonists, and enslaved people of African descent, while a handful of cases from eighteenth-century Suriname involved Indigenous Americans as suppliers of roots and herbs.[75] The knowledge of the Indigenous peoples was not only practical for Africans and their descendants in the Americas—that is, which plants in this new environment were efficacious for which ailments—it also had the power of autochthony. The significance of autochthonous knowledge and rituals binding newcomers to firstcomers in a land has been discussed extensively by historians of early Africa.[76] Incorporating Indigenous ideas and practices could therefore be a particularly potent way for practitioners of African descent to compose their wealth in knowledge.

In addition to exchanges of knowledge about specific plants, there is evidence of influences and convergences of ideas about health and healing that sometimes extended well beyond periods of extensive contact. For example, by the eighteenth century very few Indigenous Kalinago remained on Martinique. However, in a poison case from 1768 and treatises on poisoning from 1775 and 1844, the Kalinago word *piaye* (sometimes spelled *pialle*), translated as "shaman who talks to spirits," appeared in the words of African-descended enslaved people to describe both health practitioners and the objects they sold for cures.[77] By the latest of these attestations, the definition of *piaye* had evolved to include objects sold by African and African-descended healers to white duelists to ensure success; *piayes* also often appeared as primary pieces of evidence in the Cour Prévôtale poison trials of the 1820s.[78] The adaptation of this word is particularly intriguing for the conceptual link to communication with spirits as part of healing practice.

For many healers of African descent, the dead were the greatest source of knowledge and power. As "invisible agents," spirits have had a profound impact on African religion and politics—most importantly religion *as* politics.[79] The agency and knowledge of the dead was particularly significant for practitioners, clients, and wider communities trying to identify the causes of and solutions to affliction. Practitioners of African descent in slave societies often communicated with spirits through divination practices to diagnose illnesses, determine their root causes, and prescribe the best course for treatment.[80] Adaptations from Atlantic Africa often involved a wide range of specific practices, including spirit possession and contacting the spirit world using ritual objects for divination. However, healing was the common goal of these diverse practices, and many practitioners in the Americas, regardless of their region of origin or descent, bridged differences between them by incorporating, adapting, and creating new elements.[81]

The content of divination practices varied, and they were not mutually exclusive. In Bahia, *calundú* dances in the eighteenth century involved the ritual possession of the practitioner by a member of the spirit world, often indicated by a changed voice and behavior. For example, two women identified as "Mina"—from Lower Guinea—were accused of making cures in 1745 Bahia by speaking in the voices of their deceased sons (interpreted by the denouncer, a white woman, as demonic possession).[82] Several cases of the *watermama* or *Minje mama* dance in the Dutch Guianas involved divinatory practices. Like *calundú* in Bahia, *watermama* was primarily a collective dance where spirits possessed ritually prepared participants for the purposes of public healing—though this dance specifically centered on seeking the aid of a powerful water spirit connected to Ijo practices.[83] In Stedman's 1796 narrative, he described "watra Mama" as a name used by enslaved people in Suriname to indicate both a powerful and dangerous "mermaid" and their "Sybils" who communicated with her.[84] The *watermama* identified in the 1742 trial of the enslaved man April in Suriname—April himself being tried for allegedly purchasing an object to poison others from a practitioner at the Fort Nieuw Amsterdam construction site—was known as an expert in herbs to kill or cure.[85] Conjure doctors in the nineteenth-century US South also used divination to identify sources of affliction causing "tricks."[86] Finally, children were an important part of several divinatory rituals. Both the case of Hans in 1819 Berbice and of Jacques in 1767 Martinique had key roles for young girls in identifying the source of illness on respective plantations. In the former, Hans had a nine-year-old girl hold the pot where incriminating evidence against the suspected poisoner suddenly appeared; in the latter, a girl of three was instructed to place a branch of the *medecinier* tree on the skin of the accused, causing convulsions and a confession to having poisoned other enslaved people.[87]

Fame and prestige were important for practitioners of African descent to bind power through networking. A brief examination of one of the most well-known and successful of these practitioners—Gramman Quassi in Suriname—underscores common networking strategies adopted by Ignacia, Paulo Gomes, and others trying to navigate their profession as healer-diviners. Like Ignacia, Quassi was born in West Africa and had been enslaved for part of his life. Through his skill as a *lukuman*, he obtained his freedom and was well known for his preventive and therapeutic practices by the 1740s.[88] By the 1770s he was well traveled and famous in the Dutch Atlantic. Over several decades, Quassi had amassed a vast network of clients for his services, particularly in the creation and distribution of *obis*, small amulets of ritually powerful objects (shells, hair, feathers, among others) that offered protection to the wearer. His *obis* were so popular that almost all the colony's Black Rangers—enslaved men freed on condition of fighting with the Dutch against the Maroons—went to him to buy theirs. Quassi's clients were not restricted to the rangers: like many other practitioners of African descent, he was often hired by white enslavers and paid handsomely for his services in identifying perpetrators of various alleged crimes on plantations.[89]

Like Quassi, there were several very successful healers of African descent who were able to maintain a high profile without finding themselves on trial. Usually, these individuals were recognized by the government for special services performed for the colony in question. Quassi was a key ally of the Dutch colonial government in the 1750s Maroon Wars, both in his work as a spy and for supplying the rangers with *obis*.[90] His status within the colony as a powerful and much-needed ally was apparently high enough to insulate him from allegations in at least one poison case that he had been a supplier of a packet allegedly used to poison enslaved people at Plantagie Pérou on the Cottica River.[91] In the early eighteenth-century British North American colonies, colonial authorities manumitted several enslaved people in exchange for their much-desired healing knowledge.[92] Many enslaved healers in Virginia worked within the legal bounds of sanction—made possible by the loophole in the 1748 ban on medical practice by enslaved people that allowed for such practice with the knowledge and consent of all slaveholders involved.[93] Here the limitations of trial records as a source base are starkly apparent, as they capture only those practitioners who were unfortunate in their risk-taking to build networks of clients and knowledge.

Building prestige through networking over a wide geographic area was a common strategy for both free and enslaved practitioners of African descent, though the challenges to doing so varied widely with circumstances. Like Quassi, Paulo Gomes and Ignacia actively built a diverse network, offering a wide range of services to a wide range of clients—attendees at their rituals on the farm included "people of all quality." Gomes advertised his skills to his neighbors. One "gravely ill" white widow recalled to the commissioner that Gomes, whom she had known for twelve years, as they lived on the same street, had tried to persuade her many times over her long illness that she should come to his farm to be healed; she had declined his offer.[94] In Virginia, several runaway advertisements from the eighteenth century described the "great acquaintance," in some cases in counties across the colony, held by enslaved men who went by "Doctor."[95] Poison trials from the colony's county courts reveal that many practitioners crossed plantation and county lines to perform healing services and attract new clients. A recurring detail in the otherwise rather limited trial summaries was that practitioners of African descent exhibited their wares—making their services and objects used for healing known to potential clients.[96] Robert Carter's letters from the 1780s requesting the services of enslaved healers to come treat strange illnesses frequently noted how these practitioners were well known and specifically requested by the afflicted individuals for their reputation. These requests highlighted the ways in which prestige sustained and expanded a practitioner's clientele.[97] The networks of enslaved healers and their clients in Suriname can be traced like a spider web over the colony's numerous waterways: the neatly marked plantation boundaries on property maps stopped neither health practitioners' reputations nor their practices.

If networks of people and knowledge were a source of power, they were also a source of risk; binding power could make an individual morally ambiguous, and the same practices that were necessary for success could quickly lead one to being accused of causing illnesses through poisoning. A core idea from Atlantic African discussions of power centered on the morality of its use: well-known practitioners could elicit mixed feelings within communities precisely because they had access to powers and could possibly use those powers for noncommunal ends. In poison cases across these slave societies, a practitioner's reputation sometimes came up as either damning evidence or the initial cause for suspicion when people or livestock became sick.[98]

Increased visibility from the cultivation of networks could put healing practitioners at great risk for accusations of poisoning. Three interconnected trials from Suriname in 1741 illustrate well the precarious position of practitioners while also shedding light on how such networks of clients, suppliers, and knowledge could operate. In the early months of 1741, the Suriname Court of Policy and Criminal Justice began their first examination against La Rocke at Fort Zelandia, overlooking the Paramaribo parade and execution ground. At this meeting, La Rocke either confessed or confirmed an earlier confession made to his enslaver to having purchased one "poison" (vergift) from Samson to kill three enslaved women on his plantation and another from André to cure the pains in the arm of another enslaved woman working at Fort Nieuw Amsterdam. La Rocke had been identified by several people on the plantation as the one responsible for a series of misfortunes, including the illnesses of Apollo and Codjo—the former following a confrontation in the capacity of Apollo's position as the driver, the latter as part of a dispute involving Codjo's wife. The vergift to kill was a black powder with a little white inside a small cloth bag, while that to cure was a red substance packed inside of a horn. La Rocke paid for these items, in the case of the latter specifically with a bundle of bananas and a string of "papa gelt."[99] When asked for his motives for killing the women, La Rocke cited a personal dispute: during the coffee harvest, he claimed that they had repeatedly taken his coffee away and abused him, resulting in a thrashing each time he returned to the plantation shorthanded. While he insisted in the early examinations that the vergift (in the court's words) he had purchased from André was to "restore" the fourth woman, and not to harm, by his final interrogation he had changed his answer to the court's repeated questions to say that the red substance was a "poison" used to kill.[100]

Following La Rocke's three examinations, the case turned toward André. André, as well as several enslaved people from La Rocke's plantation, had been conscripted from his plantation on the Commewijne River to assist with the construction of Fort Nieuw Amsterdam. According to La Rocke's testimony, André had shown him his red vergift, advertising that it would be effective for a year, after which La Rocke purchased the substance. Apparently, he was not André's only client: André confirmed to the court that he had also performed healing services for another enslaved woman working at the fort, as well as for a man named Louis—who worked temporarily at the fort but lived on the same plantation as La Rocke. André confessed, apparently freely, to selling La Rocke the red substance in the horn to treat pains in the hands. He also instructed La Rocke on its use: to be mixed with animal fat and applied externally to the injured limb. However, André strenuously and repeatedly insisted that this substance was not a "poison" and not for killing. During André's fourth examination in early February, the court brought in La Rocke himself to confront André's testimony. When La Rocke repeated his claim that André had in fact given him poison to kill, the two men erupted into a heated exchange that ended with André striking La Rocke over the bar.[101]

La Rocke's testimony initiated a third case against the enslaved man Samson, though Samson was not convicted until the spring. Unfortunately, only the concluding summary of Samson's trial has survived, so it is unclear what Samson said in his own defense. According to this summary and La Rocke's testimony, Samson and an unnamed free Indigenous American woman—who also lived and presumably worked in Samson's enslaver's house in Paramaribo—were well known in the area as merchants of "pernicious and poisonous herbs," making and selling *vergift* to enslaved people working at Fort Nieuw Amsterdam. La Rocke claimed that Samson had shown the poison that La Rocke later purchased to Louis, the man from his plantation who had been working at the fort, indicating that Louis was a further link of information between La Rocke's Commewijne plantation, the fort, and Paramaribo. While the court investigated and acquitted two other enslaved people suspected of being connected to Samson's supply network, there is no surviving evidence that Louis was ever tried or arrested.[102] Each of the three trials ended in a gruesome public execution in the capital: La Rocke was hanged, André beheaded, and Samson broken on the wheel. The court ordered the heads of each man to be mounted on a spike in the river as a warning to others.[103]

This series of cases is particularly rich as it touches on many of the common themes of poison cases involving practitioners of African descent. Immediately striking is the geographic spread of both the connections between enslaved communities and the reputations of the health practitioners. The three defendants, La Rocke, André, and Samson, had different enslavers and lived in different parts of the colony—La Rocke on a plantation on the Commewijne River; André on a different plantation on Hooikreek, an offshoot of the same river; and Samson in a house in the city of Paramaribo. As with several other poison cases from the early 1740s, the construction site of the new fort at the meeting of the Suriname and Commeijne Rivers served as a hub.[104] André and Samson were well known at the fort, and all three had developed a reputation there for healing services. La Rocke also had a reputation for social confrontations. The exchanged red and black powders, and payments rendered for them, formed additional connections in a web of healing practice that operated largely beyond the knowledge or control of enslavers. It was along these same lines that accusations of using or selling "poison" flowed.

The accusations also highlight the moral ambiguity of binding power and the risks taken by practitioners to claim it. While details in the testimony differed—and, in the case of La Rocke, changed over the course of the investigation—these interconnected cases suggest the multiple roles of practitioners and their practices for healing and harm. La Rocke acquired multiple substances from other practitioners and seems most likely to have used them for distinct purposes. That La Rocke was both a healer, treating pains in a woman's arm, for example, and the primary suspect for illnesses, deaths, and misfortunes on his plantation, was not a coincidence. La Rocke occupied a precarious position, both morally in the eyes of the enslaved community and socially as his reputation for power put him at greater risk of accusation. While no one accused André of directly causing physical harm with poison, it was his reputation for healing and making and selling empowered substances that put him in contact with La Rocke as a client—both widening his network and increasing his risk. From Paramaribo, Samson and his unnamed Indigenous partner also expanded their clientele by selling substances to enslaved people at the fort and, through these connections, to people on other plantations—again increasing the likelihood that their practices would come before the criminal court. These three men would have been aware of the risks: while their cases were among the first of the early 1740s boom, heads of enslaved people convicted of poisoning loomed over the Suriname River outside of Paramaribo for several years before their trials. That these men conducted healing practices at all, despite knowing the risks of poison accusations, and that many more continued to do so long after the public and gruesome executions speaks volumes of the importance of binding power to practitioners of African descent.

Communal Institutions

In the late eighteenth and nineteenth centuries, the formation of new Afro-Caribbean and Afro-Brazilian religious institutions altered the landscape for ritual healing practitioners. Historians have debated the origins and formative processes of Vodou, Santeria, Candomblé, and related religions for decades, with the most recent of these works examining therapeutic practices offered by individual practitioners as simultaneous rather than in an evolutionary relationship with communal worship.[105] In terms of poison, these new institutions were also sites of fear for enslavers terrified by the prospect of rebellion—especially in the post-Haitian Revolution Atlantic world.

In Brazil, while investigations by the Inquisition dropped significantly toward the end of the eighteenth century, local courts turned their attention to early spaces of ritual worship. An important 1785 investigation involved self-identifying *Jeje* freedmen and enslaved people (*Jeje* being a Brazilian ethnic term for people affiliated with the Gbe-speaking area of the Bight of Benin) at a *calundú* in Cachoeira. Responding to a denunciation, police raided a gathering of six people. Their leader, Sebastião de Guerra, had already once been accused of *feitiçaria* and was publicly known for curing *feitiços*, dancing *calundús*, and leading worship in the *Jeje* language.[106] Unlike the *calundús* denounced earlier in the eighteenth century—which primarily focused on services rendered through divination and both preventive and therapeutic treatments of illnesses—the confiscated leaves and objects in the *Jeje* Cachoeira *calundú* were suggestive of a shrine, offerings, and congregational worship.[107]

The 1785 case was part of a transition, both in the institutionalization of healing cults with increasingly complex ritual practices among African-descended Bahians and in government efforts to repress these practices. Early nineteenth-century raids of *terreiros*—healing houses—had more to do with police fears of rebellion than complaints of these *terreiros* causing harm. In the first recorded use of the term Candomblé, in a raid in 1807 near Santo Amaro, the accusation centered not on healing or causing harm through *feitiços* but of assisting runaways and holding gunpowder and arms.[108] The police saw Candomblé practitioners and their *terreiros* as a threat not as a den of poisoners but as a place for potentially rebellious gatherings of Africans and people of African descent. This trend continued in the early nineteenth-century revolts, as some enslaved participants wore *bolsas de mandinga* as protective amulets for battle.[109] Police began to identify any African-associated object as a potential threat and sign of rebellion—but not necessarily connected to "poison."[110] Keeping in mind the relative scarcity of documentation of healing practices and practitioners in the first half of the nineteenth century, it appears that accusations of poison/*feitiçaria* had temporarily disappeared. The police investigations into "poison" that did appear in these decades were completely divorced from their raids of Candomblé houses that were increasingly institutionalized with specific rituals, initiations, and spiritual affiliations.[111]

However, by the mid-nineteenth century, investigations into "poisoning" became an avenue for policing Candomblé practitioners. In the 1850s and 1860s, police received repeated calls for greater crackdowns on the popular and burgeoning Candomblé houses. These calls from both the Catholic press and newspapers run by free people of color framed the activities at Candomblé *terreiros* as superstitions, dangerous not for their efficacy but for their perceived potential to hold Brazil back from modernity.[112] A chief source of fear was of the number of "civilized" people attending and even joining Candomblé congregations to seek solutions for their problems.[113] However, under the laws of the empire, "superstition" alone was not a crime.[114] Police instead justified their raids on *terreiros* as following noise complaints or claims that Candomblé leaders had received stolen goods as payment for various services.[115]

In Martinique, poison accusations from the early nineteenth century suggest the possible formation of new social and religious institutions with initiation practices. A critical eye is necessary, as many of these records were of chain cases and confessions extracted through torture. However, recurring details—such as the emphasis on grave dirt and social networking of participants—are suggestive of communal practices distorted by enslavers' anxieties. Surviving records from Villaret's wartime special tribunal and the cases, investigation, and correspondence surrounding the Cour Prévôtale from 1822 to 1827 frequently discussed "cults of poisoners."[116] The 1766 case of Jean Baptiste with the alleged meetings of a poisoning society at the house of Jacques Pain was an early example of this idea, but it only became a recurring feature of poison accusations in the early nineteenth century.[117] In an 1807 case at Basse Pointe, forty-two enslaved people across seven plantations were accused of participation in a poisoning society that involved an initiation ceremony and "poisons" allegedly made from the dug-up and powdered bones of children.[118]

Discussions of initiations and grave digging continued in the 1820s Cour
Prévôtale cases. The court explicitly and anxiously discussed the "sect of poisoners" across cases as 368 free and enslaved people of African descent were
caught in the frenzy. The stated purpose of the Cour Prévôtale was to un-
earth what Governor Donzelot called a "society of poisoners," well-organized
with "chiefs, secret signs, sacramental sermons, [and] a form of initiation."[119]
In the context of the development of new religious institutions in this period
across the Caribbean, there may have been some truth in the idea of secret
societies of African-descended "poisoners"—though perhaps not as enslavers in these cases understood it. However, for slaveholders, the potential threat
of a network of "poisoners" to plantation society had taken on new heights
with the specter of the Haitian Revolution in recent memory.[120] The idea of
a network of conspiracy was not always a figment of slaveholder fear, as
Ada Ferrer's work on José Antonio Aponte's movement in 1812 Cuba (which
also involved an abundantly creative composition of knowledge) can attest.
This concept reflects how central ideas of binding power could continue to
resonate even as the context and circumstances of slavery in the Americas
transformed.[121]

*　*　*

There was no clear resolution to the case of Paulo Gomes and Ignacia. Having collected denunciations and testimony from their neighbors over the
course of a month, the Inquisitorial commissioner sent the package to Lisbon. It would have been months, possibly longer, before he heard back.[122] As
with most accusations of *feitiçaria* directed at people of African descent, the
Lisbon Inquisitors decided the case was not worth the expense and declined
initiating a full trial. Instead, they neatly copied the documents for the record into volume 109 of the *cadernos do promotor*, and that was that. It is possible that Gomes and Ignacia were brought before the secular court, which
had joint jurisdiction over *feitiçaria* cases. Such was the case for the denunciation of Miguel and Maria Monjola; while the Inquisition declined to open
a trial, the secular courts were already in the process of trying the two healers when a dissatisfied neighbor denounced them to the commissioner.[123]
However, in the absence of surviving documentation, it is impossible to know.
While the fates of Gomes and Ignacia are unknown from this record, many
other poison trials of practitioners ended with concrete finality. For La Rocke,
whose head the Suriname court mounted on a pike in the river; and Jupiter,

the healing practitioner whose body the Martinique court burned at the stake; and Dido, an enslaved woman whom the Virginia Cumberland County Court hanged in 1756 for making and distributing "poisonous medicines," the risks of healing practice were very real and the results dire.

It was an irony that the strategies of binding power used by eighteenth-century practitioners to become successful—courting new clients, expanding networks of knowledge, building reputations for power and prestige—increased their risk of accusation from enslavers, enslaved communities, and other practitioners. African and African-descended healers built their professions on the composition of wealth in knowledge: from methods of contacting the dead, to the use of power objects proven through experience, to the social knowledge necessary to identify the work of other practitioners. It would have been difficult for them to have been unaware of the risks of their work, especially during the mid-eighteenth-century peaks of poison trials; yet they continued their practices and continuously worked to expand them. To be a healer—whether a *savant*, *calunduzeiro/a*, *lukuman*, or simply "doctor"—was to hold a position, however precarious, of power and prestige. Many paid for that power with their lives.

CHAPTER 6

Creating Narratives About Poison

On January 30, 1800, Martha Jefferson Randolph wrote to her father, Thomas Jefferson, about the mysterious death of Jupiter, the fifty-six-year-old enslaved coachman at Monticello. Jupiter regularly drove Jefferson the sixty-five miles to Fredericksburg, where Jefferson caught the coach to Philadelphia.[1] That January, Jefferson paid for Jupiter to stay overnight at an inn in Fredericksburg, as he had been ill. Martha Jefferson Randolph described in her letter what happened on Jupiter's return:

> To your enquiries relative to poor Jupiter he too has paid the debt to nature; finding himself no better at his return home, he unfortunately conceived him self poisoned & went to consult the negro doctor who attended the George's. He went in the house to see uncle Randolph [Randolph Jefferson, Thomas Jefferson's brother] who gave him a dram which he drank & seemed to be as well as he had been for some time past; after which he took a dose from this black doctor who pronounced that it would kill or cure. 2 ½ hours after taking the medecine [sic] he fell down in a strong convulsion fit which lasted from ten to elevin [sic] hours, during which time it took 3 stout men to hold him, he languished nine days but was never heard to speak from the first of his being seized to the moment of his death.[2]

In this same letter she gave news on the state of Ursula Granger, the enslaved head cook at Monticello. Ursula had also gone to see Sam, the "black doctor" who had come to Monticello months earlier to treat Ursula's late husband, George (the overseer), and son George Jr. (the smith). According to her, "Ursala [sic] is I fear going in the same manner with her husband & son, a constant puking shortness of breath and swelling first in the legs but now extending itself," adding that "the doctor I understand had also given her means as they term it and upon Jupiter's death has absconded." She concluded, "I should think his murders sufficiently manifest to come under the cognizance of the law."[3] By April, Ursula was dead. In a letter to his father-in-law, Thomas Mann Randolph ascribed all four deaths to the "poisons of the Buckingham Negroe conjuror."[4]

While it did not result in a trial, the case at Monticello offers a window into the ways different actors interpreted and built narratives of poisoning events. Enslavers—as plantation owners, judges, legislators, physicians, and clergy—experienced poisoning events as moments of profound and frightening usurpations of power and, perhaps more alarmingly, as a shattering of illusions over the completeness of their control over free and enslaved people of African descent. Their responses to poisoning cases were numerous: establishing new laws and ordinances to police the activities of health practitioners, conducting their own investigations and punishments on plantations, or inserting themselves into the ritual activities of these practitioners. Identifying, assessing, and theorizing about poison, poisoners, and motives through narratives became ways to try to make poison knowable and therefore conquerable. The "common knowledge" narratives that enslavers developed diverged in several significant ways from the cases that were actually being tried—let alone from the perspectives of healers of African descent and enslaved communities. Some of these divergences were in the details of supposed poisoning methods, while others included slaveholder speculation on the motives and targets of so-called poisoners. While the language and contours of slaveholder discourse on poisoning changed from the eighteenth to the early nineteenth century, the central problem of control was a constant. Enslavers built their own narrative imaginary of "poisoning," sometimes divorced from reality, and this imaginary ironically did little to ease their minds.

Through sources created by enslavers, such as these letters from Monticello, historians can catch glimpses of significantly different interpretations from the perspectives of the enslaved. It was Jupiter who first "conceived himself poisoned," and it was Jupiter and Ursula together who then took matters into their own hands, seeking out a well-known local healing practitioner. Notably, Jupiter hedged his bets and visited Randolph Jefferson for good measure. It was presumably Ursula, since Jupiter reportedly did not speak after suffering his convulsions, who told Martha Jefferson Randolph of their encounter with the "black doctor," who had warned that his remedy would "kill or cure." The conditional nature of "the means, as they call it," suggests that there was more at play in the narrative of affliction that Sam, Jupiter, and Ursula made together than Martha Jefferson Randolph understood or discussed in her letter to her father.

Crucially, enslavers were not the only ones creating narratives about poison; through their actions and words people within enslaved communities also shaped poisoning events into narratives that reflected their own conceptions of responsibility, morality, and justice. The key to understanding alleged poisoning events from the perspective of the enslaved is to see them in the wider scope of healing processes, where multiple parties—including patients, practitioners, and powerful intermediaries like spirits—came together over the series of events in an illness to collaboratively craft a narrative about the causes of and solutions to the affliction.[5] As healing practitioners and clients, people of African descent in slave societies developed their own interpretations about what—or who—was responsible for "poisoning" in ways that sometimes overlapped and sometimes came into conflict with the rendering made by slaveholders of European descent. The diverse actors involved in poison cases constructed detailed narratives that talked past each other while at the same time converging into a shared narrative of "poisoning" as a dire threat.[6]

Contested and Collaborative Narrative Building

In interactions with their clients, healers of African descent constructed narratives of their afflictions that pointed toward practical demonstration of solutions. The removal of various objects from the bodies of the afflicted was a recurring feature of demonstrative healing practice.[7] In one of the earliest descriptions of *obeah* in Barbados, Thomas Walduck described witnessing an "Obia" man in 1712 remove bones, shells, "and such odd things . . . that I have admired att [sic] it" from the bodies of enslaved people who had been "bewitched."[8] In eighteenth- and nineteenth-century Virginia, a common sign of a conjure affliction was the sensation of something crawling under the skin; the objects removed by conjure doctors often included insects, worms, or small reptiles.[9] Objects expelled from the body, usually referred to with the same term used for a practitioner's objects—*feitiços*—appeared in several trials of health practitioners originating in Bahia. In the case of Miguel and Maria Monjola, the former removed a long list of objects, allegedly placed by the latter, from the bodies of the afflicted. As part of his treatment of the white sergeant-major in his care, Miguel pulled from his body small bones, goat hairs, rags, butterflies, roots, and a small bag of insects.[10] Even when the objects themselves were not specified in testimony, the verb *tirar* (to pull out, take out, remove) came up frequently to describe healing actions taken by practitioners in Bahia. Joanna Maria, a free creole living in Salvador, was denounced in 1752 for using certain little pots to pull objects from the bodies of women; about a half century earlier, an enslaved African man named Sebastião was accused of pulling objects out of the bodies of other enslaved people following divination.[11]

The physical removal of objects from the afflicted body offered a practical demonstration of the efficacy of the healing practitioner's work and in doing so contributed to practitioners' narratives on their powers. While the precise content of these objects and works were flexible, the central focus on the creative manifestation of physical proof through ritual was key to legitimacy. The sensory and visible claims of health practitioners in these eighteenth-century cases were in continuity with testimonies of their work in the seventeenth-century Caribbean.[12] They also connect to idioms and practices in Atlantic Africa. Numerous judicial ordeals involved the consumption of a conditionally efficacious "poison" followed by analysis of the results expelled from the body through vomiting. In Angola, Francisco Buitrago's description of the work of *nganga* using the bark of the *nkasa* tree to "pull out" poison or other "malignant things" contributed to his conviction that it would also be efficacious for forcing patients suffering from demonic possession to vomit them out.[13]

The case of Paulo Gomes and Ignacia in 1740s Salvador stands out for the detailed description of the objects expelled by the afflicted and removed by other practitioners as signs of their alleged *feitiçaria*. One of the afflicted, a white woman and former lover of Gomes, had begun to throw up charcoal, insects, fish spines, and a pig's tooth—strong indications to her neighbors that she was "enfeitiçada" (ensorcelled). One of the most detailed descriptions of bodily expulsions and their position in healing practices came from João Roiz da Silva, the white painter and neighbor of Gomes. His unnamed wife was dying in the Hospiçio dos Religiosos de Jerusalem, where they gave her some medicines that had little effect. An enslaved man there told them that the illness was caused by *feitiços* and that the physician's medicine at the hospital would not work; the woman was "enfeitiçada," as evidenced by her swollen chest. Together they then took her to get some "mediçinas do preto" (Black medicines). The African practitioner they visited, who had died by the time of Roiz da Silva's testimony, proceeded to remove various "filth" from the woman's body, including fish spines, chicken feathers, lemongrass, and, again, a large pig's tooth. Roiz da Silva asked the doctor if he knew who had made the *malefício*; at first he said he did not, as Roiz da Silva's wife did not have known enemies. The practitioner assisted Roiz da Silva in carrying his wife home and then proceeded to use divination to identify the culprit. Roiz da Silva's wife died shortly thereafter.[14]

The details of Roiz da Silva's account point to another key part of how African and African-descended healers built narratives of affliction and cure: identifying the work of other practitioners. Whether called in to assist with a communal crisis or consulted by an individual, practitioners determined suspects after building an understanding of the social relationships involved.[15] It is unclear from the above case whether the unnamed "curador" (healer) assisting Roiz da Silva had asked around the neighborhood before conducting his divination, but it is significant that he did not venture to suggest a culprit before spending some time there. It would not have been difficult for him to learn about Paulo Gomes's reputation: indeed, the success of Gomes and Ignacia as powerful health practitioners depended on public knowledge of their identities. Conjure doctors in nineteenth-century Virginia conducted similar quiet investigations into personal relationships to accompany their divination and discoveries of "conjure packets"—pouches of power objects causing the affliction—to identify culprits.[16] It is important that practitioners' discovery, whether genuine or possibly staged, of objects indicative of poison in the homes of suspects usually occurred *after* these individuals had already been identified through public opinion and divination. In the case of Hans in 1819 Berbice, it was only after a period of ritual dancing and communal possession, during which members of the enslaved community identified Frederick as a poisoner, that Hans found a ram's horn and bones under Frederick's bed.[17] In both eighteenth-century Bahia and nineteenth-century Virginia, healers were considered capable of turning the affliction back on the *feitiçeiro/a*, or conjuror, who caused it. Roiz da Silva noted that shortly after his wife's death he received a concerned visit from Paulo Gomes's mother. She wanted to know whom he had seen in his effort to treat his wife, as she prayed that no *malefício* had been turned on her son.[18] Relationships between practitioners and between practitioners and wider African-descended communities were central to the narratives they constructed about poisoning.

In developing their own narratives about alleged "poisoning" events, en-slavers frequently invoked the idea of common knowledge. "Common knowledge" is not really common but is specific to time, place, and perspective; a consensus on narratives about poison—or even on a stable definition of what "poison" was—embedded in its invocation did not actually exist. Close analysis of the correspondence of sugar planter Pierre Dessalles in 1820s Martinique illustrates how enslavers collectively built narratives around alleged poisoning events.[19] Dessalles was well informed on the numerous cases that rocked Martinique in that decade; he was a member of the Conseil Supérieur. In one of his letters, he told his mother how he spent the previous day "interrogating the guilty" in that capacity at Mme. Levassor's plantation.[20] Many of his letters included tallies of recent losses of enslaved people and livestock incurred by his neighbors.[21] Similar to the conversations at Monticello, Dessalles's information came from speaking and writing with other slaveholders in a form of collaborative narrative building. One night in July 1824, a neighbor, M. Catala, was over for dinner when several of Dessalles mules were discovered sick. Dessalles had recently claimed that the plantations all around him had been suffering severe losses of enslaved people and livestock but that so far his constant vigilance had prevented any losses of his own.[22] Catala told Dessalles that he had observed the same symptoms in his own mules that had died, and that night they gathered the enslaved community on Dessalles plantation and spoke to them. When they discovered a mule dead the next day, Dessalles and Catala opened the mule's body for an amateur autopsy. They claimed to have "acquired the most certain proof of his illness; it is poison that killed him."[23] He also wrote his cousin, a M. Lasalle, sharing with him the extreme measures he had taken to deter and terrorize would-be poisoners on his plantation, including random whippings and forbidding enslaved people to enter their cabins except to sleep.[24] As the Cour Prévôtale continued, Dessalles related discussions on the "scourge."[25] He told his mother of a case in Robert about ten miles away, where it was now "widely believed that the current poison [came] from free people of color, who give bad advice to the slaves."[26] Dessalles furiously rejected a counternarrative suggesting that the livestock deaths were the result of disease and not "poison."[27] Dessalles was in constant contact with the other enslavers in his neighborhood and beyond, and poisoning in the early 1820s was a constant source of discussion that was rooted in claims of direct experience. From the dinner table to his seat on the court to his writing desk, Dessalles positioned himself as an expert, consuming and contributing to a narrative of conspiracy that required terrifying violence to stop.

Travel accounts, histories, and natural histories were also avenues for Europeans and European-descended enslavers to declare their expertise on "poison" and to spread tropes that became part of their ever-changing "common knowledge" about it. The well-known authors of these works rested their claims to authority on their extensive experience in the slave societies of the Americas, whether or not they were enslavers themselves.[28] Jesuit André João Antonil spent thirty-five years from the 1680s to 1710s living in Bahia—precisely during the period when denunciations regarding *feitiçaria* began to increase—before writing *Cultura e opulencia do Brasil por suas drogas e minas* (1711).[29] Labat, who was residing in Martinique at about the same time that Antonil traveled in Brazil, had more direct experience than Antonil with poisoning cases as he lived at the Saint-Jacques sugar plantation for over a decade—the same plantation that later shocked Pierre Clément de Laussat in the early nineteenth century with the private prison for suspected poisoners.[30] His descriptions of the practices of African "sorcerers" in *Nouveau voyage aux iles de l'Amerique* (1722) had a major impact on later British and French colonial writings on *obeah*, *vaudou*, and poisoning, including direct references in the works of enslavers Edward Long (1774) and Bryan Edwards (1792).[31] John Gabriel Stedman's *Narrative of a Five Years' Expedition* (1796) on his firsthand military experiences in Suriname in the 1770s was also widely read—going into three English editions in 1796, 1806, and 1813 and rapidly translated into Dutch, French, and German by 1800—and contained abundant discussions with enslavers, free people of color, and enslaved people on poisoning. These works spread and perpetuated slaveholders' "common knowledge."

As an example, these works contained a recurring trope that "poisoners" had direct connection to training in Africa—and that there was a causal link between Africanness and "poisoning." The relationship between poison and Africa was a given in these works, even though trials of alleged poisoners and the work of African-descended health practitioners involved people born both in Africa and the Americas. Officials and missionaries stationed in Portuguese Angola in the seventeenth and eighteenth centuries discussed Africa as a "poisoned landscape," filled not only with the flora and fauna of a treacherous climate but also people highly skilled and trained in "poisoning."[32] Enslavers in the Americas also made links to degrees of "Africanness" when discussing poisoning.[33] The slaveholders interviewed by Antonil during his travels in the late seventeenth century shared their opinion that the enslaved people who allegedly killed with poison had among them many "Masters distinguished in this Art."[34] Labat similarly claimed that almost all of the adult men from Africa in Martinique had at least some knowledge of "sorcery and poison."[35] Nearly a century later, and writing on Saint-Domingue, Moreau de Saint-Méry claimed that a quarter of the enslaved people brought from Africa were "sorcerers" proficient in "the odious art of poisoning."[36] Even those who were skeptical about the veracity (and legality) of the eighteenth-century peaks in poisoning trials, like Raymond de Laborde, took as a given that the expertise of alleged enslaved poisoners was linked to their Africanness. Laborde even referenced voyagers who assured him that "in their country there are schools where one teaches this infernal art."[37]

The alleged connection between poisoning and Africanness was so strong that during the British occupation of Martinique in 1814, Governor Charles Wales wrote to his superiors that although "native" Africans were "addicted" to "that nefarious practice of Obiah, witchcraft or Poisoning (all of which may be here called synonymous)," he could happily report a decrease in poisoning cases in relation to the ending of the transatlantic slave trade. Wales connected his triumphant satisfaction at the ending of the transatlantic slave trade, "no less conducive to Humanity than to the interest of the Planters," to the improvement of the colony that had previously been "depopulated" by poisoning. Wales here referred to not only "the loss of those actually poisoned, but also of many innocent victims who fell sacrificed to suspicion, occasioning brutal acts of cruelty and a mutual want of confidence between the master and his slave."[38] There is a lot to analyze in this remarkable letter. Wales had no problem eliding *obeah*, witchcraft, and poisoning, reflecting the ways that people recognized similar practices and concepts under different labels.[39] Wales also narratively framed the Martinique poison trials themselves and the distrust they engendered as a social ill being cured by Britain's ending of the transatlantic slave trade. Wales's prediction that poisonings would decline with the shrinking proportion of Africans in the population did not hold; many creoles were accused of poisoning in the eighteenth and nineteenth centuries, and Martinique had yet to experience its most convulsive and final major wave of poisoning accusations in the 1820s. Most significantly for discussion here, Wales repeated what was a widely shared idea on the causal connection between poison and Africanness.

Slaveholders' tropes about "poison" were not as stable as the invocation of "common knowledge" would make them seem. For example, in the late eighteenth and nineteenth centuries, narratives about poison more frequently included claims that everyone knew about specific plants that the enslaved allegedly used to poison. For example, brinvilliers (*Spigelia anthelmia*), an herb native to the Caribbean that was allegedly used by the Marquise de Brinvilliers to murder her relatives in a sensational 1676 French case, began to appear in discussions of poison by colonial officials in Martinique in the early nineteenth century.[40] French American physician Jean-Baptiste Ricord-Madianna was so convinced of the "fatal passion" of female *gardiennes d'hôpitaux* (enslaved workers at plantation hospitals) secretly and spitefully administering these herbs to kill their patients that he issued a dire warning: "Planters of the Antilles! . . . You are surrounded by a thousand poisons and a thousand malefactors, it is true; learn to know the weapons of your enemies."[41] For all the herb's prevalence in Ricord-Madianna's writing—taking up more than fifty pages of his work—it did not appear in any of the poison cases from the Cour Prévôtale or any earlier cases. Late eighteenth-century authors also increasingly pointed to the cassava, or manioc, root (*Manihot esculenta*) as part of enslaved poisoners' alleged arsenal. Cassava does contain small amounts of cyanide and requires careful preparation to be safe to eat.[42] While Europeans had long noted the importance of this preparation and the potential for accidents, it was only in the last quarter of the eighteenth century that they began to list this root as a substance allegedly used intentionally to poison.[43] By Laussat's time, in a diary entry listing poisons from 1807, he confidently described it as a "very common poison" when mixed with verdigris.[44] In a counternarrative rejecting the plausibility of cassava juice as an effective tool for alleged poisoners, Étienne Rufz de Lavison explained that it required a large quantity of fresh juice to kill a steer—so large that his experiment to do so required multiple assistants to hold the poor animal and force-feed it. To "poison" a single animal, maybe—"but organized and multiple mass poisonings, to the point of imitating an epizootic, impossible!"[45]

Confronted with deadly afflictions, people developed explanations and solutions that resonated with their own ideas about health and healing. A close analysis of the reactions to Jupiter's illness at Monticello tracks some of the contested and collaborative ways people constructed poison narratives. The enslavers at Monticello sought to make the strange deaths knowable, framing them as the result of improper care and irrational behavior of the enslaved. Pointedly ignoring his daughter's description of Jupiter's strange convulsions, Jefferson repeatedly described his death as the result of an ordinary, if severe, illness exacerbated by exhaustion and culminating in Jupiter's "imprudent perseverance in journeying" to Randolph Jefferson's plantation.[46] For Jefferson, Jupiter's death was the unfortunate result of irrational stubbornness. Martha Jefferson Randolph and Thomas Mann Randolph ascribed first the illnesses of Jupiter and Ursula, then the deaths of all four of the afflicted, to a concrete cause in the "poison" administered by an enslaved practitioner. For Martha Jefferson Randolph, the "poisonous" medicine of enslaved practitioners was a menace, tantamount to murder or at least malpractice that prevented the operation of a true cure. In describing the impact of the "poison" on Ursula, Thomas Mann Randolph used an image of an unraveling body, its "fibers" and "threads" unstrung by the power of the poison, rendering the afflicted listless, undone.[47] He mused, "The poisons of the Conjurer have the most astonishing effect in producing melancholy & despair—perhaps greatly operative in the catastrophe."[48] In this rendering, Ursula's listlessness and Jupiter's inability to speak in the days leading up to his death become the emotional effects of superstition and evidence of the dangerous power men like the "conjuror" could have on the minds of other enslaved people.[49] This explanatory idea was shared in the perceived psychological powers of practitioners of African descent over enslaved communities more broadly.[50]

Though filtered through the Monticello letters, the reported speech and actions of Jupiter, Sam, and Ursula offer insights into the ways that practitioners and clients built their own narratives of the case. It was Jupiter who first "conceived him self [sic] poisoned" and when he sought healing from the "black doctor," Sam instructed him that the "means as they term it"— would "kill or cure."[51] The "means" was a significant term as it emphasized the inherently practical nature of Sam's work: enslaved people like Jupiter and Ursula sought out "means" because they expected it to *do* something.[52] That these "means" could have opposite effects—to "kill or cure"— suggests that they and Sam saw the operation of his practice as going beyond physical effect. There are echoes here of conditionally efficacious oath draughts used in Atlantic Africa and in numerous instances in the slave societies of the Americas.[53] Whatever the outcome and whatever the conditions might have been, the actions of Sam were intended to produce a definitive result. This narrative was less about rendering an event explainable so it could be safely put out of mind and more about a clear demonstration and resolution to the affliction.

Finding and Defining Proof: Investigations,
Ordeals, and Trials

Afflicted bodies were important sites of evidence of poisoning for both enslavers and physicians trained in western medicine—though they were not
always in agreement. Records of poisoning cases describe autopsies and tests
of suspicious substances claimed to be poison, sometimes ordered by the
court and sometimes conducted before the trial by enslavers as amateurs. At
the heart of these investigations was the idea that the poisons were physical
substances that, while currently unknown to slaveholders, could be known;
to make them knowable was to diminish their power. Autopsies and tests
were ways to uncover, in the words of the Martinique Conseil Supérieur, "the
Science of their [African practitioners'] detestable art."[54] In the 1781 case of
Masongoe in Suriname, suspected of poisoning through the use of *obis*, doctors hired by the court first tested the *wiriwiri* Masongoe claimed were only
used to treat illnesses—finding nothing harmful—and then performed an autopsy on the body of his deceased patient, an enslaved man named Mingo.
Apparently, the presence of blood in Mingo's lungs was convincing enough
for the court to convict Masongoe.[55]

Martinique stands out for the legal requirements established for autopsies during the acceleration and peak of poisoning cases in the mid-eighteenth
century. Here, the colonial government considered autopsies so essential for
establishing proof that they passed an ordinance in 1749 requiring enslavers
to have a surgeon open the bodies of enslaved people or livestock suspected
of having been poisoned; said surgeon then had to submit a report as evidence to the court.[56] The language of the ordinance was dire, warning that
"we can no longer ignore that this crime is real and even common among
the slaves," and that action must be taken to "not only stop the spreading [of
poisonings], but extirpate [it], if possible, to the root."[57] Both this ordinance,
and a 1758 update reaffirming it, were printed and posted to church doors
throughout the colony.[58] The fact that the council had to repeat the mandate,
stressing the necessity of the presence of a trained surgeon, suggests that
slaveholders conducted their own autopsies—or not—as they pleased and
were confident enough to bring cases to the court without the required official autopsy.[59] Raymond de Laborde, a fierce critic of the way enslavers "neither competent nor capable" handled poisoning cases, noted in 1775 that in
all his time as a doctor in Martinique, Saint-Domingue, and Cayenne over

the past two decades not once was he called to the court to perform an autopsy.[60] Even without formal ordinances, enslavers sometimes made use of autopsies and various tests as part of their efforts to create knowledge on poisoning events. On at least two occasions Pierre Dessalles—who was not a doctor— opened the bodies of livestock he suspected to have been poisoned and was satisfied that his examination proved that poison was responsible.[61]

Intriguing as these tests were, they did not often matter for the outcome of cases in courts. In fact, autopsies and chemical tests of suspected poisons were described much more in correspondence and reports on poisoning than in actual cases, only explicitly appearing in nine cases in my dataset. The low number of cases that describe such tests is likely more reflective of the material conditions of the records than necessarily an infrequency of such tests. Interestingly, none of these nine cases precisely identified the substance in question—whether the *wiriwiri* herbs and "obias" used by Masongoe in 1781 or the powdered roots Mustapha carried about in a cane in 1787—as a physically harmful substance after the investigation. However, two of the cases ended in executions anyway, while Masongoe was condemned to convict labor at Fort Nieuw Amsterdam for life and Mustapha to a painful and humiliating form of corporal punishment known as the "Spanish Buck."[62] Similarly, while a Virginia court in 1744 investigating Tom's "Poysonous Powders Roots Herbs and Simples" determined that he was not guilty of poisoning someone with this powder, they decided to transport him from the colony anyway as a potential threat.[63]

For the two cases that ended in executions, one from Martinique and one from Suriname, the surgeon's reports did not affect the court's conviction of the guilt of the accused and did not outweigh other "evidence." This evidence primarily consisted of the confession extracted on the plantation by a gang of slaveholders in the case of Jean Baptiste (1766) and the accusations of other enslaved people in the case of Coffij and La Rose (1779). Jean Baptiste confessed to attending assemblies of "black poisoners" at the house of Jacques Pain, a free person of color, and that Pain sold Jean Baptiste and others around the island poisons to kill enslaved people and livestock. A "great quantity of poison" was subsequently found at Jacques Pain's house. However, after experimenting with these substances on a range of animals "in different fashions and quantities," the surgeons hired by the court testified that the results were inconclusive. Their testimony was not mentioned again, and the court continued to refer to these substances as "poison." While Jean Baptiste died in jail after testifying, the case expanded based on the names he gave to include thirty additional defendants—twenty-four enslaved people and six free people of color—and resulted in two executions and twenty-eight other punishments ranging from a branding and whipping to being forced to assist with the burning alive of Jacques Pain.[64] In the case of Coffij and La Rose in 1779, a doctor testified that the hair found in the food of their mistress—allegedly sprinkled there to cause death—was "not positively poisonous"; the court decided that it was the intent to "poison" that mattered and sentenced them to beheading and their heads and right hands mounted on display as a warning for others.[65] The act of testing for enslavers was more important for creating narrative control over the event than it was for actually proving by their own standards that the substances in question were physically capable of doing the harm described.

Proof was not only embedded in the afflicted body but also could be located in empowered objects as external sources of poison. Poison accusations directed at healers of African descent and evidence for trials often centered on the discovery of such objects used in their work. A close examination of some of the described objects recorded in trials suggests some of the context of their suspected use. A common element in public accusations within enslaved communities was the searching of the suspected poisoner's living space. Such searches were often followed by efforts of the accused to explain the uses of suspect items. When the enslaved people on the plantation of Andre Gomes de Medina searched the cabin of Simão in 1688, following a communal ritual presided over by a famed practitioner, they found what they considered to be damning evidence in the form of powders made from snake heads. Simão explained to the Inquisitors in Lisbon that these powders—composed, yes, of dried snake heads, along with leaves from an "erva de sangue" (herb of health)—were solely for the treatment of snakebites, to be mixed in flour, oil, and garlic and consumed by the patient.[66] While the powders of Simão did not appear to have been hidden, many other cases noted concealed locations of practitioners' supplies and objects: secreted in chests, buried under the floor, or placed in roof thatching.[67]

In some cases, the "poison" itself was conceived of as a hidden object. Among the accusations directed against Paulo Gomes from his Salvador neighbors was the murder of a man named Copme Pacheco—allegedly so Gomes could spend more time with Pacheco's wife. According to witnesses, Pacheco died from profuse bleeding from the mouth after "catching" the small pot of *feitiços* that had been placed in his door. In another accusation from the same case, a woman accused Gomes of causing the deaths of enslaved people in her household by hiding a small pot of *maleficio* in her bed.[68] Indeed, part of the enslaved practitioner Coffij's claim to fame at the Suriname Fort Nieuw Amsterdam construction site in 1742 was his stated ability to locate and remove all of the hidden poison-calabashes—their presence being the cause of a series of illnesses and misfortunes. The testimony at Coffij's trial did not describe these objects as calabashes (that is, containers) *of* poison, but referred to the same objects as both calabashes *and* poison (that is, the hidden objects themselves *were* the "vergift").[69]

Such hidden objects were believed to be capable of causing afflictions even without physical contact. The surviving fragment of the trial of Quashie in 1731 Suriname focused on a paper packet—containing herbs, gum, and a root—that had been found buried in the path.[70] In Martinique, Jean Baptiste confessed in 1766 not only to being part of a network distributing "poisons" around the island but also to making his owner impotent by hiding a special baton—also purchased from an expert health practitioner—in the corner of the sugar mill.[71] In a later case from Suriname, the court tried three enslaved people for poisoning their enslaver through "superstition"—in this case by burying small bags of coals in the plaza of the house for him to walk over.[72] Similarly, in nineteenth-century Virginia several overseers reported enslaved people being afraid to enter plantation yards, as they claimed walking over a conjuror's buried roots could be enough to conjure or poison them.[73]

Ritual ordeals to identify poisoners—or for accused poisoners to try and prove their innocence—were powerful mechanisms for communities to build narratives about alleged poisoning events. Ordeals and the use of spirit power had long had an important judicial role in Atlantic Africa. In one of the early Portuguese accounts of their interactions with Mande speakers, Valentim Fernandes observed in 1500 the use of "some *maleficio*" to identify thieves.[74] Seventeenth- and eighteenth-century European accounts discussed corpse interrogation to identify causes of death and poison ordeals whereby those accused of crimes—such as abusing extraordinary powers for selfish ends (witchcraft), adultery, and murder—could attempt to clear their name. Forms of corpse interrogation were common from the Gold Coast to the Bight of Biafra.[75] According to Bosman, following a death on the Gold Coast, the relatives of the deceased launched an inquiry into the causes: had the deceased perjured or broken an oath? Did the person have any "powerful Enemies, who may have laid *Fetiche's* [sic] in his way"? During this interrogation, the body would move to indicate affirmative answers to questions. "If there be no suspicion of Poyson," the next investigation would be into whether the household was deficient in any way in the performance of offerings and rites, until people were satisfied that the cause of death had been properly identified.[76]

In Atlantic Africa, those accused by such rituals or other forms of divination as the cause of death or the perpetrator of another crime generally had recourse to prove their innocence through a poison ordeal as a form of oath draught: the consumption of a substance believed to cause death if and only if the oath taker lied.[77] This conception of "poison" as conditionally efficacious depending on the morality and truthfulness of the consumer was very different from the way late seventeenth- and eighteenth-century Europeans discussed and thought about poison. According to Bosman's informants on the Gold Coast, "They believe the perjured Person shall be swelled by that Liquor till he bursts; or if that doth not happen, that he shall shortly dye [sic] of a Languishing Sickness."[78] The words Ewe and Twi speakers used for these ordeals made a semantic connection between empowerment objects and the agency of spirits; these poison ordeals and oaths were understood to have the power to strike down liars because they were connected to the spirit world, not because of the physical properties of the substance consumed.[79] Described by Europeans as "red Water," "bitter water," "Oath-Draught," and "edible Fetish," I suspect that the substance West Africans used to conduct these ordeals was bark from *Erythophleum suaveolens*—the same tree whose vomit-inducing properties attracted Francisco Buitrago's attention in Angola.[80] Called the "red water tree," "bois rouge," and "ordeal tree" in West Africa today, *E. suaveolens* has a natural distribution from coastal Senegambia through the tropical forests and wooded savannas of West, West Central, and Central Africa.[81] An oath draught using the bark of *E. suaveolens* was but one of many kinds of ritual ordeals Atlantic Africans used to identify and resolve questions on affliction—ordeals that they and their descendants translated to new contexts in the Americas.

Ritual ordeals in slave societies, usually led by a specialist practitioner but requiring participation from the wider community, were often adapted from these Atlantic African judicial procedures to plantation contexts. The coffin ordeal was common, where a diviner interrogated a corpse to reveal the cause of death and the body then pulled coffin-bearers to the guilty party.[82] Another common practice in the Americas involved the accused willingly taking an oath and consuming a substance to prove their innocence—with a grisly death to follow if they lied.[83] While some judicial practices, like the boiling water ordeal in a 1688 Bahian *feitiçaria* accusation, were remark-

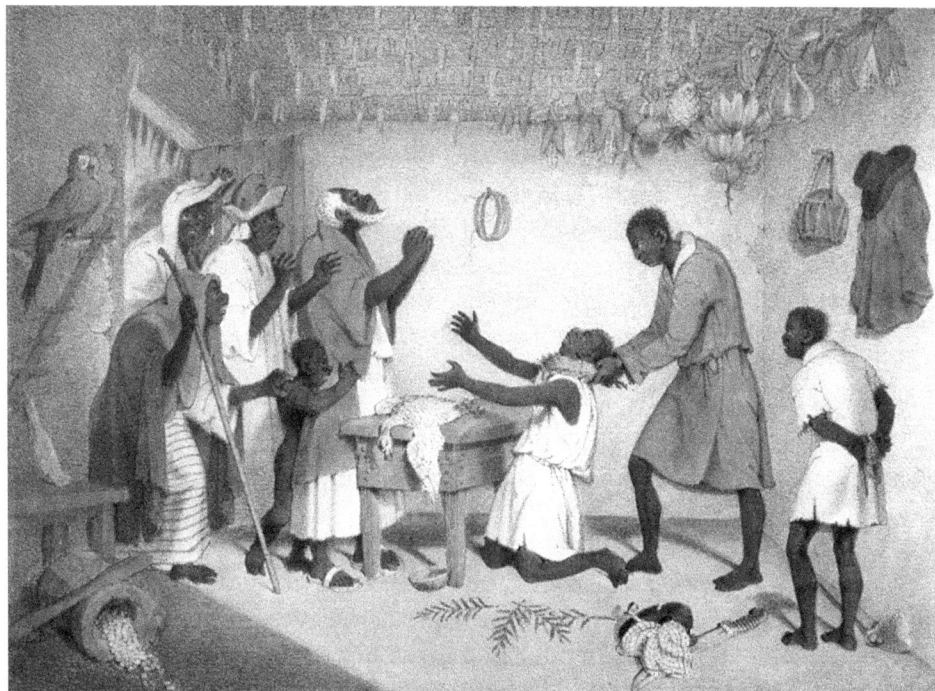

Figure 6. This image from Richard Bridgens's travels to the West Indies in the 1820s and 1830s depicts a ritual ordeal to identify a thief from a set of suspects: lying under oath would allegedly cause the prepared band of herbs to tighten around the neck of the guilty party. Note the engagement and responses of the crowd to the left. Jerome Handler and Kenneth Bilby also discuss this image in detail. "An Obeah Practitioner at Work, Trinidad, 1836," *Slavery Images: A Visual Record of the African Slave Trade and Slave Life in the Early African Diaspora*, accessed August 11, 2023, http://www.slaveryimages.org.

ably similar to contemporaneous practices in Atlantic Africa, their adaptation to the specific contexts of power in the Americas often led to changes.[84] For example, the Saramaca Maroons incorporated torture to extract confession for poison cases—part of Dutch judicial proceedings but absent from known evidence of contemporary Atlantic African proceedings. Similarly, early nineteenth-century poison and *obeah* investigations run by enslaved communities in Berbice included extreme forms of violence as part of ordeals to identify culprits that were more a part of the plantation world than African antecedents.[85]

The 1775 case of Quacoe in Suriname, as described in a letter to the Suriname court from the overseer H. C. Dorfeld, illustrates well the active participation of the crowd at multiple stages of an investigation. Following the death of an enslaved woman, who had suffered great pains in her belly and wasted away over several weeks, the enslaved community as a group went to Dorfeld to accuse Quacoe of poisoning her and request that he be put in irons. In addition to being the head carpenter, the text of Dorfeld's letter suggests that Quacoe was a health practitioner; the enslaved community believed that Quacoe had had the power to cure Quamina but had refused to do so. At Quamina's funeral, held in the living quarters of the enslaved, the gathered crowd conducted a coffin ordeal that involved running past the cabins led by Quamina's coffin, which they then vehemently flung at Quacoe's door. The crowd then searched Quacoe's living space for "Wisschy" (*wissi*) but found nothing. They then washed Quamina's dead body and gave the water to Quacoe to drink as another ordeal: if guilty, he would die. Dorfeld noted to the court that he did not interfere, as Quacoe willingly drank the water to try and prove his innocence. However, this was not the end of the case. Some time later, still convinced that Quacoe was responsible for Quamina's death, four men went to Quacoe's cabin and began beating him; several young women with sticks joined in. There is some dispute between the account of Quacoe, who said that the men dragged him from his hut and began beating him, and that of the other men, who claimed instead that Quacoe had come out on his own and that a shouting confrontation had escalated into a brawl. In any event, Dorfeld was alerted to the incident when Quacoe stumbled into the main house, "half dead" and covered with blood, and fainted on the floor.[86] At every step of this investigation—going in a group to the overseer, the coffin and oath-drinking ordeals, the public beating—enslaved men and women from Quacoe's plantation were not only active participants but driving forces enacting what they saw as justice against a perceived poisoner. Their narrative of his alleged guilt was strong enough to incorporate multiple forms of finding and defining proof.

The courthouse was a key site of narrative building about poison. In each trial colonial governments—often made up of the enslavers in these slave societies—claimed and asserted narrative control over alleged poisoning events, defining the terms of procedure, determining the outcomes, and choosing how and what information to record. The imbalance of power between enslavers and the enslaved in producing court records was dramatic and should not be forgotten. However, close reading of the cases themselves reveals a range of ways in which enslaved people participated in the narrative construction of cases, including evidence that enslaved people sometimes brought their own investigation results to slaveholders, knowing that they would provoke a trial.

It would be misleading to imply that enslaved people initiated most or even a majority of poison cases. There were many cases where enslaved people on plantations were anything but instigators or willing participants in poison investigations. For example, in a well-known Suriname case, a white overseer named Benjamin Pousset at the Sinabo sugar plantation was tried for accusing and personally whipping, torturing, and beheading an enslaved woman he believed to be a poisoner over the objections and pleas of the Sinabo enslaved community who were forced to watch. A similar incident occurred on Pierre Dessalles's plantation in Martinique in 1824 and 1825, when he reduced rations, set curfews, separated men and women, increased beatings, and instituted random jailing until the community produced a culprit responsible for the series of deaths among livestock.[87] However, as Natalie Zemon Davis has argued concerning Suriname, internal systems of justice within enslaved communities coexisted with the plantation rule of enslavers and the criminal justice of the colonial government.[88] Ritual ordeals and court trials alike were fundamentally about contested narratives.

Enslaved witnesses had an important role in poison trials beyond the subset of cases that explicitly originated within enslaved communities; their testimony helped construct narratives in individual court cases. In my dataset, courts recorded specifically named enslaved individuals as witnesses directly testifying in court in thirty-two cases.[89] This number does not include numerous cases where defendants were forced to act as witnesses by naming alleged accomplices and testifying against them. I treat these cases as distinct from those where none of the witnesses were on trial, and they could produce large "chains" of cases similar to those seen in the early modern European witch hunts.[90] In Martinique and Suriname, the enormous pressure on defendants to confess and name names was amplified by the legal use of torture. Even in cases where the witnesses were not on trial themselves, it is also often unclear the degree of coercion involved in requiring enslaved people to testify against each other. When the Suriname court examined Hendrick, Coffie, Quassie, and Alida about the activities of Francies, a man from the same plantation, all but Hendrick denied having any information; their testimony suggests that they were suspected of having information and had been brought before the court, not that they volunteered.[91] However, initial denunciations made by enslaved people to the Inquisitorial commissioner in Bahia were by their nature supposed to be voluntary and secret. Vicente Francisco de Britto, an enslaved man owned by a Capitão Mor in São Gonçalo parish, not only voluntarily went to the Inquisition to denounce the freed healer Simão but likely did so against the wishes of his enslaver.[92] What the records I have do suggest is that the testimony of the enslaved against each other could carry significant weight in court; in most of these cases, they were the only witnesses, and their testimony was often the only evidence against the accused.

The information that can be gleaned from witness testimony depended significantly on the legal structure and record-keeping of the court in question. Slave codes in Virginia, Martinique, and Suriname allowed enslaved people to act as witnesses only in trials of other enslaved people. For the Lisbon Inquisition, the commissioner in Bahia could discreetly interview anyone—free or enslaved—likely to have information regarding the case, though the testimony of enslaved people was sometimes instead filtered through an interview with the enslaver. Such was the case in the interview of Josefa Maria da Incarnação, who told the commissioner what people in her household had been saying about the activities of practitioners of African descent in the neighborhood.[93] Bahia was also unusual in that free people of color also frequently made denunciations or were interviewed for testimony by commissioners in their investigations. In Suriname, the court usually examined witnesses separately but sometimes brought them in during the examination of the defendant for a dramatic direct confrontation: such was the case of Quassie, brought in during the examination of Samsam to claim that Samsam carried *vergift* in a horn—a charge that Samsam insisted was false.[94] The Suriname records frequently included vivid detail from witness testimony, such as Dosoe's description of the discovery of a jaw bone allegedly planted by Coffiee under the cabin of a man to make him ill, or the recollection of Fortuijn, Coridon, Cupido, and Willem of how Isaac had collapsed while digging a ditch and how together they carried him back to his cabin.[95] While both the Virginia and Martinique courts examined enslaved witnesses, the summaries of these cases that have survived rarely recorded any detailed information on the names, backgrounds, or often even the legal status of the witnesses. In one of the more detailed Virginia summaries, the record only states that a man named "Africa"—so named for an African birth?—testified against Boatswain, an enslaved healer on another plantation, in 1764 for "Preparing and administering Poisonous medicines," testimony that contributed to a conviction.[96]

Evidence from the early nineteenth century suggests a shift in the ways enslaved people made use of both colonial courts and the law of slaveholders on their plantations, focusing instead on building narratives of poisoning events through internal investigations only. While communities of the enslaved had specifically brought several cases to enslavers during the mid-eighteenth-century peaks of trials, likely influencing many more as slaveholders sought general opinion from the enslaved to identify suspected poisoners, by the nineteenth century they increasingly conducted divinations, ordeals, and punishments of suspected poisoners in secret. It is important not to overstate this shift and to recognize that we may never know the scope of actions taken secretly by the enslaved precisely because of their secret nature. The rituals to identify poisoners that many enslavers had sanctioned and participated in began to shift at the same time that the number of poison cases tried by the courts declined; court officials also increasingly classified efforts to root out suspected poisoners through magical means as dangerous "superstitions" to be stamped out. While someone like Maskree in 1744 had the full support of the overseer Versteegh and the enslaved community at Plantagie Jagtlust, by the early nineteenth century, practitioners like him were at just as high a risk of being arrested for conducting an ordeal to find a "poisoner" as they were for "poisoning." It was during this same period that—with the Martinique Cour Prévôtale as an important exception—poison trials overall declined, and in courts including the Cour Prévôtale, the proportion of healers among the accused also declined.[97]

Evidence suggests that some enslaved people seeking to conduct poison investigations in the early nineteenth century actively—and prudently—tried to avoid the involvement of their enslavers. The handful of cases related to poisoning investigated by the Office of the Fiscal of Berbice in the 1810s and 1820s focused on actions taken to identify sources of illnesses, not on those who allegedly caused illnesses themselves. For example, in two cases of health practitioners, Hans (1819) and Willem (1823), enslaved people on the respective plantations hired them to identify individuals believed to be responsible for causing illnesses and deaths with poison.[98] In both cases, the primary concerns of the court were not the alleged poisonings but the fact that the enslaved drivers within each community had secretly organized illegal divination rituals that resulted in injuries and, in the case of Willem, the beating and death of the suspected culprit.[99] A British colony from 1815, Berbice was subject to the series of anti-*obeah* legislation of the British Caribbean; "poison" became less significant than the practice of *obeah*, which included attempts to identify poisoners.[100] In Jamaican *obeah*, the 1820s was a pivotal decade, during which the *obeah* practitioners who were prosecuted were no longer tried for allegedly causing harm but for conducting healing rituals, which may have included efforts to divine and identify poisoners as threats to community health.[101] The Berbice cases appear to have been part of a similar crackdown.

Data from Suriname cases, which had the most detailed trial records—and correspondingly the most cases that clearly identified accusations originating within enslaved communities—suggest that enslaved people sought to involve enslavers or courts less frequently in their investigations of poisoners after the 1770s. While the total number of poison cases did drop significantly in the 1780s and 1790s, cases with enslaved instigators fell disproportionately, with only two such cases in these decades.[102] The high proportion of cases instigated within enslaved communities in the earliest poison trials makes sense in the context of enslaved Africans contributing major foundations to ideas of what made a "poisoner" in the Americas. Likewise, as trials took on a life of their own and slaveholders began to see poisoning everywhere, it is not surprising that the total number of cases dwarfed those identified as beginning with investigations by the enslaved. The difference between the eighteenth-century case summaries from the Conseil Supérieur and the detailed cases in the Cour Prévôtale suggest a similar pattern. The former, while short on details in many of the cases, identified at least one as having specifically originated in accusations by the enslaved, while in the thirty highly detailed cases of the latter, not a single case described such an initial investigation.[103]

Trials and the narratives they generated could take on a life of their own, and the infrastructure created specifically to investigate and punish alleged poisoners could create a narrative engine that fed on itself. A close analysis of the creation and development of Martinique's special tribunals culminating with the Cour Prévôtale highlights this process. Deeming a 1724 edict from the crown on poison insufficient to handle the particular circumstances of poisoning in the colony, two years after its passage the Conseil Supérieur of Martinique proposed the creation of special itinerant courts specifically to try poison cases directly on the plantations where accusations were made. The goal of such a court was swift trials and executions, with no opportunity for appeal, and its existence would have symbolically shifted the site of judicial power from the urban tribunals to the plantations themselves. With no official response, the proposal died; however, its central ideas would feed into the creation of special rules and tribunals for poison cases in the future.[104]

Even with the mandated autopsies from 1749 onward, trials in Martinique did not meet legal expectations for sufficient proof; the solution of the legislature was to repeatedly bypass their own rules of evidence that they claimed made poison cases too difficult to prosecute. They first did so in 1753 with the creation of an extraordinary commission specifically to try poison cases. Unlike the ordinary tribunal courts in Saint-Pierre and Trinité, where free and enslaved people were tried and then sent on an automatic appeal for felony crimes to the Conseil Supérieur in Fort Royal, these special poison tribunals were mobile, meeting on the plantations where the accusations originated; they had a lower standard of proof for conviction (automatic appeals still went to the council in Fort Royal and were recorded as summaries).[105] The number of cases per year leapt forward after 1753, peaking with ten cases in 1755 alone.[106] In addition to enabling the 1750s peak, the establishment of special rules for poison cases set an important legal precedent that allowed for further waves of cases in the early nineteenth century.

The next special tribunal of 1803 to 1809, established by Captain-General Louis Thomas Villaret de Joyeuse, operated in the context of the Napoleonic wars in the years between the first and second British occupations of the island and in the immediate aftermath of the Haitian Revolution. Villaret directed his attention to the alleged poisoning deaths of enslaved people and livestock as an urgent crisis to be dealt with—along with acts of arson and runaways stealing canoes to escape to British islands. Building on the 1753 precedent, he established an itinerant tribunal, made up of both government officials and local notable slaveholders, to swiftly try these three kinds of cases. Executions, usually burning at the stake for poisoning, were held on site immediately following the trial, with no opportunity for appeal.[107] Within two years Villaret reported success in that the "blight of poisonings," both "terrible and too familiar to Martinique's plantations," was being diminished thanks to the special tribunal.[108] The tribunal itself had become a key part of the narrative about alleged poisoning as a necessary form of protection from "blight" through extreme violence.

Villaret's tribunal obtained results, with many poison trials and executions. An exact recording of the numbers involved has not survived, but the contemporary journal of colonial prefect Pierre-Clément de Laussat contained about a dozen detailed anecdotes of cases from this tribunal involving alleged conspiracies with networks of healers.[109] The frequency and severity of the trials did not stop the alleged epidemic of poisoning, and trials continued right up to start of the second British occupation in

February 1809.[110] Nor did the occupation stop poison prosecutions; the new British governor continued the tribunals and the prominent role of local enslavers in their prosecution.[111] Investigating and punishing alleged poisoners—and the construction of narratives around poisoning events that these trials engendered, particularly with the heightened concern about alleged conspiracy—was so important to enslavers in the colony that it continued through the context of war and foreign occupation. With the war over, preparation for a new special court began only a few years after the return of Martinique to French hands.

The Cour Prévôtale, a special tribunal operating from 1822 to 1827 exclusively for trying free and enslaved people of African descent for poisoning, was a machine that both perpetuated the narratives about poisoning crisis from past tribunals and established new tropes on the "common knowledge" of who was a poisoner. Repeating the idea that too many suspected poisoners could escape justice in the ordinary courts and explicitly drawing from the legal precedent of Villaret's tribunal, Governor Donzelot called for the implementation of extraordinary measures "to satisfy justice" and "produce a beneficial terror."[112] Relaxing the rules of evidence resulted in a staggering number of defendants and convictions: across thirty cases—most operating as omnibus trials covering multiple defendants from a single area—the court tried 368 people for poisoning, resulting in 289 convictions and 104 executions.[113] The proportion of health practitioners among the accused had sharply declined, amounting to only 7 percent, and there was only a single case involving no target.[114] Instead, a significant proportion of the accused were identified as the most loyal or favored among the enslaved, with a connotation for enslavers of betrayal; this connection was presented as common knowledge in Donzelot's report on the foundation of the tribunal.[115] References to *maléfice* decreased, appearing in only three trials, while together mineral poisons appeared in 40 percent of the cases: arsenic in particular was enough of a concern for Donzelot to issue new restrictions on its legal sale.[116] Patterns of cases where the accused were more likely to be female, used mineral poisons, and were connected to positions of the greatest proximity to enslavers—especially enslaved domestics—replaced that of the predominantly male African-descended health practitioner.

Enslavers wielded the narrative of the "most trusted slave" as a sharp critique of the antislavery movement and calls for amelioration. A year into the Cour Prévôtale, Governor Donzelot wrote to the metropole to justify the court's existence. Donzelot asserted that it was "almost always the richest blacks, the best treated by their owners, the domestics enjoying all their confidence" who were the leaders of poisoning plots.[117] Donzelot went on to make a connection between the "gentleness" of the treatment of the enslaved in Martinique compared to the British islands—which he claimed did not have a poisoning problem—and further blamed liberal philanthropists for inflaming enslaved communities with their antislavery discourse.[118] The idea continued to persist in slaveholders' letters defending and calling for the reinstatement of the court after its suppression. One letter from 1827 argued that poison was not the "fruit" of "barbarous treatment" by enslavers, as "each time" the culprits were the best-treated enslaved people—the "favorites."[119]

The Cour Prévôtale did not dissolve or fade away slowly. Instead, planters' use of the tribunal for a deliberate campaign of terror against what they described as an epidemic of poison ended in late 1826 with a suppression order from the metropole.[120] Baron Delamardelle had been sent to report on the Cour Prévôtale in 1823. Although he conceded that "poisonings" were a serious problem and that convictions were difficult to obtain under normal proceedings, his conclusions were highly unfavorable on points of legality. This court had swift and closed proceedings, with no lawyer for the accused. Furthermore, it was organized on the basis of color rather than status and was therefore in Delamardelle's assessment fundamentally against the modern French judicial system.[121] The suppression was met with protest: from the governor, who reluctantly disbanded the tribunal while predicting that poisonings would soon be back on the rise, to A. Rivière, a planter and former prosecutor on the Cour Prévôtale, who, within six months of the suppression, argued that the ravages of poison, "the scourge most strongly opposed to prosperity," was worse than ever and now included his own plantation.[122]

The collapse of the Cour Prévôtale was in many ways the result of a clash of narratives about poison, this time between colonial enslavers and metropolitan observers. People like Donzelot and Rivière held tightly to the narrative of poison as the gravest threat faced by the colony, a story of poison that had been reinforced over and over by the precedent of extraordinary tribunals and the violence they meted out against alleged poisoners. Delamardelle did not reject the idea that poisoning by free and enslaved people of African descent was a serious problem; instead, his narrative prioritized the concerns and judicial norms of the metropole over what he saw as dangerous innovations by colonists. Poison trials in the colony had become self-perpetuating, even as the content of the so-called "common knowledge" that enslavers constructed around poison had changed from the eighteenth to the nineteenth century. The story of the court shows how narratives through the infrastructure of institutions could take on lives of their own.

* * *

Narratives about poison were flexible; the specific forms of accusations and ideas about "poisoners" could change while remaining embedded within the core idea of poison as either the weapon of the weak or the abuse of power by the strong. People built narratives around what they saw to conform to what they expected to see, to their preconceived notions of the world; these narratives in turn gradually altered those preconceptions.[123] The problem of focusing on one narrative of poisoning in any specific case or across the wider phenomenon of poisoning cases is not that it is necessarily wrong but rather incomplete.

The efforts of enslavers to assert narrative control over poisoning cases—through trials, through the circulation of news, through tropes and flexible claims on the methods of so-called poisoners—highlight the enormous power they wielded in slave societies; however, they also reveal the fragility of that control. In a fundamental way these efforts all failed, even when they resulted in public awareness through printed circulation, the gruesome executions of alleged poisoners, and the terrorizing of enslaved communities. The actions that enslavers took to ease their minds were self-defeating: trials heightened unease and increased the likelihood of more trials in a region, and both the use of hired African-descended practitioners to perform rituals and the snowballing repetition of tropes on alleged methods emphasized the idea that these practitioners had access to terrifying powers beyond enslavers' control.[124]

As for the 1800 case at Monticello, the flight of Sam to parts unknown left the case unresolved. Thomas Jefferson, Martha Jefferson Randolph, and Thomas Mann Randolph discussed their theories, making the events that resulted in the deaths of Jupiter, Ursula, and the Georges comprehensible to themselves; then they moved on. While Sam and his alleged targets gradually disappeared from their correspondence, the poisoning event briefly revealed both a tear in the enslavers' sense of control over the healing work of enslaved people and the careful effort they undertook to try to stitch it back together again.

"The Taken-for-Granted Must Cease to Be So"

In 1846 and 1847, the final years of slavery in Martinique, enslaver Joseph Havre stood trial for imprisoning three people—the driver Jean Baptiste, the hospital head Angèle, and the chief refiner Elie—in an attic for three years on suspicion of "poisoning." Havre was not the first slaveholder tried for abusing and torturing alleged poisoners.[1] However, the wider context of Havre's trial in the years just preceding emancipation in 1848 was unique. By the time the royal prosecutor found out about Havre's actions, by means of an anonymous tip, Elie had died of dysentery and Jean Baptiste and Angèle could no longer walk. This case was also unusual for the quantity of detail that was recorded and survived. Tucked away in a folder in a box in the Archives Nationales d'Outre-Mer are sixteen letters circulating between the Procureur Général, two governors, and two Ministères de la Marine back in Paris. Most remarkably, in one of these letters the prosecutor attached clippings from multiple issues of the *Courrier de la Martinique* newspaper reporting on the dramatic trial, including transcripts of speeches from the witness stand, crowd reactions, and the prosecutor's own penciled marginalia.[2] The prosecution's case rested on the legal limits of slaveholders' authority to imprison enslaved people, as well as the lack of concrete proof that any "poisoning" as they understood it had actually occurred. The defense's case, which was ultimately successful with a jury of slaveholders, was that Havre did what was necessary to counter the very real and dangerous threat of poisoning on his plantation. During the sensational trial, at least twenty-three enslaved people testified as witnesses: though called in as witnesses for the defense, their testimony different significantly in the details and emphasis they placed on aspects of the case.

According to Havre's testimony at his trial in Saint-Pierre, from 1840 to 1842, eighteen enslaved people and numerous mules and horses had died on the plantation. The whole plantation said that the deaths were caused by "poison," confirmed for Havre by the autopsy of a woman who had a suspiciously quick death, and—according to Havre—all pointed to Jean Baptiste as the poisoner. Once arrested and interrogated by Havre—through unspecified means—Jean Baptiste allegedly claimed that he, Angèle, and Elie had been poisoners together. Havre's suspicions of Angèle were apparently confirmed the next day when some water she gave to him tasted strange as he feared she had put something into it. The defense pointed to the fact that the "epidemic" of illnesses had stopped "as if by enchantment" after Havre's actions as justification for them.[3] Several white witnesses from Grand-Anse, including the Abbé Jacquier, testified that everyone in the neighborhood knew about the poisonings at Havre's plantation and the extreme measures he took to stop them. The mayor of Grand-Anse gave a vigorous defense of Havre's actions, rebuffing the prosecutors' push for scientific proof of poison by claiming that poisons are very difficult to detect and citing cases from the 1820s Cour Prévôtale. Havre's uncle continued this line of reasoning by arguing that since the government would not act without proof that was impossible to obtain, slaveholders had to take the law into their own hands.

Havre's arguments intertwined with long-simmering tensions over who had the authority in colonial slave societies to define and deal with alleged poisoning events. The Havre case came twenty years after the efforts of slaveholders to claim control through a "beneficial terror" by means of the Cour Prévôtale no longer aligned with the interests of the metropole, resulting in the court's suppression.[4] Enslavers like Pierre Dessalles frequently expressed their frustration that people in the metropole and officials sent from there did not understand the danger enslavers faced from poisoners.[5] In a series of letters fervently attempting to persuade the newly appointed governor to reinstate the Cour Prévôtale, former prosecutor A. Rivière insisted that poisonings had to be judged differently in Martinique than in France as slaveholders in Martinique faced "an organized system of destruction." Rivière concluded this 1827 letter with a warning that public opinion was resoundingly negative toward the metropole, as enslavers had come to believe that it did not understand Martinique and its needs.[6] While Rivière's efforts were unsuccessful, his letters exuded the frustration shared by Dessalles and others with the metropole's check on their ability to haul alleged poisoners to court. Similar opinions quickly surfaced among the slaveholders who testified as defense witnesses and were affirmed by an acquittal given by a jury of the same: Rivière himself contributed a written deposition in support of Havre.[7]

Havre's defense drew directly on key concepts and tropes about poison that had roots in European thought and had been circulating and mutating among enslavers in the Americas for centuries. His lawyer's final statement framed Jean Baptiste's alleged actions as a "usurpation" of power motivated by emotional fury at Havre ending his "despotic rule over the other slaves." He argued that "in our colonies, the black man . . . proceeds by means proper to his weakness; he proceeds above all by poisoning."[8] In this rendering, enslaved people of African descent turned to poison as "weapons of the weak" and a tool of usurpation to overthrow the natural order of things. It was "common knowledge" among enslavers in Martinique and elsewhere that enslaved people were natural "poisoners" who used such weapons to enact vengeance on their enslavers—and that this "poisoning" was the assumed cause of any deaths of livestock or other enslaved people on a plantation.

By casting doubt both on the supposed efficacy of the "poisons" of enslaved people and on the legitimacy of enslavers' unfettered power on their plantations, the prosecution's arguments were part of an increased European skepticism of the ideas of both slaveholders and people of African descent.[9] A doctor in Martinique for eight years, Étienne Rufz de Lavison researched and published in 1844 a thorough critique and debunking of Martinican slaveholders' claims on poisoning. To conduct his work, he collected anecdotes from enslavers and published theories and tested them with a series of experiments on animals. He indignantly shared an anecdote he had observed in the assizes courts of a local doctor called to testify in an 1842 poisoning case. When a magistrate asked him if enslaved people possessed any substances capable of producing pulmonary tuberculosis, the doctor replied, "As a doctor, I know of no substance which has this property; as a creole, I believe the blacks so wicked, that they are capable of anything!"[10] For Rufz de Lavison, this doctor's self-identification as a creole—in this context a person of European descent born in the Americas—rendered his judgment on the capabilities of alleged poisoners suspect. While mainly chastising Martinican enslavers, Rufz de Lavison also employed the same paternalistic language on the "superstitions" of the enslaved and a palpable contempt for their healing knowledge. Countering the argument that practitioners of African descent had knowledge of plants unknown to Europeans, he claimed with confidence that "there is not a sprig of herb in our fields, in our forests, which is not only known, but classified, drawn, studied, [and] ordered."[11] Even as he critiqued enslavers and their investigations of poisoning, Rufz de Lavison was also drawing on transformations in European medical discourse that

disdained the work of all healers who were not licensed physicians as ineffective and unscientific.

Looking past the core arguments between the prosecution and defense,
a close read of this case also highlights complex contestations and convergences in the narratives about "poisoning" from the perspective of the approximately two dozen enslaved people who spoke before the court. They
were witnesses for the defense who had been called on specifically to support Havre's case that his actions against Jean Baptiste, Angèle, and Elie were
justified. For example, Dogué the carpenter told the court that Jean Baptiste
prepared "poison" that he gave Angèle to put into the herbal teas consumed
by the sick in the plantation hospital. However, most of the testimony repeatedly contradicted Havre's assertion that the three individuals had been
"poisoners" intent on causing harm. While Alexis, the man in charge of the
plantation's livestock, acknowledged that "people said" that several cows had
been poisoned, he claimed that he never heard anyone in the quarters point to
Jean Baptiste and Angèle specifically as the poisoners. More sensational—
marked in the newspaper transcript as causing an audible reaction from the
crowd—was Césaire the cook's claim that Elie had discussions with a man
from another plantation on how to put something in Havre's food so "he
would have become good to everyone." Césaire described a possible taming
practice, interpreted by Havre as giving him "packets for sorcery" as "poison."[12]
Through their testimony, these witnesses painted a complex portrait of the
work of healing practitioners that neither Havre nor the wider court understood as anything but a threat to Havre's control over the plantation and by
proxy the order of the slave society.

Jean Baptiste and Angèle gave their own interpretation of the events of the
past several years as the trial that was ostensibly about Havre quickly became
one of their alleged poisonings as well. They each spoke in excruciating detail
about the violence and humiliations of their years of confinement in the attic,
including the conditions of Elie's death by dysentery and a time when Havre
met their request for more water by forcing a man named Alphonse to uri-
nate in a vase for them. Both vehemently denied being "poisoners" and offered their own interpretations on why they had been accused. Jean Baptiste
based his statement on the difficulties of his position as a driver, claiming
that Havre did not like him because he did not beat people hard enough and
that other enslaved people resented him because of his position. He also
noted that he had been saving money for years with a dream of purchasing
his manumission and had been in the process of negotiating with Havre on

the subject when Havre arrested him. In contrast, Angèle specifically blamed Jean Baptiste for her imprisonment. While Jean Baptiste insisted that he had never accused anyone of poisoning, Angèle called him a liar from the stand and continuously claimed that Jean Baptiste had accused her. Both insisted that there was no "poison" on the plantation—that the deaths in the enslaved community had been the result of natural illness rather than any deliberate attack.[13]

The result of this explosive case—Havre's acquittal—was not surprising. After the acquittal, the prosecutor complained that this outcome exposed problems with the "creole character" and that men of "weak spirit" who believe in "poison" in the face of evidence because "all the world around [them] professes this belief" would continue to acquit their peers.[14] Despite this conclusion of the case, there were several consequences for Havre. At the prosecutor's advice, the governor concluded that it would not be safe for Jean Baptiste and Angèle to return to Havre, forcing him to sell them to a temporary guardian. They were soon freed, and the prosecutor also made a point in February 1848—only a few months before the abolition of slavery in the French empire in the context of the 1848 Revolution—to inform the new governor of "this important case."[15] While the Havre case is captivating in its own right, for the purposes of this book it particularly highlights the multiple and contested ideas about poison and how they were articulated and rendered through moments of alleged poisoning events. Through the tangled web of accusations and counteraccusations, everyone involved in the case made interpretive claims that drew on a range of ideas about poison.

"Poison" is as much an idea as it is an action, one that is neither timeless nor universal. Ideas about poison and relationships between poison, healing, and power mutated over time, and contemporary actors in poisoning events had different interpretations of what they saw and experienced in the same historical moment. This book has explored poisoning cases from the perspectives of African and African-descended healing practitioners, enslaved communities, and enslavers, tracking durable ways of discussing poison along with trials as sites of both the evolution of these ideas and the consequences thereof. The implications of this investigation go beyond a greater understanding of the phenomenon of poison cases. The contested ideas about health and power revealed through poison trials show how the ideas of Africans in the Atlantic world had an impact that transcended imperial boundaries, shaping convergences across locales. Bahia, Martinique, Virginia, and the Dutch Guianas were very different places, yet they each had a connection to Atlantic African moral philosophies through the engine of the transatlantic slave trade. Europeans understood what they saw from the earliest cases through their own idioms of "poison" and shaped a new engine of poison trials accordingly. These cases became self-perpetuating, but in dialogue with the actions and ideas of both enslavers and the enslaved. Even in the extreme disparity of power in these slave societies, the concerns, hopes, fears, and dreams of Africans and their descendants—and the actions they took to improve their lives—had an enormous impact on the relationships, lives, and laws of people in these locales. We cannot hope to understand the Atlantic world without understanding the role of Africans in shaping it.

People from Western Europe and Atlantic Africa had developed different idioms and ways of understanding the relationships between poison, healing, and power. They carried these ideas with them and adapted them to new circumstances in the slave societies of the Americas. At the same time, they continued to transform their own ideas. Europeans in the early modern period had developed a discourse of poison as a "weapon of the weak," a tool used to usurp power from the powerful. It was a gendered crime linked to women or "womanly" men. In contrast, people in Atlantic Africa in the early modern period built their discourse of poison around the idea of it being an abuse of power committed by the strong. Healers and rulers—and rulers *as* public healers—could be dangerous, "poisonous," threats precisely *because* they were powerful. Understanding the circulation and interaction of ideas in the Atlantic basin is necessary for understanding poison cases in the Americas.

Durable key concepts rooted in Atlantic Africa and Western Europe shaped the development of poison trials in the slave societies of the Americas; their forms and expression mutated as narrative logics of poisoning cases took on lives of their own. While the social context and violence of life under slavery was distinct, these extremes heightened many of the core issues of African moral philosophy on the intentions and uses of power. The specifics of the fraught position of enslaved drivers, for example, and other relationship conflicts may have been embedded in the context of slavery, but they were also specific instances for wider community discussion on the morality of power. Instead of seeing social conflict as the "real" issue and accusations of "poison" as merely a front, this book has taken seriously the concept that negative emotions and antisocial abuses of power *were* "poison" and tracked how this idea played out for diasporic Africans. The core work of healing practitioners of African descent—of tying and binding—incorporated these community concerns as well as the networking and physical work of creating empowered objects. The power held by extraordinary practitioners—the power whose use or abuse so concerned wider communities of African descent—came from composition and communication with sources of knowledge across communities of the living and the dead. European core concepts also had a key role, as it was enslavers and colonial officials of European descent who shaped the infrastructure for the laws, investigations, and trials. They transferred their gendered associations with poison to newly racialized ones. While slaveholders often relied on healers of African descent, their uneasy discourse centered on how to control these practitioners as perpetually "illegitimate" wielders of power. The idea of taming evoked special horror less because of fear of physical harm and more as it represented the ultimate inversion of what they saw as the natural order of things.

The social history of ideas in this book was made possible through embracing comparative historical linguistics as a key method used by historians of early Africa; combining this method with close social historical analysis offers avenues forward in the study of the intellectual and cultural history of the African Atlantic. As Kathryn de Luna explains in her recent introduction of the method to Atlanticists, "Words are as much historical sources as political treatises or court testimony because language is a product of the history of its speakers and words bear the content of that contested history."[16] In exploring ancient and widespread roots about empowerment, tying/untying, and health, many of the paths I walked on are well trodden by scholars of Africa. However, investigating the specific nuances and changes over time in words like *-gàng- has opened up new avenues of analysis in the fraught colonial archive from the slave societies of the Americas. Problematic as they are, trial records can contain fragments of African idioms, sometimes expressed in African words but more often in European vernacular. Close attention to the *way* that people of African descent spoke about affliction, relationships, and power—even when using European words—and reading them alongside the word histories from Atlantic Africa allows for a clearer understanding of how and why people understood, suspected, or used "poison." It is my hope that this book will serve in part as a proof of concept for other Atlanticists interested in the possibilities of comparative historical linguistics to adopt this method for creating deep-scale histories of ideas. The variety of potential subjects is limited only by the creativity of human language. If this method can yield insights on how diasporic Africans thought about poisoning events, what other aspects of their lives and experiences could it help Atlanticists understand?

The idea that "poison" meant different things to different people at different times—that the "taken-for-granted must cease to be so"—is not merely a curious detail from the past.[17] The differences in how people in the Atlantic world saw and interpreted "poison" and its relationship to health and power were matters of life and death. Poison was connected to central concerns of life: to securing well-being in this world for oneself and one's relatives; to concerns about the morality and use of power; to the complex and fraught relationships that bound people together. These "poisoned relations" shaped the lives of thousands.

APPENDIX A

An Introduction to Comparative Historical Linguistics

Comparative historical linguistics—a method that has been used by Africanists for decades—requires further explanation to understand how it works and what kinds of insights it can (and cannot) offer. The basic idea of the method is that languages are archives.[1] Words have histories, as human speakers of languages have created new words and changed the meanings of existing words over time. By paying close attention to the diachronic phonology of words—how the shape and structure of sounds within words have changed over time—and to the distribution of meanings across related languages, historians who use this method can reconstruct histories of word roots. While the method makes frequent use of dictionaries and ethnographies created in the nineteenth and twentieth centuries—both for attestations of words and for descriptive content that can expand on what speakers meant when making these attestations—historical linguistics is *not* simply the imposition of modern meanings of words onto the past.[2] The end goal of such word reconstruction is roughly comparable to that of a word history created through a text-based philological analysis—though the results, by the indirect nature of their reconstruction, are inherently more provisional.[3]

A drawback of using language as a source—that it cannot provide information on the lived experiences of individuals—is also a source of strength. The archive of words in a language is a much broader source of information than a body of documents only produced by a small segment of the elite in a society.[4] Historians cannot know the conversations of individual speakers of a protolanguage in the way that they could by examining personal letters or recorded testimony, but they can track changes in words over time that reflect hegemonic ways of speaking.[5] It is very difficult for an individual to create a new word and have it last in a spoken language without other individuals finding it useful and using it. Any subject discussed by speakers of human languages has the potential to be analyzed using this method. By building archives of reconstructed words, historians have been able to track interactions between groups over time and explore what people talked about. While the early works of historians using historical linguistics—pioneered by Jan Vansina and Christopher Ehret in the 1960s—focused on population movements, technologies, and political organization, in the past twenty years historians have taken the field in new directions by applying this method to metaphysical questions. New works focused, for example, on ideas about motherhood and fame relating to skilled hunters show the possibilities of using historical linguistics to track abstract ideas.[6] The word histories reconstructed through comparative historical linguistics help build social histories of ideas.

Creating an "archive" of words through comparative historical linguistics has four major steps: building a classification of related languages; determining each language's regular sound change rules; building a lexicon of words connected to roots of interest; and constructing the histories of roots based on differences in the vocabulary web.[7] Languages have "genetic" relationships to each other that can be mapped in a classification tree. A key principle is that, over an extended period, as speakers of a shared language come into less and less frequent contact with each other, languages diverge into two (or more) daughter languages that share grammatical cores, with the "mother" (or proto-) language ultimately ceasing to exist.[8] One can therefore derive root forms in protolanguages by looking at shared roots in branches of the language family tree. Linguists use several methods to determine whether and how two languages are related, including lexicostatistics (calculating the shared percentage of cognates from core vocabulary lists), the comparative method (examining possible cognates through regular sound correspondence rules), and a new phylogenetic classification method developed in the last decade that uses computer modeling. Historians using historical linguistics often combine lexicostatistics—which is the fastest method but has flaws—with analyses of grammar and common innovations in the comparative method.[9]

Diachronic phonology—the study of change over time in sound patterns in a language—helps linguists track chronological depth due to patterns in how speakers of a language change the sounds they use. Regular sound correspondence follows the principle that within each language these sound changes follow consistent rules across that language. For example, the proto-Bantu root *bantu (meaning "people") became over time the Swahili word watu and the Gikuyu word andū—"b" softened to "w" in one branch of the "family tree" while disappearing entirely in another. The root is the same.[10]

As my source base for this project was dictionaries—many of which did not use diacritic marks to indicate tone—rather than attestations collected in fieldwork, I was not able to reconstruct tone. I have therefore used early forms and tone symbols of each root when referring to the root in its descendant iterations, even though changes in tones may have occurred.[11] As for the consonants, I used the dictionaries to create spirantization and diachronic phonology charts to track regular sound changes. Many of the consonants in the roots I chose to investigate were quite stable, especially *k (with k > k across all the Njila languages I investigated). Another fairly stable consonant in the Njila family is *b, though b > Ø occurs in several of the Kwanza languages. A common phonological change across the Njila languages was d > l, with d > r as an exception in the Okavango branch. Also common was g > Ø; however, addition of the nasal (for example, nganga) before the g appears to have stabilized it.

By determining the regular sound changes for languages and their protolanguages and mapping them onto the frame of the classification tree—often drawing from the work of linguists engaged in this data processing—historians can then start to track and interpret the implications of changes in roots over time. They can also determine from this evidence if a word was inherited from a linguistic ancestor, innovated as a new word, or borrowed from speakers of another language with different regular sound correspondences: each tells a different story about that word and the speech communities that used it. When we say a daughter language inherited a word from a mother language, what we mean is that speakers of the daughter language continue to use the same word in the same way that speakers in the protolanguage above them on the family tree did. Inherited words point to stories of durability; when linguistic descendants no longer find a word useful to speak about their world, they stop using it. Innovated words are acts of creation, with speech communities fashioning new words from inherited vocabulary through derivation—for example, developing an adjective to describe a noun or, for Bantu languages, adding a new noun class prefix that changes the semantic domain of a noun. Not every instance of creative word-play lasts, but new words that people find useful can endure and be passed down or borrowed. Borrowed or loan words offer historical insight on the relationships between speakers of different languages. Different kinds of borrowing suggest different kinds of relationships. At one extreme, the borrowing of a single word from another language points to the probable conclusion that the item indicated by the word was adopted: for example, a new kind of tool. At the opposite end of the spectrum, the borrowing of a large group of words at once could indicate the assimilation of speakers of one language into speakers of another.

Politics of prestige and influence can also result in borrowing well beyond the geographic area of speakers of a language; for example, there is evidence of speakers of languages outside of the borders of the Kingdom of Kongo borrowing prestigious Kikongo words in the sixteenth and seventeenth centuries.[12] Multilingualism also complicates these stories, as any one individual past or present could be part of multiple speech communities.[13]

The next step requires amassing as many attestations as possible in as many languages within the language family as possible around the idea(s) of interest and from that semantic web mapping commonalities and divergences in meaning onto that linguistic family tree. A key principle here is "words and things"—the premise that if speakers of a protolanguage used a word (as determined through reconstruction), then that word had meaning for them in reference to an object or idea.[14] For my research, after an initial round of sampling to find about a dozen roots relating to healing and harming, I pulled every word I could find containing these roots from dictionaries for twenty-nine currently spoken languages in the Njila family and three languages in the related and geographically adjacent Kikongo Language Cluster (KLC). In doing so, I created a dataset of over 2,500 words. I also tracked attestations of the root words in Bantu languages and protolanguages outside of the Njila and KLC families to determine the antiquity of root changes.[15] I was then able to conduct my analyses on distributions of attested meaning and grammatical forms to build my root word histories.

While the reconstruction of the form of words as a group of sounds is relatively straightforward (though it does take considerable time and effort), the problem of meaning is thornier. How can we know what speakers of a protolanguage *meant* when they used or heard words, especially when working with languages that do not have a deep history of written documentation?[16] The attestations—specific utterances of words—that make up the initial dataset of words, whether collected through fieldwork in the present or in the bulk of dictionaries and ethnographies that were created by missionaries in the colonial late nineteenth and early twentieth centuries, were not elicited in a vacuum. Historians must always be wary not to uncritically project meanings—whether from the present or the nineteenth century—into the deeper past.[17] Working comparatively with attestations across many languages (ideally a combination of interviews from fieldwork, dictionaries, grammars, collections of proverbs, and so forth) helps mitigate this issue. A greater volume of data can give greater confidence of patterns of how words were used and the distribution of meanings; distributions of meaning attached to the same groups of sounds mapped onto a linguistic family tree can point to the probable antiquity of word meanings. As Kathryn de Luna and Jeffrey Fleisher put it, it is "more likely that the meaning 'tree' adhered to the proto-Bantu *-tí than that the meaning 'tree' was invented hundreds of times independently for the same cluster of sounds."[18] Furthermore, the geographic distribution of words in the present or recent past can give historians clues about the movement and genealogy of languages.[19] By exploring the relationships between words and their surrounding vocabulary— both horizontally through similar words contemporaneously spoken and vertically through the reconstructed linguistic chronology—one can track how a word has changed over time and the context in which it may have been used. Morphology—studying the forms of words—can also help historians provisionally reconstruct changes in word usage and meaning: consider the implications, for example, of speakers of a language taking an existing verb and innovating from it a new noun used as a political title.[20]

Africanist David Lee Schoenbrun has said that to tell stories of the early past, historians have to use historical imagination—not the same thing as fiction—to "bridge the islands of knowledge about the world of the people who made what is now known to what we readers know to be true about existing in the world."[21] The insights I draw from comparative historical linguistics, though inherently provisional, help to tell stories of Atlantic African moral philosophy and ideas about power that developed in the slave societies across the Atlantic—ideas expressed in complex ways during "poisoning" events.

APPENDIX B

Language Classification Trees

For each of the following classification trees, I have only included the languages I worked with, not the full collection of languages in the classification.

Romance and Germanic Classification Trees (Indo-European Family)

Both of the following trees are from Glottolog 4.2.1, an online reference for world language classification using hundreds of linguistic sources. See "Family: Romance," Glottolog (accessed 23 June 2020), https://glottolog.org/resource/languoid/id/roma1334; and "Family: Germanic," Glottolog (accessed 23 June 2020), https://glottolog.org/resource/languoid/id/germ1287.

ROMANCE

LATIN

1. Italo-Western Romance
   a. Gallo-Rhaetian
      i. Old French (c. 840–1400)
         1. Anglo-Norman (heavy influence on Middle English)
         2. Middle French (c. 1300–1700)
            a. Modern French (c. 1700 to present)
   b. Ibero-Romance
      i. Galician (c. 870–1400)
         1. Portuguese (c. 1400 to present)

GERMANIC

PROTO-GERMANIC

1. Northwest Germanic
   a. West Germanic
      i. Old High German
      ii. Old Dutch (c. 400–1150)
         1. Middle Dutch (c. 1150–1500)
            a. Modern Dutch (c. 1500 to present)
      iii. Anglo-Frisian

1. Old English (c. 450–1100)
   a. Middle English (c. 1100–1500)
      i. Modern English (c. 1500 to present)

Kikongo Language Cluster and Njila Classification Trees (Bantu Family)

The KLC classification is from de Schryver et al., "Introducing a State-of-the-Art Phylogenetic Classification of the Kikongo Language Cluster," *Africana Linguistica* 21 (2015): 87–162. The Njila classification tree is taken from Vansina, *How Societies Are Born*. Since the Southern Moxico languages split recently and are very closely related, I follow Jan Vansina in using the same dictionary for Lucazi, Nyemba, Mbwela/Nkoya, and Ngangela. I use the alpha-numeric Guthrie coding system for ease of identification; for languages that do not have a specific Guthrie number, I added a lowercase letter. Malcolm Guthrie, *Comparative Bantu: An Introduction to the Comparative Linguistics and Prehistory of the Bantu Languages* (London: Gregg International, 1971).

KIKONGO LANGUAGE CLUSTER

1. Proto North Kikongo
2. Proto South, Central, East, West Kikongo
   a. South, Central, East Kikongo
      i. H16 Kikongo
   b. West Kikongo
      i. H16d Kikongo-Fiote
      ii. H12 Civili

NJILA

PROTO-NJILA

1. Northern Unit
   a. Kwilu
      i. H40 Mbala
      ii. L10–L20 Group
         1. L11 Pende
         2. L101 Sonde
         3. L12 Holo
   b. Kwanza
      i. H20 Group
         1. H21 Kimbundu
         2. H23 Libolo
         3. H22 Kisama
      ii. H24 Songo
      iii. Hb Mbui
2. Southern Unit
   a. Eastern
      i. Lunda Block
         1. Nuclear Rund Group
            1. L53 Rund

        2. L51 Sala
        3. Ld Mpasu
        4. L21 Kete-Ipila
  ii. Moxico
      1. Northern Moxico
        1. K14 Lwena
        2. K11 Cokwe
      2. Southern Moxico
        1. K13 Lucazi
        2. Ka Nyemba
        3. K17 Mbwela/Nkoya
        4. K12b Ngangela
b. Kunene
  i. Umbundu-Okavango
      1. Umbundu
        1. R11 Umbundu
        2. Okavango
          1. K33 Kwangari
          2. K332 Dcrirku
  ii. Cimbebasia
      1. Nyaneka-Nkhumbi
        1. R13 Nyaneka
        2. R14 Nkhumbi
      2. Kwanyama Branch
        1. R21 Kwanyama
      3. Herero Branch
        1. R31 Herero

APPENDIX C

Word Roots

adj. = adjective
n. = noun
v.t. = transitive verb
v.i. = intransitive verb
NC = noun class (for Bantu languages)

ROMANCE AND GERMANIC ROOTS

Information on the Latin roots are directly from the Oxford Latin Dictionary, while the Germanic roots are from the Oxford English Dictionary online, Friedrick Kluge's *Etymological Dictionary of the Germanic Language,* the online database of the *Deutsches Wörterbuch von Jacob Grimm und Wilhelm Grimm,* and the *Etymologiebank NL* online database. Each dictionary/database is listed in full in the bibliography.

1. gëban

Language: Old High German

Definition: v.t. to give

> Major derivatives: gift n. 1. a present; 2. a poison; firgift n. poison; fargiftjan v.t. to inflict poison

2. pōtō

Language: Latin

Definition: v.t 1. to take as a drink; 2. to swallow (liquid), to drink; 3. (v.i.) to drink to quench one's thirst; 4 (v.i.) to drink intoxicating drinks.

> Major derivatives: pōtiō 1. the act of drinking, 2. a drink, 3. a potion (given as a medicine or given to procure death, enchantment, etc.)

3. uenēnum

Language: Latin

Definition: n. 1. a potent herb or other substance used for medical, magical, etc. purposes, or a supernatural influence; 2. a poison, the use of poison, poisoning; 3. something physically harmful or destructive, or pernicious moral influence, or malicious speech; 4. a dye

Major derivatives: uenēno v.t. 1. to bewitch, enchant; 2. to imbue or infect with poison; 3. to treat, imbue (with a dye); uenēficus adj. 1. of or concerned with sorcery, (—person) a sorcerer/sorceress; 2. (—person) a poisoner. uenēficum n. 1. the use of magical arts, sorcery, or a potent substance; 2. the act of poisoning, or a poisonous substance, poison

RECONSTRUCTED KIKONGO LANGUAGE CLUSTER AND NJILA ROOTS

Information on the root form, protolanguage, and gloss are from the Bantu Lexical Reconstructions online database (BLR-3). I have included the BLR-3 index number as well as the number from Malcolm Guthrie's Comparative Series (C.S.). The listed languages under "Attestations" are from my own research in dictionaries (listed in the bibliography).

1. *-bánd-

Protolanguage: Proto-Bantu

Gloss: v.t. to split[1]

BLR-3: 87

C.S.: 50–51

KLC Attestations: Kikongo, Kikongo-Fiote, Civili

Njila Attestations: Pende, Holo, Kimbundu, Libolo, Mbui, Lwena, Cokwe, Lucazi, Umbundu, Nyaneka-Nkhumbi, Herero

2. *-dèmb-

Protolanguage: Proto-Bantu

Gloss: v.i. to be tired, be weakened

BLR-3: 919

C.S.: 555

KLC Attestations: Kikongo, Kikongo-Fiote, Civili

Njila Attestations: Pende, Kimbundu, Rund, Lwena, Cokwe, Lucazi, Umbundu, Kwangari, Dcrirku, Kwanyama

3. *-dòg-

Protolanguage: Proto-Bantu

Gloss: v.t. to bewitch, to curse

> Major derivatives: *-dògì (Noun Class [NC] 14) witchcraft, spell, poison; *-dògì (NC 1/2) witch

BLR-3: 1100

C.S.: 644–647

KLC Attestations: Kikongo, Kikongo-Fiote, Civili

Njila Attestations: Pende, Kimbundu, Mbui, Lwena, Cokwe, Umbundu, Kwangari, Dcrirku, Nyaneka-Nkhumbi, Kwanyama

4. *-gàng-

Protolanguage: Proto-Bantu

Gloss: v.t. to tie up. Variant: *-kàng-

Major derivatives: *-gàngà (NC 14) medicine; *-gàngà (NC 1/2, 9/10) expert, healer-diviner

BLR-3: 1331–1332

C.S.: 785–788

KLC Attestations: Kikongo, Kikongo-Fiote, Civili

Njila Attestations: Pende, Holo, Kimbundu, Mbui, Rund, Lwena, Cokwe, Lucazi, Umbundu, Kwangari, Dcrirku, Nyaneka-Nkhumbi, Kwanyama, Herero

5. *-kác-

Protolanguage: Proto-Bantu

Gloss: v.i. to dry up, coagulate, be hard

BLR-3: 1646

C.S.: 972

KLC Attestations: Kikongo, Kikongo-Fiote, Civili

Njila Attestations: Kimbundu, Rund, Lwena, Cokwe, Lucazi, Umbundu, Kwangari, Kwanyama

6. *-kítì (NC 3/4)

Protolanguage: Proto-Bantu. Inherited by Proto-KLC speakers, but not Proto-Njila speakers.

Gloss: fetish, charm, spirit—especially nature spirits[2]

BLR-3: 1819

C.S.: 1072–1073

KLC Attestations: Kikongo, Kikongo-Fiote, Civili

Njila Attestations: Kimbundu, Mbui, Rund, Lwena, Umbundu, Kwangari

7. *-kód-

Protolanguage: Proto-Bantu

Gloss: (Homophonic cluster) 1. v.i. to be strong, be hard, be difficult; 2. v.t. to take, to touch

Major inherited derivative(s): *-kód- v.t. to intoxicate, from 1; *-kódè (NC 1/2) captive, booty, from 2

BLR-3: 1874, 6999

C.S.: 1104, 1107, 1110

KLC Attestations: Kikongo, Civili

Njila Attestations: Pende, Kimbundu, Mbui, Rund, Lwena, Cokwe, Lucazi, Umbundu, Dcrirku, Nyaneka-Nkhumbi, Kwanyama

APPENDIX D

Geographic Overview of Poisoning Cases

Table 2 summarizes the timing and distribution of my dataset of 542 poison cases from Bahia, the Dutch Guianas, Virginia, and Martinique from 1680 to 1850.

The form and organization of each colonial court system affected how cases appeared and were tried. Cases in Bahia were handled by the Inquisition. Unlike the Inquisition in the Spanish empire, with independent regional offices in American cities like Lima and Cartagena, the Lisbon Inquisition handled all cases in the Portuguese overseas empire from the metropole. Individuals wishing to make a confession or denunciation went to the regional Inquisitorial commissioners—for Bahia, based in Salvador—who conducted an initial investigation and sent their findings to Lisbon. If the Inquisitors chose to pursue the case, the commissioner would arrest the accused, gather additional testimony, and send both across the Atlantic to be tried in Lisbon. If not, the initial report and testimony were instead copied into the *cadernos do promotor*, the prosecutor's notebooks: a repository of the cases that were not pursued. The Inquisition was far more interested in accusations of judaizing or heresy then *feitiçaria* and related crimes, usually declining to undertake the expense of trying *feitiçaria* cases.[1] In Suriname and Berbice, the respective Courts of Policy and Criminal Justice, made up of appointed local elites, conducted these trials. They were both the main criminal courts and the respective colonies' legislative bodies, responsible for issuing ordinances.[2] Most of the members of each court had no legal education, and this system had neither jury nor defense lawyers. The Suriname criminal court was made up of thirteen planter elites appointed for life by the governor, who presided over the meetings himself. One of the councilors on the court doubled as the *fiscaal*, a public prosecutor who conducted the initial investigations into complaints and decided whether cases would go to court.[3] Until 1869, Suriname's legal system operated under the 1532 Constitutio Criminalis Carolina and Philip II's 1570 Criminal Ordinance, along with Roman slave law. These law codes had been replaced in the Netherlands by Napoleon's penal reforms at the end of the eighteenth century, but the reforms were not applied to the colonies.[4] The Carolina, passed by Holy Roman Emperor Charles V, allowed for the use of torture to extract confessions and established the forms for prosecuting witches.[5] County courts in Virginia as both a colony and a state had jurisdiction over civil cases and only criminal cases with enslaved defendants. The men who served as appointed commissioners on these courts of *oyer and terminer* were local elites who were usually enslavers—and who often brought enslaved people to trial themselves. For an example of a commissioner appearing in multiple roles, in Cumberland county, slaveholder George Carrington was a judge in the respective trials of Isaac and Quash (1759), Peter and Mingo (1763), and Frank and Dick (1769); the enslaver of a woman named Dido, who was hanged for allegedly preparing and attempting to administer "poisonous medicines" in 1756; and one of the plaintiffs in the 1773 case against Caesar, accused of preparing and exhibiting a "poisonous medicine" to an enslaved woman named Jenny.[6] White colonists accused of crime were instead

Table 2. Total Poison Cases, 1680–1849

	Bahia	Dutch Guianas[a]	Virginia	Virginia (Brunswick, Cumberland)	Marti- nique	TOTAL
1680–1689	6	—	—	—	—	6
1690–1699	6	—	—	—	—	6
1700–1709	15	—	0	—	—	15
1710–1719	4	—	0	—	—	4
1720–1729	2	0	0	—	—	2
1730–1739	4	16	1	—	1	22
1740–1749	22	41	4	0	6	73
1750–1759	24	1[b]	30	5	36	91
1760–1769	6	27	56	7	4	93
1770–1779	1	28	65	5	2	96
1780–1789	1	5	23	6 [3]	—	32
1790–1799	3	8	—	[4]	—	15
1800–1809	0	c	—	[5]	3[d]	8
1810–1819	—	c	—	[6]	—	6
1820–1829	4	2	—	[0]	30	36
1830–1839	1	—	—	[0]	27	28
1840–1849	—	—	—	[1]	8	9
TOTAL	99	128	179	39 [19]	117	542

For this table, I have included both full trials and investigations. Bahia cases include all *feitiçaria* cases (under the same criteria used to make the table on Bahia demographics). A dash mark (—) indicates that I have no data for this period and place. The second column on Virginia refers to data I collected from Cumberland and Brunswick Counties—data that is included in Philip Schwarz's accounting of poison cases in Virginia from 1704 to 1785. I extended my analysis in these two counties up to 1839. For the total poison cases, I do not include the pre-1785 Brunswick and Cumberland cases in the "total" tallies (as these numbers are included under "Virginia"). I have placed the numbers for nonduplicate cases in [brackets] for tallying purposes.

[a] Data from the Dutch Guianas predominantly from Suriname, with four poison cases from Berbice in the 1770s. This table does not include poison cases from British Guiana (formerly Berbice, Demerara, and Essequibo) after 1815.

[b] Several volumes of the Raad van Politie records are missing for this decade, so this number may be inaccurately low.

[c] Locations and period where trial data does exist, but I have not conducted research.

[d] The poison cases I have for this decade are only those forwarded to the Ministère de La Marine by Villaret as an illustration of his tribunal. There were many more cases from this tribunal, but these are the only ones that have survived.

Sources: ANTT Inquisição Lisboa Series 30, Cadernos do Promotor, and Series 28, Processos; APEB Seção Judiciário, Devassas; Schwarz, *Twice Condemned*, Table 10, p. 96 (for the Virginia data); NADH Raad van Politie en Criminele Justitie; NA-Kew CO 116 British Guiana, Berbice Records of the Court of Policy and Criminal Justice; ANOM Série F3 Collection Moreau de Saint-Méry, Annales du Conseil souverain de la Martinique; ANOM Dépôt des papiers des colonies, greffes Martinique, Cour d'assises de Fort-de-France et Saint-Pierre; ANOM Série C8 Correspondance à l'arrivée en provenance de la Martinique (for cases from Villaret's tribunal, 1806–1808); ADM Série U7 Cour Prévôtale.

tried at the General Court in Williamsburg. County courts were sites of affirmation for slave-holders' social standing, and a rotating cast of Virginia gentry tried enslaved people in poison cases in the second half of the eighteenth century.[7] In Martinique, the Conseil Supérieur was an appeals court that covered criminal and civil cases of all individuals. Cases would have first been tried in the regional tribunals; however, all cases involving crimes with the potential for capital punishment—including poisoning—were automatically appealed to the council.[8] The earliest surviving collection of trial summaries from the Conseil Supérieur starts in 1726, but there are several reports of earlier instances of poisoning in the governors' correspondence.[9]

Before the mid-eighteenth century, laws in Bahia, the Dutch Guianas, Virginia, and Martinique did not make specific connections between poison and healing practitioners of African descent.[10] However, early poison *cases* from the 1680s to the 1740s *did* begin to make these links; poison legislation followed experiences shaped by these early trials. The timing of the emergence of poison cases coincided with the massive growth of each colony's enslaved African population tied to respective plantation booms. West and West Central Africans brought their ideas about the ambivalent powers of health practitioners across the Atlantic; along with European anxieties toward growing enslaved populations, these ideas helped coalesce a particular concern with "poison."[11] With the acceleration of plantation slavery in the late seventeenth and early eighteenth centuries, poison became a crime linked to people of African descent, especially enslaved people, and with the particular importance of healers. As the number of enslaved Africans increased, so did the number of poison cases and the connections between them. Demographic changes in these colonies impacted not only European perceptions of Africans as a growing potential threat to their enslavers, but also the transmission and transformation of Atlantic African moral philosophies navigating fraught power and social interactions.

Once early trials and poison laws in each of these locations had established connections between poison, healing, and enslaved Africans, the number of cases accelerated to peaks in the mid-eighteenth century. The 1740s was a decade of transition, as a common and growing sense of crisis led to the creation of new laws to control both African practitioners and enslavers for their increasing extrajudicial punishments of alleged poisoners on their plantations.[12] As cases became intertwined with new legal regimes, they began to take on a life of their own. Trials operated in a feedback loop as poison cases built on each other—either directly through chains of trials or indirectly through the circulation of knowledge about specific cases, as they reinforced slaveholders' ideas about who poisoners were and how they operated. Trials in these peak decades were fairly consistent and remarkably similar between locations, as the associations that had been forged during the period of emergence perpetuated and sustained themselves.

With variations in the duration and timing, slaveholder investigations connecting poison, healing, and people of African descent accelerated to a mid-century peak. Half of the twelve full Inquisitorial trials originating in Bahia from 1680 to 1802 came from the decades between 1740 and 1769, as did forty-six of the eighty-one *feitiçaria* investigations (57 percent) in the *cadernos do promotor*. The number of investigations per year reached a peak with eight cases in 1750 alone.[13] The proportion of *feitiçaria* accusations in the *cadernos* to the total reflects increased local concern, as it rose from 26 percent between 1700 and 1739 to 51 percent between 1750 and 1759.[14] Poison trials peaked in Suriname in the 1740s but remained at a high plateau that only began to falter after the mid-1770s. The immediate aftermath and impact of the 1745 government ordinance on poison is difficult to detect, as volumes for trials in 1746, 1749, and most of the 1750s have not survived. The robust number of cases in the 1760s and early 1770s do suggest continued concern with poison. Surviving trial data for eighteenth-century Berbice is much more limited than for Suriname, but the poison cases for the colony are suggestive of similar patterns. Berbice's criminal court records from 1764 to 1792 contained four poison cases, with none after 1775.[15] Poison cases in Virginia after 1748 also accelerated dramatically. From 1730 to 1748, there were only five poison cases in the colony; in the 1750s this number shot up to thirty cases, then fifty-six cases in the 1760s, and a peak of sixty-five cases in the 1770s. Over the eighteenth century in Virginia, more enslaved people were accused of poisoning than for any other crime except theft.[16] Martinique poison cases accelerated to their first peak in the mid-1750s, with thirty-six cases in that decade alone.[17] The infrastructure built by Martinique's colonial government to swiftly try and convict alleged poisoners among the enslaved contributed to a unique secondary peak in the 1820s.

From the late eighteenth to the mid-nineteenth century, these four locations broadly shared a pattern of decline in the numbers of poison cases and shifts in relationships between poison and healing that had shaped cases during the peak decades. In Suriname, the relative position of poison cases in the context of all trials diminished over time from the 1770s onward.[18] Poison trials in Suriname did not disappear as completely as they did in Berbice, but after 1775 the steady number of cases per year dropped to a sporadic trickle.[19] In Virginia, the decades-long rise and peak only began to drop in the 1780s, with twenty-three cases from 1780 to 1784.[20] Changes in the infrastructure for trying cases, such as reforms within the Lisbon Inquisition for Bahia and the suppression of the Cour Prévôtale—a special tribunal that tried the 1820s wave of cases in Martinique—contributed significantly to declines of cases in these regions. *Feitiçaria* denunciations to the Inquisition in the *cadernos do promotor* had largely disappeared by the end of the eighteenth century, and the Lisbon Inquisition itself was disbanded in 1821. Few investigations by Bahia's secular courts and limited official correspondence from the eighteenth and early nineteenth centuries have survived; those records that have survived predominantly, and unsurprisingly, focused on other problems. The first thirty-five years of the nineteenth century was a period of near constant conflict and rebellion in Bahia, exemplified by a series of uprisings of free and enslaved Africans organized by ethnic affiliations: poison was not a relative concern. The major political changes of this period included the relocation of the Portuguese court to Rio de Janeiro following the French invasion of the Iberian peninsula in 1808 and the formation of the independent Empire of Brazil in 1822.[21]

Laws from the first half of the nineteenth century also ceased to explicitly link poison and the work of healers of African descent, shifting from European fears of the efficacy of their practices to designations of "superstition" if mentioned at all.[22] In Bahia, legal links between poison, healing, and people of African descent were also absent in the new imperial Criminal Code of 1830. In fact, the only mention of poison in the entire code was as part of a list of aggravating circumstances for crime; the only mention of medical practice was in a section forbidding abortions. For British Guiana, formed from the former Dutch colonies of Berbice, Demerara, and Essequibo after the Napoleonic Wars, a significant part of this shift can be attributed to the separation of poison and *obeah* into separate legal categories. With the 1830s and emancipation as a key turning point, from a legal perspective *obeah* shifted from a crime of causing physical harm and/or inciting rebellion to a crime of fraud, defined as preying on superstition. In Virginia, colonial laws regarding enslaved people and poison remained on the books until the 1840s, and county courts of *oyer and terminer* continued to try postrevolution cases involving enslaved people. Shortly after the suppression of the Cour Prévôtale in 1827, changes in Martinique's slave codes also began to break down the connections between poison and "sorcery" that had held sway among enslavers for the better part of the last century. By a royal ordinance in September 1828, France applied the 1810 Napoleonic Code Pénal to her remaining Caribbean colonies, a code that mentioned poison only as an example of voluntary homicide, and punished "superstitious" practices, such as divination, with the relatively light punishment of a fine and several days in jail. In 1831, the Martinique council assembled a project for how to apply the new laws to the enslaved population. This report contained traces of white lawmakers' particular concerns about poison: specifically, how to root out alleged societies of enslaved cultists organized with the express purpose of poisoning people and livestock. The code even added a new element, by classifying the killing of one's enslaver by any means, including poison, as parricide. However, the 1831 code did mark a significant shift in the prosecution of poison cases, as it separated the practice of alleged "sorcery" and medicine from poison. Enslaved people convicted of conducting "spells, enchantments, or other superstitious practices," including grave robbing to make and operate *maléfices*, were condemned to work in chain gangs. For practicing medicine or preparing remedies of any kind, the code likewise sentenced the enslaved to three months in prison or convict labor; those who sold, distributed, or possessed "false beverages" with "dangerous ingredients," including compositions made for "superstitious purposes," were sentenced to a whipping and time in the public stocks. Not even the possession or sale of "substances to kill," as long as they were not used, would result in the gruesome capital punishments from less than a decade earlier. The overlap between "sorcery," healing, and poison could now only legally occur with "attempts on the life" of a person or "useful" animal with a "substance that can give death." Only enslaved people accused of using a "real" poison—as defined by the government as a physical substance proven to cause physical harm, such as arsenic—with malicious intent could be tried as a poisoner. Practices that were once enough to convict and sometimes execute enslaved people in the eighteenth century, such as composing and distributing drugs or *maléfices*, were no longer capital crimes.[23]

Along with numeric decline, the content of these nineteenth-century cases shifted as well. They contained a higher frequency of accusations involving mineral poisons, such as arsenic, as well as a greater concern with "superstition" than "sorcery." While courts continued to police the healing practices of people of African descent, the figure of the healer as poisoner was replaced in enslavers' imaginations and trials by that of the enslaved domestic; at the same time, enslaved women made up an increasing proportion of the accused. The degree of dissociation of the elements in earlier poison cases, as well as the pace of decline in the frequency of trials, varied between locations. However, by the mid-nineteenth century the period of poison trials centered on African practitioners had come to an end.

APPENDIX E

Demographic Data

Over the late seventeenth and early eighteenth centuries, an important shift in the scale and demographics of the transatlantic slave trade across the Atlantic—driven by the insatiable demand for enslaved labor from plantations and supply of captives from rising conflicts in Atlantic Africa—corresponded with an expansion of concern about Africans and their connections to poison. The number of Africans brought to these four locations rose dramatically in the late seventeenth and early eighteenth centuries, overlapping with the emergence of poison cases. In Bahia from 1660 to 1730 and Martinique from 1680 to 1730, the number of Africans disembarking in each colony rose exponentially. The number of disembarking Africans in Bahia rose from 1,032 in the 1660s to 5,624 the following decade, then 11,896 in the 1680s and 43,958 in the 1690s. The number of disembarking Africans in Martinique also rose dramatically: 2,250 in the 1680s; 3,639 in the 1690s; 6,705 in the 1700s; 13,328 in the 1710s; and 22,681—the second highest decade total for the colony's entire history—in the 1720s.[1] The rises for the Dutch Guianas and Virginia in the late seventeenth century were less dramatic but still significant. Numbers of disembarking Africans in the Dutch Guianas show an increase from 6,048 in the 1670s to 11,120 in the 1680s. In Virginia, 1,144 Africans disembarked in the 1690s and 8,831 in the 1700s. The peak decade for Virginia's entire history was the 1730s, with 17,838 people disembarking.[2]

Though imperfect, census data from each location also points to a large and growing proportion of Africans and people of African descent within each population in the late seventeenth and early eighteenth centuries. In Martinique, the 8,967 enslaved people identified by the 1683 census made up an already high 66 percent of the population: many most likely worked on the colony's 122 sugar plantations. By 1726, the number of sugar plantations had nearly quadrupled, and the enslaved population had risen to 40,403 (77 percent). With an emergent free Black population of 1,304, the total population of African descent in this year outnumbered white *habitants* four to one. In Suriname, the 4,137 enslaved Africans and creoles of African descent in 1684 made up 81 percent of the population—a significant compositional shift from the proportion of 55 percent at the peak of the English colony in 1663. By the 1701 census, the population of African descent—including 8,500 enslaved people and approximately 1,000 Maroons—dwarfed the 700 Europeans in the colony. That proportion would only increase with the boom of the enslaved population over the first half of the eighteenth century; by 1752 the 37,835 recorded enslaved people—most of whom had been born in Africa—made up a staggering 95 percent of the population. The total population from the 1684 census also included 144 enslaved Indigenous Americans. Virginia never came close to such radically skewed proportions between enslaved and free populations; however, over the first half of the eighteenth century, the proportion of enslaved people did increase significantly. The enslaved population grew from 3,000 people (7 percent of the total population) in 1680 to 16,390 (28 percent) two decades later in 1700. By 1750 that population and its relative proportion had further increased to 107,100 (46 percent)—the highest proportion from 1680 to 1840. Unfortunately, general census figures for seventeenth-century Bahia—though ordered by the crown—either were not conducted or have not survived.

Table 3. Number of Africans Disembarked, 1580–1850

	Bahia	Dutch Guianas	Martinique	Virginia
1581–1590	166	0	0	0
1601–1610	236	0	0	0
1611–1620	105	0	0	0
1621–1630	1,189	0	0	0
1641–1650	4,094	0	0	0
1651–1660	1,032	2,095	856	344
1661–1670	1,302	4,265	4,529	85
1671–1680	5,624	6,048	1,000	1,788
1681–1690	11,896	11,120	2,250	1,564
1691–1700	43,958	10,411	3,639	1,144
1701–1710	48,297	11,144	6,705	8,831
1711–1720	70,212	9,619	13,328	6,478
1721–1730	84,021	13,205	22,681	13,565
1731–1740	86,846	18,496	17,013	17,838
1741–1750	86,754	27,398	25,941	9,514
1751–1760	70,708	29,064	19,450	10,717
1761–1770	62,740	44,496	6,849	8,498
1771–1780	74,141	29,290	5,362	2,393
1781–1790	76,989	5,918	2,439	0
1791–1800	90,709	12,010	20,863	0
1801–1810	95,972	22,129	4,974	30
1811–1820	114,980	706	5,412	0
1821–1830	96,854	1,479	10,908	0
1831–1840	19,377	0	181	0
1841–1850	65,024	0	0	0

Table 4. Number of Africans Disembarked from the Bight of Benin, 1680–1750

	Bahia	Dutch Guianas	Martinique	Virginia
1681–1690	8,826	3,714	1,329	0
1691–1700	29,168	4,884	305	0
1701–1710	43,292	5,963	3,145	315
1711–1720	44,182	6,449	7,874	0
1721–1730	52,747	4,123	12,595	0
1731–1740	50,831	6,307	8,582	380
1741–1750	48,005	478	8,666	0

Table 5. Number of Africans Disembarked from West Central Africa, 1680–1750

	Bahia	Dutch Guianas	Martinique	Virginia
1681–1690	1,296	5,095	0	0
1691–1700	7,745	4,854	500	0
1701–1710	1,436	2,568	351	92
1711–1720	9,060	1,202	2,051	146
1721–1730	24,007	1,853	5,455	1,116
1731–1740	30,110	258	3,367	2,966
1741–1750	35,541	9,095	6,361	640

Table 6. Number of Africans Disembarked from the Gold Coast, 1680–1750

	Bahia	Dutch Guianas	Martinique	Virginia
1681–1690	768	514	0	0
1691–1700	412	453	305	0
1701–1710	0	1,068	482	404
1711–1720	3,411	325	419	391
1721–1730	2,547	6,812	269	1,199
1731–1740	1,206	11,097	1,656	558
1741–1750	0	1,801	2,768	226

Table 7. Number of Africans Disembarked from the Bight of Biafra, 1680–1750

	Bahia	Dutch Guianas	Martinique	Virginia
1681–1690	294	1,125	0	174
1691–1700	5,209	0	304	525
1701–1710	3,081	0	450	2,267
1711–1720	8,217	0	1,593	2,743
1721–1730	3,225	0	0	4,547
1731–1740	3,867	0	230	4,094
1741–1750	2,276	0	426	4,559

The first solid data I have is from a 1724 ecclesiastical census. According to it, by 1724 the 45,482 enslaved Africans made up 57 percent of Bahia's population. However, this census did not distinguish between the free white and free African population; anecdotal evidence from early eighteenth-century travelers suggests that the latter were a large portion of the Salvador population.[3]

The following tables are of data obtained from Voyages: The Transatlantic Slave Trade Database (accessed 5 May 2022).

NOTES

Introduction

1. Proces van Quashie, 28 July 1731, Nationaal Archief (NADH) Oud Archief Suriname: Raad van Politie (RVP), vol. 787, n.p.; Trial of Peter, 23 May 1765, Library of Virginia (LVA) Cumberland County Court Order Books (CCOB), vol. 1764–67, pp. 124–125; Procès de Zéphir, September 1768, Archives Nationales d'Outre-Mer (ANOM) Série F3 Moreau de Saint-Méry Collection, Seances du Conseil Souverain, vol. 246, pp. 516–518; D. Fernando José de Portugal to Martinho de Melo e Castro, 24 December 1789, Arquivo Historico Ultramarino (AHU) Administração Central Bahia, Bahia-CA, box 70, f. 13366.

2. Wyatt MacGaffey, "Dialogues of the Deaf: Europeans on the Atlantic Coast of Africa," in *Implicit Understandings: Observing, Reporting, and Reflecting on the Encounters Between Europeans and Other Peoples in the Early Modern Era*, ed. Stuart Schwartz (Cambridge: Cambridge University Press, 1994), 249–267.

3. Denúncia de Paulo Gomes e Ignacia, 21 October 1749, Arquivo Nacional Torre do Tombo (ANTT), Inquisição de Lisboa (IL) Series 30 Cadernos do Promotor, vol. 109, pp. 153–160; Proces van Goliath en Prins, 4 August 1742, NADH RVP, vol. 795, n.p.; Procès de Jean François, January 1742, ANOM Série F3, vol. 244, pp. 363–366; Trial of Tom, 9 June 1744, LVA Caroline CCOB, vol. 2, pp. 288–290.

4. Peter Geschiere, *Witchcraft, Intimacy, and Trust: Africa in Comparison* (Chicago: University of Chicago Press, 2013), xv, 16–17, 29. Geschiere compares witchcraft accusations from early modern European villages, nineteenth-century Candomblé houses, and his own forty years of fieldwork in Cameroon with the central argument that witchcraft discourse addresses a common human issue—fear of attack from within—and that the links between witchcraft and intimacy in Africa were not unique. See also Sharla M. Fett, *Working Cures: Healing, Health, and Power on Southern Slave Plantations* (Chapel Hill: University of North Carolina Press, 2002), 87; Alison Games, *Witchcraft in Early North America* (Plymouth: Rowman & Littlefield, 2010), 54.

5. Fett, *Working Cures*, 6, 37, 56, 87, 95–106; James H. Sweet, *Recreating Africa: Culture, Kinship, and Religion in the African-Portuguese World, 1441–1770* (Chapel Hill: University of North Carolina Press, 2003), 139; John M. Janzen, *Lemba, 1650–1930: A Drum of Affliction in Africa and the New World* (New York: Garland, 1982).

6. Michael A. Gomez, *Reversing Sail: A History of the African Diaspora*, 2nd ed. (Cambridge: Cambridge University Press, 2020), 70.

7. Yvan Debbasch, "Opinion et droit: Le crime d'empoisonnement aux Iles pendant la période esclavagiste," *Revue française d'histoire d'outre-mer* 50, no. 179 (1963): 137–188; Pierre Pluchon, *Vaudou, sorciers, empoisonneurs de Saint-Domingue à Haïti* (Paris: Éditions Karthala, 1987); Douglas B. Chambers, *Murder at Montpelier: Igbo Africans in Virginia* (Jackson: University Press of Mississippi, 2005); Caroline Oudin-Bastide, *L'effroi et la terreur: Esclavage, poison et*

sorcellerie aux Antilles (Paris: Éditions La Découverte, 2013); Diana Paton, *The Cultural Politics of Obeah: Religion, Colonialism and Modernity in the Caribbean World* (Cambridge: Cambridge University Press, 2015). For works that discuss poisoning cases but are not primarily focused on them, see Philip J. Schwarz, *Twice Condemned: Slaves and the Criminal Laws of Virginia, 1705–1865* (Baton Rouge: Louisiana State University Press, 1988); Carolyn E. Fick, *The Making of Haiti: The Saint Domingue Revolution from Below* (Knoxville: University of Tennessee Press, 1990); Fett, *Working Cures*; Karol K. Weaver, *Medical Revolutionaries: The Enslaved Healers of Eighteenth-Century Saint Domingue* (Urbana: University of Illinois Press, 2006); Luiz Mott, *Bahia: Inquisição & Sociedade* (Salvador: EDUFBA, 2010); Natalie Zemon Davis, "Judges, Masters, Diviners: Slaves' Experience of Criminal Justice in Colonial Suriname," *Law and History Review* 29, no. 4 (Nov. 2011): 925–984; Randy M. Browne, *Surviving Slavery in the British Caribbean* (Philadelphia: University of Pennsylvania Press, 2017).

8. Diana Paton and Maarit Forde, eds., *Obeah and Other Powers: The Politics of Caribbean Religion and Healing* (Durham, NC: Duke University Press, 2012); Diana Paton, "Witchcraft, Poison, Law, and Atlantic Slavery," *William and Mary Quarterly* 69, no. 2 (Apr. 2012): 235–264; Trevor Burnard and John Garrigus, *The Plantation Machine: Atlantic Capitalism in French Saint-Domingue and British Jamaica* (Philadelphia: University of Pennsylvania Press, 2016), 102–122; John Garrigus, "'Like an Epidemic One Could Only Stop with the Most Violent Remedies': African Poison Versus Livestock Disease in Saint Domingue, 1750–88," *William and Mary Quarterly* 78, no. 4 (2021): 617–652.

9. Gwendolyn Midlo Hall, *Social Control in Slave Plantation Societies: A Comparison of St. Domingue and Cuba* (Baltimore: Johns Hopkins University Press, 1971), 41, 62; Schwarz, *Twice Condemned*, 97; Fick, *Making of Haiti*, 61–73; Barbara Bush, *Slave Women in Caribbean Society, 1650–1838* (Bloomington: Indiana University Press, 1990), 50–52, 73–75; Rudi Otto Beeldsnijder, *"Om Werk Van Jullie te Hebben": Plantageslaven in Suriname, 1730–1750* (Utrecht: Instituut voor Culturele Antropologie te Utrecht, 1994), 224–228; Bernard Moitt, *Women and Slavery in the French Antilles, 1635–1848* (Bloomington: Indiana University Press, 2001), 139–146; Weaver, *Medical Revolutionaries*, 89–94. Weaver also cautions that some accusations of poisoning could reflect retaliation blaming healers for dead patients more than any intent to kill.

10. Marisa Fuentes, *Dispossessed Lives: Enslaved Women, Violence, and the Archive* (Philadelphia: University of Pennsylvania Press, 2016), 11.

11. Fuentes, *Dispossessed Lives*, 107; Jason T. Sharples, "Discovering Slave Conspiracies: New Fears of Rebellion and Old Paradigms of Plotting in Seventeenth-Century Barbados," *American Historical Review* 120, no. 3 (2015): 817; Sasha Turner Bryson, "The Art of Power: Poison and Obeah Accusations and the Struggle for Dominance and Survival in Jamaica's Slave Society," *Caribbean Studies* 41, no. 2 (2013); Browne, *Surviving Slavery*.

12. Browne, *Surviving Slavery*, 4.

13. For example, see Weaver, *Medical Revolutionaries*; Londa Schiebinger, *Secret Cures of Slaves: People, Plants, and Medicine in the Eighteenth-Century Atlantic World* (Stanford, CA: Stanford University Press, 2017).

14. Todd Lee Savitt, *Medicine and Slavery: The Diseases and Health Care of Blacks in Antebellum Virginia* (Urbana: University of Illinois Press, 1978).

15. See Rhys Isaac, *Landon Carter's Uneasy Kingdom: Revolution and Rebellion on a Virginia Plantation* (Oxford: Oxford University Press, 2004); Rana A. Hogarth, *Medicalizing Blackness: Making Racial Difference in the Atlantic World, 1780–1840* (Chapel Hill: University of North Carolina Press, 2017); Deirdre Cooper Owens, *Medical Bondage: Race, Gender, and the Origins of American Gynecology* (Athens: University of Georgia Press, 2017). On the differences between societies with slaves and slave societies, see Ira Berlin, *Generations of Captivity: A History of African American Slaves* (Cambridge, MA: Harvard University Press, 2003). For more on slaveholders' ideas about medical treatment, see Fett, *Working Cures*, 20–21, 25, 28. For more

on violence and survival in slave societies, see Browne, *Surviving Slavery*; Fuentes, *Dispossessed Lives*.

16. Savitt, *Medicine and Slavery*, 171, 175–176; Sweet, *Recreating Africa*, 60; Isaac, *Landon Carter's Uneasy Kingdom*, 117–118, 315; Susan Scott Parrish, *American Curiosity: Cultures of Natural History in the Colonial British Atlantic World* (Chapel Hill: University of North Carolina Press, 2006), 259, 283, 285; Weaver, *Medical Revolutionaries*, 41–42; James H. Sweet, *Domingos Álvares, African Healing, and the Intellectual History of the Atlantic World* (Chapel Hill: University of North Carolina Press, 2011), 56, 69–70; Pablo F. Gómez, *The Experiential Caribbean: Creating Knowledge and Healing in the Early Modern Atlantic* (Chapel Hill: University of North Carolina Press, 2016), 125.

17. For exceptions that do explore these tensions and relationships in detail, see Fett, *Working Cures*, 87–88, 107; Davis, "Judges, Masters, Diviners," 949, 956, 971; Browne, *Surviving Slavery*, 4, 134.

18. For example, relating to obeah accusations, see Bryson, "Art of Power," 72, 83. For a comparative look at intimate spaces as locales conducive to witchcraft accusations, see Geschiere, *Witchcraft, Intimacy, and Trust*.

19. Brian P. Levack, *The Witch-Hunt in Early Modern Europe* (London: Longman, 1987), 18; Stuart Clark, *Thinking with Demons: The Idea of Witchcraft in Early Modern Europe* (Oxford: Clarendon, 1997), 4–8.

20. Games, *Witchcraft in Early North America*; Fernando Cervantes, *The Devil in the New World: The Impact of Diabolism in New Spain* (New Haven: Yale University Press, 1994); Laura de Mello e Souza, *The Devil and the Land of the Holy Cross: Witchcraft, Slavery, and Popular Religion in Colonial Brazil*, trans. Diane Grosklaus Whitty (Austin: University of Texas Press, 2003); Sweet, *Recreating Africa*; John K. Thornton, "Cannibals, Witches, and Slave Traders in the Atlantic World," *William and Mary Quarterly* 60, no. 2 (Apr. 2003): 273–294; Sweet, *Domingos Álvares*; Paton, "Witchcraft, Poison, Law"; Gómez, *Experiential Caribbean*.

21. For more on spirits, "witchcraft," and power in African history, see Wyatt MacGaffey, *Kongo Political Culture: The Conceptual Challenge of the Particular* (Bloomington: Indiana University Press, 2000); David M. Gordon, *Invisible Agents: Spirits in Central African History* (Athens: Ohio University Press, 2012); Geschiere, *Witchcraft, Intimacy, and Trust*; Jan Vansina, *How Societies Are Born: Governance in West Central Africa Before 1600* (Charlottesville: University of Virginia Press, 2004). John Thornton's work in particular has explicitly made connections between ideas and concerns about witches in Atlantic Africa—especially in the Kingdom of Kongo—and the history of the transatlantic slave trade. See John K. Thornton, *The Kongolese Saint Anthony: Dona Beatriz Kimpa Vita and the Antonian Movement, 1684–1706* (Cambridge: Cambridge University Press, 1998); Thornton, "Cannibals, Witches, and Slave Traders." See also the work of anthropologist Rosalind Shaw on Sierra Leone, in "The Production of Witchcraft/ Witchcraft as Production: Memory, Modernity, and the Slave Trade in Sierra Leone," *American Ethnologist* 24, no. 4 (1997): 856–876; Shaw, *Memories of the Slave Trade: Ritual and the Historical Imagination in Sierra Leone* (Chicago: University of Chicago Press, 2002).

22. Kevin Dawson, *Undercurrents of Power: Aquatic Culture in the African Diaspora* (Philadelphia: University of Pennsylvania Press, 2018); Herman L. Bennett, *African Kings and Black Slaves: Sovereignty and Dispossession in the Early Modern Atlantic* (Philadelphia: University of Pennsylvania Press, 2019); Mary E. Hicks, "Blood and Hair: Barbers, *Sangradores*, and the West African Corporeal Imagination in Salvador da Bahia, 1793–1843," in *Medicine and Healing in the Age of Slavery*, ed. Sean Morey Smith and Christopher D. Willoughby (Baton Rouge: Louisiana State University Press, 2021).

23. For examples of more recent scholarship moving past the creolization debate, see Akinwumi Ogundiran and Paula Saunders, eds., *Materialities of Ritual in the Black Atlantic* (Bloomington: Indiana University Press, 2014); Gómez, *Experiential Caribbean*.

24. Benjamin Breen, *The Age of Intoxication: Origins of the Global Drug Trade* (Philadelphia: University of Pennsylvania Press, 2019); Kalle Kananoja, *Healing Knowledge in Atlantic Africa: Medical Encounters, 1500–1850* (Cambridge: Cambridge University Press, 2021).

25. For an example of a historian using a similar approach, see Hicks, "Blood and Hair," 62, 64–69.

26. MacGaffey, "Dialogues of the Deaf," 259–260.

27. While largely taken up by Africanists, the origination of this framework involved medical anthropologists studying cases from very different locales—from Kongo to Quebec—and discussing their work together at an influential McGill seminar in 1971. See John M. Janzen, "Therapy Management: Concept, Reality, Process," *Medical Anthropology Quarterly* 1, no. 1 (1987): 68–84; Janzen, with the collaboration of William Arkinstall, MD, *The Quest for Therapy in Lower Zaire* (Berkeley: University of California Press, 1978).

28. For two examples of works focused on public healing, see Janzen, *Lemba*; Neil Kodesh, *Beyond the Royal Gaze: Clanship and Public Healing in Buganda* (Charlottesville: University of Virginia Press, 2010).

29. Steven Feierman and John M. Janzen, eds., *The Social Basis of Health and Healing in Africa* (Berkeley: University of California Press, 1992).

30. Historians grapple with this issue in different ways. Pablo Gómez, for example, chooses to use an Indigenous American term, *Mohán/Mohanes* (translated in several Inquisition cases as "a master of sorcerers") to describe Black ritual practitioners rather than the terms of accusation like *brujas*, sorcerers, and witches. See Gómez, *Experiential Caribbean*, 11.

31. For strong introductions to each location as a slave society, see Rhys Isaac, *The Transformation of Virginia, 1740–1790*, 2nd ed. (Chapel Hill: University of North Carolina Press, 1999); Stuart B. Schwartz, *Sugar Plantations in the Formation of Brazilian Society: Bahia, 1550–1835* (Cambridge: Cambridge University Press, 1985); Alex van Stipriaan, *Surinaams contrast: Roofbouw en overleven in een Caraïbische plantage economie, 1750–1863* (Amsterdam: Centrale Huisdrukkerij Vrije Universiteit, 1991); Caroline Oudin-Bastide, *Travail, capitalism et société esclavagiste: Guadeloupe, Martinique (XVIIe–XIXe siècle)* (Paris: Découverte, 2005).

32. For examples, see Weaver, *Medical Revolutionaries*; Philip D. Morgan, *Slave Counterpoint: Black Culture in the Eighteenth-Century Chesapeake and Lowcountry* (Chapel Hill: University of North Carolina Press, 1998); Jerome S. Handler and Kenneth M. Bilby, *Enacting Power: The Criminalization of Obeah in the Anglophone Caribbean, 1769–2011* (Jamaica, Barbados, Trinidad and Tobago: University of the West Indies Press, 2012); Paton, *Cultural Politics of Obeah*; Gómez, *Experiential Caribbean*; Fuentes, *Dispossessed Lives*.

33. For examples, see Cervantes, *Devil in the New World*; Kris Lane, "Taming the Master: Brujería, Slavery, and the Encomienda in Barbacoas at the Turn of the Eighteenth Century," *Ethnohistory* 43, no. 3 (1998): 477–507; Laura A. Lewis, *Hall of Mirrors: Power, Witchcraft, and Caste in Colonial Mexico* (Durham, NC: Duke University Press, 2003); Nicole von Germeten, *Violent Delights, Violent Ends: Sex, Race, and Honor in Colonial Cartagena de Indias* (Albuquerque: University of New Mexico Press, 2013); Gómez, *Experiential Caribbean*.

34. Lewis, *Hall of Mirrors*, 12; Cervantes, *Devil in the New World*, 17.

35. Lewis, *Hall of Mirrors*, 38.

36. Gómez, *Experiential Caribbean*, 59–67, 70–78, 130–132; von Germeten, *Violent Delights, Violent Ends*, 103–107. Both Gómez and von Germeten discuss the complex and fascinating accusations and counteraccusations to the Inquisition made by two competing practitioners of African descent: Paula de Eguiluz and Diego Lopez.

37. The literature on the flow and circulation of knowledge between Iberian, British, French, and Dutch colonies is vast and has been booming for the past twenty years. For examples, see Jorge Cañizares-Esguerra, *Nature, Empire, and Nation: Explorations of the History of Science in the Iberian World* (Stanford, CA: Stanford University Press, 2006); Marcy Norton,

Sacred Gifts, Profane Pleasures: A History of Tobacco and Chocolate in the Atlantic World (Ithaca, NY: Cornell University Press, 2008); Matthew James Crawford, *The Andean Wonder Drug: Cinchona Bark and Imperial Science in the Spanish Atlantic, 1630–1800* (Pittsburgh: University of Pittsburgh Press, 2016); Ernesto Bassi, *An Aqueous Territory: Sailor Geographies and New Granada's Transimperial Greater Caribbean World* (Durham, NC: Duke University Press, 2016); Jorge Cañizares-Esguerra, ed., *Entangled Empires: The Anglo-Iberian Atlantic, 1500–1830* (Philadelphia: University of Philadelphia Press, 2018); Breen, *Age of Intoxication*; Matthew James Crawford and Joseph M. Gabriel, eds., *Drugs on the Page: Pharmacopoeias and Healing Knowledge in the Early Modern Atlantic World* (Pittsburgh: University of Pittsburgh Press, 2019).

38. "Copy of the Record Book of the Slave Trials of St. Andrew Jamaica from 17 March 1746 to 16 Dec. 1782," enc. in Charles Metcalft to Lord John Russell, 5 April 1840, National Archives (NA-Kew) Colonial Office (CO) 137/248, Jamaica Despatches. For a detailed statistical analysis of this record, see Diana Paton, "Punishment, Crime, and the Bodies of Slaves in Eighteenth-Century Jamaica," *Journal of Social History* 34, no. 4 (2001): 923–954.

39. Fuentes, *Dispossessed Lives*, 101–103.

40. Michel-Rolph Trouillot, *Silencing the Past: Power and the Production of History* (Boston: Beacon, 1995), 26.

41. Fuentes, *Dispossessed Lives*, 4–5, 8.

42. For examples, see Camilla Townsend, *Malintzin's Choices: An Indian Woman in the Conquest of Mexico* (Albuquerque: University of New Mexico Press, 2006); James H. Sweet, "Reimagining the African-Atlantic Archive: Method, Concept, Epistemology, Ontology," *Journal of African History* 55 (2014): 147–159; Fuentes, *Dispossessed Lives*; Camilla Townsend, *Annals of Native America: How the Nahuas of Colonial Mexico Kept Their History Alive* (Oxford: Oxford University Press, 2017); Sasha Turner, "The Nameless and the Forgotten: Maternal Grief, Sacred Protection, and the Archive of Slavery," *Slavery & Abolition* 38, no. 2 (2017): 232–250; Sophie White, *The Voices of the Enslaved: Love, Labor, and Longing in French Louisiana* (Chapel Hill: Omohundro Institute and University of North Carolina Press, 2019).

43. White, *Voices of the Enslaved*.

44. Surviving records from the Lisbon Inquisition (1536–1821), police investigation reports from Cachoeira in Bahia (1751–1839 [1820–1839]), Suriname (1722–1828) and Berbice (1764–1793) Courts of Policy and Criminal Justice, the Martinique Conseil Supérieur (1729–1778), and assisez court records for Fort-de-France and Saint-Pierre (1830–1848) all fit this description. Virginian county courts (1704–1865) only contained criminal trials when the defendants were enslaved; the Cour Prévôtale (1822–1826) tried enslaved people and free people of color exclusively for the crime of poison; and the Fiscal's reports from Berbice (1819–1832) and Demerara and Essequibo (1826–1834)—as part of the new British Guiana—only handled complaints by and against enslaved people.

45. Feierman and Janzen, eds., *Social Basis of Health*, 14; Lawrence M. Friedman, *A History of American Law*, 2nd ed. (New York: Simon & Schuster, 1985), 75.

46. White, *Voices of the Enslaved*, 13.

47. Isaac, *Transformation of Virginia*, 324.

48. Davis, "Judges, Masters, Diviners," 960, 976–978; Mott, *Bahia: Inquisição & Sociedade*, 115; Oudin-Bastide, *L'effroi et la terreur*, 70.

49. White, *Voices of the Enslaved*, 8.

50. Rhiannon Stephens and Axel Fleisch, "Introduction: Theories and Methods of African Conceptual History," in *Doing Conceptual History in Africa*, ed. Axel Fleisch and Rhiannon Stephens (New York: Berghahn, 2016), 12. For an example of this kind of conceptual history conducted with archaeological sources in a Native American context, see Scott G. Ortman, "Conceptual Metaphor in the Archaeological Record: Methods and an Example from the American Southwest," *American Antiquity* 65, no. 4 (2000): 613–645; Scott G. Ortman, "Bowls to Gardens:

A History of Tewa Community Metaphors," in *Religious Transformation in the Late Pre-Hispanic Pueblo World*, ed. Donna M. Glowacki and Scott Van Keuren (Tucson: University of Arizona Press, 2011), 84–108.

51. Manuscript sources in Arabic created by West African scholars in Timbuktu and Jenne are important exceptions. See Michael A. Gomez, *African Dominion: A New History of Empire in Early and Medieval West Africa* (Princeton: Princeton University Press, 2018), 19–20, 24–26. There are also important sixteenth-century documentary sources created by Africans in the Kingdom of Kongo. The letters from King Afonso I to several kings of Portugal in the early sixteenth century are particularly notable. See Linda Heywood and John K. Thornton, *Central Africans, Atlantic Creoles, and the Foundation of the Americas, 1585–1660* (New York: Cambridge University Press, 2007), 61–70, for more on Afonso I and his letters.

52. See Games, *Witchcraft in Early North America*; Paton, "Witchcraft, Poison, Law"; Davis, "Judges, Masters, Diviners"; Geschiere, *Witchcraft, Intimacy, and Trust*; Oudin-Bastide, *L'effroi et la terreur*.

53. For more on the challenges and uses of these kinds of documents, see John Thornton, "European Documents and African History," in *Writing African History*, ed. John E. Phillips (Rochester: University of Rochester Press, 2005), 254–265.

54. Robert W. Slenes, "'Malungu, ngoma vem!' Africa coberta e descoberts do Brasil," *Revista USP* 12 (1992): 48–67; Christiana Mobley, "The Kongolese Atlantic: Central African Slavery & Culture from Mayombe to Haiti" (PhD diss., Duke University, 2015), 204–206. In contrast, for works focused on the Atlantic world that do use and discuss comparative historical linguistics, see Marcos Abreu Leitão de Almeida, "Speaking of Slavery: Slaving Strategies and Moral Imaginations in the Lower Congo (Early Times to the Late 19th Century)" (PhD diss., Northwestern University, 2020); Kathryn M. de Luna, "Sounding the African Atlantic," *William and Mary Quarterly* 78, no. 4 (2021): 581–616.

55. For the culminating work of this project, see Koen Bostoen and Inge Brinkman, eds., *The Kongo Kingdom: The Origins, Dynamics and Cosmopolitan Culture of an African Polity* (Cambridge: Cambridge University Press, 2017).

56. For recent work introducing Africanists' methods to Atlanticists, see de Luna, "Sounding the African Atlantic."

Chapter 1

1. Clark, *Thinking with Demons*, 114.

2. Levack, *Witch-Hunt in Early Modern Europe*, 37, 110. For more on this idea of inversion in European witch theory, see Stuart Clark, "Inversion, Misrule and the Meaning of Witchcraft," *Past and Present* no. 87 (1980): 100–101.

3. Alisha Rankin, *The Poison Trials: Wonder Drugs, Experiment, and the Battle for Authority in Renaissance Science* (Chicago: University of Chicago Press, 2021), 17. See also Franck Collard, *The Crime of Poison in the Middle Ages*, trans. Deborah Nelson-Campbell (Westport, CT: Praeger, 2008), 94–110.

4. Thornton, *Kongolese Saint Anthony*, 42–43.

5. Vansina, *How Societies Are Born*, 190–191; J. D. Cordeiro da Matta, *Ensaio de Diccionario Kimbúndu-Portuguez* (Lisbon: Da Casa Editoria Antonio Maria Pereira, 1893), 22. This *ndembu* title is not to be confused with the Lunda polity, sometimes called Lunda-Ndembu, that later became the Lunda Empire in the Central African interior. For more, see John Thornton, *A History of West Central Africa to 1850* (Cambridge: Cambridge University Press, 2020), 145–146, 218–235. Modern convention refers to the people of the Kwanza valley using this title in the early modern period as the Dembos. For more on Dembos polities, see Thornton, *History of West Central Africa*, 23–24.

6. For example, see Schwarz, *Twice Condemned*; Fick, *Making of Haiti*; Beeldsnijder, *"Om Werk Van Jullie te Hebben"*; Robert A. Voeks, *Sacred Leaves of Candomblé: African Magic, Medicine, and Religion in Brazil* (Austin: University of Texas Press, 1997); Rachel Harding, *A Refuge in Thunder: Candomblé and Alternative Spaces of Blackness* (Bloomington: Indiana University Press, 2000); Moitt, *Women and Slavery in the French Antilles*; Chambers, *Murder at Montpelier*; Weaver, *Medical Revolutionaries*. The emphasis on resistance has been stronger in literature focused on continental North America than in Latin American scholarship.

7. de Luna, "Sounding the African Atlantic," 585–586, 590.

8. For a discussion of tone and consonants, see Appendix A.

9. Marcos Abreu Leitão de Almeida, "African Voices from the Congo Coast: Languages and the Politics of Identification in the Slave Ship *Jovem Maria* (1850)," *Journal of African History* 60, no. 2 (2019): 177–178.

10. For more on noun classes and Bantu languages, see Mark Van de Veld, "Nominal Morphology and Syntax," in *The Bantu Languages*, ed. Mark Van de Veld, Koen Bostoen, Derek Nurse, and Gérard Philippson (New York: Routledge, 2019), 237–269.

11. P. G. W. Glare, *Oxford Latin Dictionary* (Oxford: Clarendon, 1982), 1418.

12. Glare, *Oxford Latin Dictionary*, 2027.

13. Glare, *Oxford Latin Dictionary*, 2027.

14. Fritz Graf, *Magic in the Ancient World* (Cambridge, MA: Harvard University Press, 1999), 46–47.

15. "poison, n.," "poison, v.," "poisoner, n.," *Oxford English Dictionary (OED) Online*, 2015, www.oed.com (accessed 30 June 2016); "empoisonner," "empoisonneur, euse," *Trésor de la Langue Française (TLFi)*, Université de Lorraine, http://atilf.atilf.fr (accessed 8 July 2016).

16. For more on the major Bantu divergences, see Rebecca Grollemund et al., "Bantu Expansion Shows That Habitat Alters the Route and Pace of Human Dispersals," *Proceedings of the National Academy of Sciences of the United States of America* 112, no. 43 (2015): 13296–13301.

17. *-bánd-* (to heal, to cure) attested in Kikongo-Fiote, Kimbundu. *-bánd-* (practice of healing, curing) attested in Kimbundu, Mbui, Lwena, Southern Moxico, Umbundu, Nyaneka-Nkhumbi. Mission de Landana, *Dictionnaire Français-Fiote* (Paris: Maison-Mère, 1890); J. D. Cordeiro da Matta, *Ensaio de diccionario Kimbúndu-Portuguez* (Lisbon: Da Casa Editoria Antonio Maria Pereira, 1893); P. António da Silva Maia, *Lições de gramática de Quimbundo (Português e Banto), dialecto Omumbuim: Língua indígena de Gabela, Amboim, Quanza-Sul, Angola, Africa Ocidental Portuguesa* (Cucujães, Portugal, 1957); Albert E. Horton, *A Dictionary of Luvale* (El Monte, CA: Rahn Brothers Printing & Lithographic, 1953); Domingos Viera Baião, Ernesto Lecomte, and José Sutter, *Dicionário Ganguela-Português: Língua falada nas regiões do Cubango, Nhemba e Luchaze, Província de Angola* (Lisbon: Centro des Estudos Filológicos, 1940); Grégoire Le Guennec and José Francisco Valente, *Dicionário Português-Umbundu* (Luanda: Instituo d'Investigação Científica d'Angola, 1972); Rev. W. H. Sanders and Rev. W. E. Fay, *Vocabulary of the Umbundu Language, Comprising Umbundu-English and English-Umbundu* (Boston: Beacon, 1885); Padre António Joaquim da Silva, *Dicionário Português-Nhaneca* (Lisbon: Instituto de Investigação Científica de Angola, 1966).

18. *-kod-* (to be in good health) attested in Kikongo, Pende, Southern Moxico, Umbundu, Nyaneka-Nkhumbi, Kwanyama. K. E. Laman, *Dictionnaire Kikongo-Français: Avec une étude phonétique décrivent les dialects les plus importants de la langue dite Kikongo* (Ridgewood, NJ: Gregg Press, 1964); Barthelemy Gusimana, *Dictionnaire Pende-Français* (Bandundu: Publications Ceeba, 1972); Baião and Sutter, *Dicionário Ganguela-Português*; Le Guennec and Valente, *Dicionário Português-Umbundu*; da Silva, *Dicionário Português-Nhaneca*.

19. Relict distributions of this meaning from *-dèmb-* are so widespread that I think it is less likely to have been a recent and rapidly expanded innovation than for it to have been very old. Innovations with *-kác-* attested in Kikongo, Civili, Kimbundu, Rund, Lwena, and Cokwe.

W. Holman Bentley, *Dictionary and Grammar of the Kongo Language, as Spoken at San Salvador* (London: Baptist Missionary Society and Trübner, 1887); Laman, *Dictionnaire Kikongo-Français*; P. Marichelle, *Dictionnaire Vili-Français* (Loango: Imprimerie de la Mission, 1902); da Matta, *Ensaio de diccionario Kimbúndu-Portuguez*; Jay Nash, "Ruund, 1996," Comparative Bantu Online Dictionary, University of California, Berkeley (accessed 21 April 2016); Horton, *Dictionary of Luvale*; Malcom Brooks MacJannet, *Chokwe-English English-Chokwe Dictionary and Grammar Lessons* (Missão da Biula, Angola: Malcom Brooks, 1949).

20. Attested in Pende, Kimbundu, and Cokwe. Gusimana, *Dictionnaire Pende-Français*; da Matta, *Ensaio de diccionario Kimbúndu-Portuguez*; MacJannet, *Chokwe-English English-Chokwe Dictionary*.

21. Attested in Pende, Rund, Lwena, and Cokwe. Gusimana, *Dictionnaire Pende-Français*; Nash, "Ruund, 1996"; Horton, *Dictionary of Luvale*; MacJannet, *Chokwe-English English-Chokwe Dictionary*.

22. Attested in Holo, Kimbundu, Libolo, Songo, Mbui, Lwena, Cokwe, Southern Moxico, Umbundu, and Nyaneka-Nkhumbi. Jan Daeleman, *Ki-Holo (notes provisoires)* (Heverlee, Belgium, 1961); da Matta, *Ensaio de diccionario Kimbúndu-Portuguez*; S. W. Koelle, *Polyglotta Africana, or a Comparative Vocabulary of Nearly Three Hundred Words and Phrases in More Than One Hundred Distinct African Languages*, 2nd ed. (Graz, Austria: Akademische Druck u. Verlagsanstalt, 1963); J. Pereira do Nascimento, *Diccionario Portuguez-Kimbundu* (Huilla, Angola: Typographia da Missão, 1903); Harry Johnston, *A Comparative Study of the Bantu and Semi-Bantu Languages* (Oxford: Clarendon, 1919); Koelle, *Polyglotta Africana*; da Silva Maia, *Lições de gramática de Quimbundo*; Horton, *Dictionary of Luvale*; MacJannet, *Chokwe-English English-Chokwe Dictionary*; Baião and Sutter, *Dicionário Ganguela-Português*; Le Guennec and Valente, *Dicionário Português-Umbunu*; Sanders and Fay, *Vocabulary of the Umbundu Language*; and da Silva, *Dicionário Português-Nhaneca*. Vansina argues that *-bàndà* (healer, diviner) instead came from a root meaning "concubine," noting that *-mbanda* practitioners in the central Angolan river valleys blended genders with their dress and talked about themselves as "wives of the spirit that possessed them." Words from *-bánd-* with marriage connotations appeared frequently in my search through KLC languages but not in terms for healer-diviners. In the Njila family similar connotations only appear in Pende (*mbanda*, "wife"); however, the 1972 dictionary notes that this term is a neologism in Pende. After consulting with Kathryn de Luna and following David Schoenbrun's work on this root, I think it is therefore more likely that the root meanings of *-bàndà* practitioners had less to do with marriage per se than with the idea to split (and its inverse, to bind). Kathryn de Luna, personal communication, 1 February 2018; David Lee Schoenbrun, *The Historical Reconstruction of Great Lakes Bantu Cultural Vocabulary* (Cologne: Rüdiger Köppe, 1997), 178; David Lee Schoenbrun, "Conjuring the Modern in Africa: Durability and Rupture in Histories of Public Healing Between the Great Lakes of East Africa," *American Historical Review* 111, no. 5 (2006): 1421. For more on discussions of *jinbanda* in Central Africa and Brazil in the seventeenth century, see Sweet, *Recreating Africa*, 54–57; Luiz Mott, "Feiticeiros de Angola na América Portuguesa," *Revista Pós Ciências Sociais* 5, no. 9 (2008): 5, 8–9, 23–24.

23. Grollemund et al., "Bantu Expansion Shows."

24. Christopher Ehret, *History and the Testimony of Language* (Berkeley: University of California Press, 2001), 3. This section focuses almost exclusively on Njila speakers, as I have not conducted the kind of historical linguistic analysis with KLC speakers to enable me to do the same with them. The dates I use in this section come from Robert Joseph Papstein and a lexicostatistic analysis of cognate percentages of core vocabulary conducted from Papstein and the work of Yvonne Bastin, André Coupez, and Michael Mann. See Robert Joseph Papstein, "The Upper Zambezi: A History of the Luvale People, 1000–1900" (PhD diss., University of California, Los Angeles, 1978); and Yvonne Bastin, André Coupez, and Michael Mann, *Continuity and*

Divergence in the Bantu Languages: Perspectives from a Lexicostatistic Study (Tervuren, Belgium: Musée Royal de l'Afrique Central, 1999). More research is needed to express greater confidence and precision with these date ranges. For now, I am layering these date estimates onto the divergences mapped out by Jan Vansina in *How Societies Are Born.*

25. Jan Vansina assembled the Njila classification I use (see Appendix B) through a combination of historical linguistics—identifying shared innovations—and archaeology, connecting these innovations to physical and very roughly datable evidence. For Vansina's classification of the Njila family and his explanation of how he came to it, see the appendix in Vansina, *How Societies Are Born,* 273–284. It is also important to emphasize that the spread of these languages was not exclusively or necessarily the result of massive sweeping migration. Language is not the same thing as population. David Schoenbrun, "Mixing, Moving, Making, Meaning: Possible Futures for the Distant Past," *African Archaeological Review* 29, no. 2/3 (2012): 301–302, 304; Almeida, "African Voices from the Congo Coast," 176–177; Vansina, *How Societies Are Born,* 53–55; Kathryn M. de Luna and Jeffrey B. Fleisher, *Speaking with Substance: Methods of Language and Materials in African History* (New York: Springer, 2018), 12–15.

26. Vansina, *How Societies Are Born,* 59.

27. For some of the most recent linguistic work on the Bantu expansion, particularly in West Central Africa, see Gilles-Maurice de Schryver et al., "Introducing a State-of-the-Art Phylogenetic Classification of the Kikongo Language Cluster," *Africana Linguistica* 21 (2015): 87–162; Grollemund et al., "Bantu Expansion Shows "; Rebecca Grollemund, "Nouvelles approaches en classification: Application aux langues bantu du Nord-Ouest" (PhD diss., Université Lumière Lyon 2, 2012).

28. For a useful analysis comparing the degree of relation between languages like Kimbundu and Kikongo, see de Luna, "Sounding the African Atlantic," 594–595.

29. "Southern Moxico" is actually the proto-language of eight languages spoken today (including Nkangala, Lucazi, and Mbunda). However, the most useful dictionary of these languages, compiled in 1939 and used by Vansina in *How Societies Are Born,* treats them as a single language. Furthermore, preliminary evidence using glottochronology and albeit limited core vocabulary data from Bastin et al. in *Continuity and Divergence* suggests that Southern Moxico only began to diverge into its daughter languages in the early nineteenth century. For the purposes of this book, I will use "Southern Moxico" to refer to these languages together.

30. Vansina, *How Societies Are Born,* 56–59.

31. Collard, *Crime of Poison in the Middle Ages,* 98. Interestingly, criminal records show that while women were disproportionately accused of poisoning more than other crimes, they were a minority of people accused of poisoning overall. Collard notes that the vast majority of people tried for all crimes were men. For more on demographics of the accused and their relationship to tropes and discourse about who was a poisoner, see pp. 94–110.

32. For more on the trope of "the poison of usurpation" and plots involving royal women in particular, see Collard, *Crime of Poison in the Middle Ages,* 146–148.

33. Collard, *Crime of Poison in the Middle Ages,* 98; and Lynn Wood Mollenauer, *Strange Revelations: Magic, Poison, and Sacrilege in Louis XIV's Court* (University Park: Pennsylvania State University Press, 2006), 57.

34. Cited in Roy Porter, *The Greatest Benefit to Mankind: A Medical History of Humanity* (New York: W. W. Norton, 1997), 130. See also Clark, *Thinking with Demons,* 129; Mollenauer, *Strange Revelations,* 57.

35. Gabriele Ferrario, "Maimonides' *Book on Poisons and the Protection Against Lethal Drugs,*" in *Toxicology in the Middle Ages and Renaissance,* ed. Peter Wexler (London: Elsevier, 2017), 39.

36. Levack, *Witch-Hunt in Early Modern Europe,* 8.

37. Clark, *Thinking with Demons,* 110–111, 133.

38. Clark, *Thinking with Demons*, 441–442; Levack, *Witch-Hunt in Early Modern Europe*, 8–9. For a well-known example exploring this gap in conceptions of witchcraft, see Carlo Ginzburg, *The Night Battles: Witchcraft and Agrarian Cults in the Sixteenth and Seventeenth Centuries*, trans. John and Anne C. Tedeschi (Baltimore: Johns Hopkins University Press, 1983).

39. Collard, *Crime of Poison in the Middle Ages*, 127; Paton, "Witchcraft, Poison, Law," 239–240; Mollenauer, *Strange Revelations*, 53.

40. Mollenauer, *Strange Revelations*, 59.

41. Clark, *Thinking with Demons*, 133.

42. Collard, *Crime of Poison in the Middle Ages*, 128, 130–131, 145.

43. David Lee Schoenbrun, *A Green Place, A Good Place: Agrarian Change, Gender, and Social Identity in the Great Lakes Region* (Portsmouth, NH: Heinemann, 1998), 91, 108, 112–113; Janzen, *Lemba*, 4–6, 21, 95. For an analysis of the relationship between healing and politics in institutional power in the Great Lakes Region, see Kodesh, *Beyond the Royal Gaze*.

44. Vansina describes the act of leadership as one of arbitration, with the title for these chiefs, *soba*, deriving from a new verb **-sompá-*, "to try, to arbitrate." Vansina, *How Societies Are Born*, 163–164, 167.

45. Vansina, *How Societies Are Born*, 188–190, 193–195; Heywood and Thornton, *Central Africans, African Creoles*, 79, 106. For more on oral traditions on the founding of the Kingdom of Kongo, see John K. Thornton, "The Origins of Kongo: A Revised Vision," in *The Kongo Kingdom: The Origins, Dynamics, and Cosmopolitan Culture of an African Polity*, ed. Koen Bostoen and Inge Brinkman (Cambridge: Cambridge University Press, 2018), 36–41. For extensive discussion of the spiritual responsibilities of the King of Kongo in a later period, see Thornton, *Kongolese Saint Anthony*.

46. MacGaffey, *Kongo Political Culture*, 12.

47. MacGaffey, *Kongo Political Culture*, 11; Wyatt MacGaffey, "A Central African Kingdom: Kongo in 1480," in Bostoen and Brinkman, eds., *Kongo Kingdom*, 53–56.

48. MacGaffey, *Kongo Political Culture*, 11–13, 16, 19, 112.

49. MacGaffey, *Kongo Political Culture*, 2; Thornton, *Kongolese Saint Anthony*, 42–43. Note the g > k sound change.

50. da Matta, *Ensaio de diccionario Kimbúndu-Portuguez*, 22.

51. Vansina, *How Societies Are Born*, 167. See also Kathryn M. de Luna, *Collecting Food, Cultivating People: Subsistence and Society in Central Africa* (New Haven: Yale University Press, 2016), "Chapter 3: Fame in the Kafue" and "Chapter 4: Of Kith and Kin."

52. See Eugenia W. Herbert, *Iron, Gender, and Power: Rituals of Transformation in African Societies* (Bloomington: Indiana University Press, 1993); Colleen E. Kriger, *Pride of Men: Ironworking in 19th Century West Central Africa* (Portsmouth, NH: Heinemann, 1999). See also Koen Bostoen, Odjas Ndonda Tshiyayi, and Gilles-Maurice de Schryver, "On the Origin of the Royal Kongo Title *Ngangula*," *Africana Linguistica* 19 (2013): 53–83.

53. Meanings of both "to be in good health" and "to make strong" attested in Pende, Southern Moxico. Gusimana, *Dictionnaire Pende-Français*; Baião and Sutter, *Dicionário Ganguela-Português*. See also Vansina, *How Societies Are Born*, 192.

54. Njila and KLC speakers in the kingdoms of middle Angola were not the only ones to make connections between ironworking, healing, and leadership in this period. For example, Southern Moxico speakers on the eastern plains began using the same root, **-band-*, for a new noun *muvandye* ("bellows") as their inherited words *tyimbanda* ("doctor-sorcerer") and *vumbanda* ("science of the sorcerer"). However, they were different in the extent of their elaboration of the responsibilities of powerful kings to use their spiritual power for public prosperity. See Baião, Lecomte, and Sutter, *Dicionário Ganguela-Português*, 26, 177.

55. Vansina, *How Societies Are Born*, 206, 209–211, 218–219, 221–222, 229–234.

56. In the east, Lwena speakers began elaborating *-kitɪ* words to describe spirits, masks, and dances connected to initiation ceremonies. While descended from a different branch of Njila than Lwena speakers, Pende speakers living in the northwestern part of the Kalahari sands also innovated words to discuss initiations from roots they had also used to discuss health and healing. With the phonology *kanga*, it seems unlikely that Pende speakers derived this word from those for *-gang-* people (all of which follow *-gàngà* spelling), but rather from *-kàng-* as a variant of *-gàng-*. See Horton, *Dictionary of Luvale*, 110–111; Gusimana, *Dictionnaire Pende-Français*, 66–67.

57. Bantu Lexical Reconstructions 3 (BLR-3), no. 976, C.S. 575.

58. For more on the *mulemba* tree and birdlime, see Vansina, *How Societies Are Born*, 239.

59. Vansina, *How Societies Are Born*, 190–191.

60. *-dèmb-* (to calm, to pacify, to tame) attested in Kikongo, Kikongo-Fiote, Civili, Kimbundu, Rund, Southern Moxico, and Umbundu. Bentley, *Dictionary and Grammar of the Kongo Language*; Laman, *Dictionnaire Kikongo-Français*; Mission de Landana, *Dictionnaire Français-Fiote*; Marichelle, *Dictionnaire Vili-Français*; da Matta, *Ensaio de diccionario Kimbúndu-Portuguez*; Nash, "Ruund, 1996"; Baião and Sutter, *Dicionário Ganguela-Português*; Sanders and Fay, *Vocabulary of the Umbundu Language*. Vansina argues that the roots for the verb "to calm" and the nouns relating to ancestors and particular trees associated with them came from different roots, respectively, *-dèmb-* (BLR-3: to be tired, to be weakened), from which I derived the Proto-Njila-KLC verb *-demb-*, "to calm, pacify, sooth, tame," and *-dìmb-* (BLR-3: to trap by birdlime), with the lime coming from the ancestor tree. Given the overlap between ideas about hunting, medical practice, and connections to both ancestors and leadership in surviving words from one or both of these roots—and inconsistencies in the recording or use of tones—I think it is plausible that Njila and KLC speakers made use of near-homophonic relationships between these roots. See Vansina, *How Societies Are Born*, 239; Almeida, "Speaking of Slavery," 125. For information on verb-to-noun derivation in Bantu, see Thilo C. Schadeberg and Koen Bostoen, "Word Formation," in Van de Veld et al., eds., *Bantu Languages*, 172–203.

61. Attested in Pende and Holo. Gusimana, *Dictionnaire Pende-Français*; Daeleman, *Ki-Holo*. See also Vansina, *How Societies Are Born*, 239, n.95. Note the d > l sound change.

62. Vansina, *How Societies Are Born*, 239–240, see n.95–96.

63. Vansina, *How Societies Are Born*, 240.

64. MacJannet, *Chokwe-English English-Chokwe Dictionary*, 49.

65. Horton, *Dictionary of Luvale*, 153.

66. Gusimana, *Dictionnaire Pende-Français*, 40, 130.

67. Vansina, *How Societies Are Born*, 69, 81–83, 149, 157.

68. Vansina, *How Societies Are Born*, 107–108, 123, 153–154, 264.

69. Based on Vansina's work on language evidence, significant changes in Herero immigration and leadership in the sixteenth century make this period a plausible candidate for such a change in leadership words. However, for -*bàndà* this idea should be taken as only a suggestive hypothesis. For more on Herero history up to the mid-nineteenth century, see Vansina, *How Societies Are Born*, 122–129.

70. Rev. F. W. Kolbe, *An English-Herero Dictionary with an Introduction to the Study of Herero and Bantu in General* (Cape Town: J. C. Juta, 1883), 11, 19, 30, 61, 65, 85, 111, 146, 148, 171, 179, 188, 254, 358, 367, 454. From the diachronic phonology chart I made, in Herero *mb > mb while *b > β. Along with the close association in the attested meanings, this sound change correspondence strongly suggests that *ouvande* shared the same root as *ombanda* and so on.

71. *Oxford Portuguese Dictionary* (Oxford: Oxford University Press, 2015); "venin," *Trésor de la Langue Française* (accessed 8 July 2016).

72. "gift, n.," *OED Online* (accessed 27 January 2019).

73. Friedrich Kluge, *Etymological Dictionary of the Germanic Language*, 4th ed., translated from the German (London: Bell, 1891), 119; "geben," "gift," "vergift," "giftig," "vergiften," "vergifter," "vergiftig," "vergiftigen," "vergeben," "ver-," *Deutsches Wörterbuch von Jacob Grimm und Wilhelm Grimm auf CD-ROM und im Internet,* Universität Trier, 2019, (accessed 27 January 2019), http://dwb.uni-trier.de/de/.

74. "gif," "gift," "vergift," "vergiftig," "vergeven," "venijn" in Marlies Philippa et al., *Etymologisch Woordenboek van het Nederlands* (Amsterdam: Amsterdam University Press, 2003–2009), accessed through *Etymologiebank.nl*, 2010 (accessed 27 January 2019), http://www.etymologiebank.nl.

75. Vansina, *How Societies Are Born,* 268–269. The literature on "witchcraft" in African history is vast. As a useful starting place from an Atlanticist's perspective, see Thornton, "Cannibals, Witches, and Slave Traders."

76. Bentley, *Dictionary and Grammar of the Kongo Language,* 289; Laman, *Dictionnaire Kikongo-Français,* 213–214.

77. For more on witches and their hunger in West Central African thought, see Thornton, "Cannibals, Witches, and Slave Traders"; Thornton, *Kongolese Saint Anthony,* 42–43; MacGaffey, *Kongo Political Culture,* 2; Vansina, *How Societies Are Born,* 268–269.

78. Glare, *Oxford Latin Dictionary,* 668–670.

79. Roger Sansi, "Sorcery and Fetishism in the Modern Atlantic," in *Sorcery in the Black Atlantic,* ed. Luis Nicolau Parés and Roger Sansi (Chicago: University of Chicago Press, 2011), 21.

80. Sansi, "Sorcery and Fetishism in the Modern Atlantic," 22.

81. Gomez, *Reversing Sail,* 43–47.

82. For more on the history of these pouches in Portuguese history, see Vanicléia Silva Santos, "As bolsas de mandinga no espaco Atlântico: Século XVIII" (PhD diss., Universidade de São Paulo, 2008).

83. Timothy D. Walker, *Doctors, Folk Medicine and the Inquisition: The Repression of Magical Healing in Portugal During the Enlightenment* (Leiden: Brill, 2005), 84.

84. For an enormously influential article in African history on this idea of the composition of networks of extraordinary people as central to leadership, see Jane I. Guyer and Samuel M. Eno Belinga, "Wealth in People as Wealth in Knowledge: Accumulation and Composition in Equatorial Africa," *Journal of African History* 36 (1995): 91–120. For more on influential ideas about porous divide between people and objects through the example of *minkisi* among the Bakongo, see MacGaffey, *Kongo Political Culture,* 1, 12–13.

85. de Luna, "Sounding the Atlantic," 609.

86. For more on these major intellectual debates more broadly, see Richard Kieckhefer, *Magic in the Middle Ages* (Cambridge: Cambridge University Press, 2000), 3–5, 9, 12, 14–17, 81, 184, 199. In developing theories of magic, intellectuals in the late Middle Ages and Renaissance also increasingly drew upon classical and Arabic sources. See Brian P. Copenhaver, *Magic in Western Culture: From Antiquity to the Enlightenment* (Cambridge: Cambridge University Press, 2015), 24, 232, 236, 444; Kieckhefer, *Magic in the Middle Ages,* 16–17.

87. Ferrario, "Maimonides' *Book on Poisons,*" 32–34, 37–38.

88. Ferrario, "Maimonides' *Book on Poisons,*" 35.

89. Ferrario, "Maimonides' *Book on Poisons,*" 39–40. For examples on the use of milk to neutralize poison, see João Curvo Semedo, *Observaçoens medicas doutrinaes de cem casos gravissimos* (Lisbon: Na Officina de Antonio Pedroso Galram, 1727), 271; Mathieu Joseph Bonaventure Orfila, *Traité des poisons: Tirés des régnes minéral, végétal et animal, ou toxocologie générale, considérée sous les rapports de la physiologie, de la pathologie et de la médicine légale* (Paris: Chez Crochard, 1814), vol. 1.1, 183–184, 186. For examples of the use of bezoars against poison, see João Vigier, *Pharmacopea Ulyssiponense, Galenica, e Chymica, que contem os principios, diffiniçoens,*

e termos geraes de huma, & outre pharmacia: & hum lexicon universal dos termos Pharamaceu-
ticos Galenicas, de que se usa neste reyno, & virtudes, & dosis dos medicamentos chymicos (Lisbon:
Na Officina de Pascoal da Sylva, Impressor de S. Magestade, 1716), 398; Semedo, *Observaçoens*
medicas doutrinaes, 271.

90. Rankin, *Poison Trials,* 39–40, 81, 109.

91. Attested in Kikongo, Kikongo-Fiote, and Civili. Bentley, *Dictionary and Grammar of the*
Kongo Language; Mission de Landana, *Dictionnaire Français-Fiote*; Marichelle, *Dictionnaire*
Vili-Français; Laman, *Dictionnaire Kikongo-Français.*

92. de Luna, *Collecting Food, Cultivating People,* "Chapter 5: Life on the Central Frontier:
The Geographies of Technology, Trade, and Prestige, 750–1700"; Vansina, *How Societies Are*
Born, 188–189, 238. For more on the origin and structure of the Kingdom of Kongo, see Thornton,
History of West Central Africa, 24–37.

93. Heywood and Thornton, *Central Africans, Atlantic Creoles,* 106.

94. Peter Brown, *The Body and Society: Men, Women, and Sexual Renunciation in Early*
Christianity, 2nd ed. (New York: Columbia University Press, 2008), xxxvii. Schoenbrun also discusses the idea of braided evidence, in "Mixing, Moving, Making, Meaning," 300, 314.

Chapter 2

1. Francisco de Buitrago, "Arvore da Vida, e thezouro descuberto da Avore Irmãa da que se
fez a Cruz da Nossa Redempção: Para livrar dos maleficios do demonio, P.A. vida e saude dos
enfeitiçados ou vexados do mesmo demonio, e outras mtas," 1731, Biblioteca Nacional de Portugal (BNP), box 13114, reel 437 (microfilm). A special thank you to Ben Breen, who very kindly
introduced me to this manuscript in the Biblioteca Nacional. Following convention, I have chosen to use the modernized spelling of his name "Buitrago" rather than as it appears in the manuscript "Buytrago."

2. Breen, *Age of Intoxication,* 85–91; Kananoja, *Healing Knowledge in Atlantic Africa,*
61–65.

3. Buitrago, "Arvore da Vida," 6–7.

4. Buitrago, "Arvore da Vida," 7–8. Giovanni Antonio Cavazzi also described the poisonous
"Cassa Vero" tree as an evergreen with leaves similar to a laurel. Cavazzi also claims that "those
who eat of [the fruit] are not subjected to certain infirmities of the country." P. Giovanni Antonio
Cavazzi, *Istorica descrittione de tre regni Congo, Matamba, et Angola* (Milan: Nelle stampe del
l'Agnelli, 1690), 1.25.

5. Buitrago, "Arvore da Vida," 2–3, 5, 63.

6. Breen, *Age of Intoxication,* 85–91, n.87; Kananoja, *Healing Knowledge in Atlantic Africa,*
62–63.

7. Conde de Ficalho, *Plantas uteis da Africa Portugueza* (Lisbon: Imprensa Nacional, 1884),
168–169; Laman, *Dictionnaire Kikongo-Français,* 712; W. Holman Bentley, *Dictionary and*
Grammar of the Kongo Language, as Spoken at San Salvador (London: Baptist Missionary Society and Trübner, 1887–1895), 380.

8. BLR-3, no. 1646, C.S. 972.

9. Herman Bennett explores how politics in Atlantic Africa and early modern Europe mutually constituted each other in the fifteenth and sixteenth centuries. See Bennett, *African Kings*
and Black Slaves, 2–7.

10. Roquinaldo Ferreira, *Cross-Cultural Exchange in the Atlantic World: Angola and Brazil*
During the Era of the Slave Trade (Cambridge: Cambridge University Press, 2012), 248. For more
on the idea of "Atlantic Creoles," see Ira Berlin, *Many Thousands Gone: The First Two Centuries of*
Slavery in North America (Cambridge, MA: Harvard University Press, 1998); Heywood and
Thornton, *Central Africans, Atlantic Creoles*; Jane Landers, *Atlantic Creoles in an Age of Revolution*

(Cambridge, MA: Harvard University Press, 2010); Toby Green, *The Rise of the Trans-Atlantic Slave Trade in Western Africa, 1300–1589* (Cambridge: Cambridge University Press, 2012).

11. Kananoja, *Healing Knowledge in Atlantic Africa*, 32, 34–35. For a broader discussion of these issues regarding religious practices, see Sweet, *Recreating Africa*, 112–117.

12. For an example of scholarship that uses historical linguistics and focuses specifically on a West African region, see Edda L. Fields-Black, *Deep Roots: Rice Farmers in West Africa and the African Diaspora* (Indianapolis: Indiana University Press, 2008). As she notes, the challenges of conducting historical linguistics with the Atlantic family of languages in coastal Guinea are significantly greater than for Bantu languages due to these languages being understudied and therefore having far fewer archaeological studies in the region to work with. See pp. 12–13.

13. For a wider exploration of this idea across the Portuguese empire in the Atlantic and Indian Ocean worlds, see Hugh Cagle, *Assembling the Tropics: Science and Medicine in Portugal's Empire, 1450–1700* (Cambridge: Cambridge University Press, 2018).

14. Green, *Rise of the Trans-Atlantic Slave Trade*, 17.

15. George E. Brooks, *Landlords and Strangers: Ecology, Society, and Trade in Western Africa, 1000–1630* (Boulder, CO: Westview, 1993), 49–50, 53–54.

16. Gomez, *Reversing Sail*, 33–37. For more on early and medieval West Africa, see Gomez, *African Dominion*.

17. Sweet, *Domingos Álvares*, 13–17. For more on the heterogeneity of Dahomey itself, see Robin Law, *Ouidah: The Social History of a West African Slaving Port, 1727–1892* (Athens: Ohio University Press, 2004), 74–75.

18. Eastern Benue-Congo is the branch that contains the entire Bantu family. Kay Williamson and Roger Blench, "Niger-Congo," in *African Languages: An Introduction*, ed. Bernd Heine and Derek Nurse (Cambridge: Cambridge University Press, 2000), 30–36. Linguists working in Africa have long debated the classification of these languages, but the modern consensus has the Atlantic and Mande groups diverging from Proto-Mande-Atlantic-Congo at a much earlier period than Kwa and West Benue-Congo, which were more closely related as they shared a mother language, East Volta-Congo. See Williamson and Blench, "Niger-Congo," 18. For a brief discussion of some of the history of linguistic debate regarding Atlantic languages, see Fields-Black, *Deep Roots*, 14.

19. Williamson and Blench, "Niger-Congo," 18, 21, 27, 30–31.

20. Luis Nicolau Parés and Roger Sansi, "Introduction," in Parés and Sansi, eds., *Sorcery in the Black Atlantic*, 10–12; Suzanne Preston Blier, *African Vodun: Art, Psychology, and Power* (Chicago: University of Chicago Press, 1995), 24, 27; Paton, "Witchcraft, Poison, Law," 245, 248; Games, *Witchcraft in Early North America*, 20–21; Shaw, *Memories of the Slave Trade*, 201, 213–216.

21. Jean Barbot, *Barbot on Guinea: The Writings of Jean Barbot on West Africa, 1687–1712*, ed. P. E. H. Hair, Adam Jones, and Robin Law (London: Hakluyt Society, 1992), 1: 274–275. Barbot plagiarized freely in the original edition of *A Description of the Coasts of North and South Guinea* (1732). Editors Hair, Jones, and Law have painstakingly combed through and identified which parts of his narrative were original observations and which were copied: I am only using the original observations.

22. Willem Bosman, *A New and Accurate Description of the Coast of Guinea: Divided into the Gold, the Slave, and the Ivory Coasts (reprint of the 1705 first English edition)* (London: Ballantyne, 1907), 151–152.

23. Blier, *African Vodun*, 4; Law, *Ouidah*, 89, 92. For more on the destruction of the snake house during the Dahomean conquest of Ouidah, see William Snelgrave, *A New Account of Some Parts of Guinea, and the Slave Trade* (London: James, John, and Paul Knapton, at the Crown in Ludgate-Street, 1734), 10–12.

24. Bosman, *New and Accurate Description*, 382.

25. Chambers, *Murder at Montpelier*, 52, 56.

26. Bosman, *A New and Accurate Description*, 383–384; Chambers, *Murder at Montpelier*, 62.

27. Barbot, *Barbot on Guinea*, 275.

28. Kananoja, *Healing Knowledge in Atlantic Africa*, 81, 114.

29. Bosman, *A New and Accurate Description*, 225.

30. Bosman, *A New and Accurate Description*, 221–222.

31. Walter Hawthorne, *From Africa to Brazil: Culture, Identity, and an Atlantic Slave Trade, 1600–1830* (Cambridge: Cambridge University Press, 2010), 210; Sweet, *Domingos Álvares*, 26; Chambers, *Murder at Montpelier*, 62; Paton, "Witchcraft, Poison, Law," 245.

32. J. G. Christaller, *Dictionary of the Asante and Fante Language Called Tshi (Twi)*, 2nd ed. (Basel: Basel Evangelical Missionary Society, 1933), 240–242.

33. R. P. B. Segurola, *Dictionnaire Fon-Français* (Paris: Cotonou, 1963), 95, 159.

34. Chambers, *Murder at Montpelier*, 62.

35. Hicks, "Blood and Hair," 66.

36. Kananoja, *Healing Knowledge in Atlantic Africa*, 10, 32, 127–129.

37. Hicks, "Blood and Hair," 62, 64, 66–68.

38. For just a few examples, see Kimbundu *múxi* ("páu, arvore, tronco"); Umbundu *uti* ("tree"); Kikongo *nti* ("tree, timber, trunk . . . may sometimes be used vaguely for plants in general, especially medicinal plants"). Da Matta, *Ensaio de diccionario Kimbúndu-Portuguez*, 114; Sanders and Fay, *Vocabulary of the Umbundu Language*, 33; Bentley, *Dictionary and Grammar of the Kongo Language*, 398. As the word "tree" is part of core vocabulary that is generally conservative, it is useful as well for illustrating regular sound changes. For example, the regular sound correspondence chart I assembled as part of my linguistic research, for H21 Kimbundu the Proto-Bantu *ti > ʃi (in Portuguese "x" is often pronounced as "ʃ" in the IPA; mu- is a noun class prefix). See also BLR-3, no. 2881.

39. Segurola, *Dictionnaire Fon-Français*, 65.

40. Segurola, *Dictionnaire Fon-Français*, 65–66; Diedrich Westermann, *Evefiala or Ewe-English Dictionary: Gbesela Yeye or English-Ewe Dictionary*, 2nd ed. (Nendeln, Liechtenstein: Kraus Reprint, 1973), vol. 1, 231–232. Fon speakers use this same root in a compound with *vodun* for the word *àtímévodu* (group of "fetiches" living in a tree). For example, in Dahomey, leopards, which hunt from trees, were considered powerful *àtímévodu* in particular association with the king of Dahomey. In Zora Neale Hurston's 1927 interviews with Cudjoe Lewis, a Yoruba-speaking man enslaved and smuggled to Alabama in 1859, Lewis described an episode from his childhood when a man was put to death for taking the whiskers from a dead leopard, as they were "poisonous" and belonged to a king. Zora Neale Hurston, *Barracoon: The Story of the Last "Black Cargo"* (New York: Harper Collins, 2018), 26–28.

41. Chambers, *Murder at Montepelier*, 56.

42. Kay Williamson, *Dictionary of Ọ̀nị̀chà Igbo*, ed. Roger Blench (Benin: Ethiope Press, 1972), 204, 240, 252–253.

43. Blier, *African Vodun*, 69; Hawthorne, *From Africa to Brazil*, 210, 218–219; Chambers, *Murder at Montpelier*, 56, 64.

44. Bosman, *New and Accurate Description*, 223–224.

45. John Atkins, *A Voyage to Guinea, Brasil, and the West-Indies* (London: Printed for Caesar Ward and Richard Chandler, 1735), 56, 79, 101.

46. John Matthews, *A Voyage to the River Sierra-Leone on the Coast of Africa* (London: Printed for B. White and Son, at Horace's Head Fleet-Street, and J. Sewell, Cornhill, 1788), 132.

47. Hawthorne, *From Africa to Brazil*, 209, 222; David Robinson, *Muslim Societies in African History* (New York: Cambridge University Press, 2004), 45; Sylviane Anna Diof, "Devils or Sorcerers, Muslims or Studs: Manding in the Americas," in *Trans-Atlantic Dimensions of Ethnicity in the African Diaspora*, ed. Paul E. Lovejoy and David V. Trotman (London: Continuum,

2003), 147. For more on the adoption and circulation of *bolsas* into the Portuguese Atlantic, see Santos, "As bolsas de mandinga."

48. Jean-Léopold Diouf, *Dictionnaire Wolof-Français et Français-Wolof* (Paris: Éditions Karthala, 2003), 169, 338, 498.

49. Matthews, *Voyage to the River Sierra-Leone*, 132.

50. Mungo Park, *Travels in the Interior Districts of Africa,* ed. Kate Fergus Marsters (Durham, NC: Duke University Press, 2000), 92.

51. Barbot, *Barbot on Guinea*, 221; Bosman, *New and Accurate Description*, 123.

52. Blier, *African Vodun*, 74, 78, 80, 92.

53. Blier, *African Vodun,* 244–246, 293–296.

54. Bosman, *New and Accurate Description*, 123.

55. Westermann, *Evefiala*, vol. 1, 26, 28; Blier, *African Vodun*, 78.

56. Blier, *African Vodun*, 26. See suite of slavery words in Segurola, *Dictionnaire Fon-Français*, 286.

57. Christaller, *Dictionary of the Asante and Fante Languages,* 214, 498.

58. Lewis, *Hall of Mirrors*, 65, 160.

59. Westermann, *Evefiala*, vol. 1, 6; Segurola, *Dictionnaire Fon-Français*, 94–95; Blier, *African Vodun*, 2, 4.

60. Christaller, *Dictionary of the Asante and Fante Languages*, 37, 41, 44.

61. Bosman, *New and Accurate Description*, 147, 153–154.

62. While Bosman in the original Dutch described the object as a "beswoorne" (conjured thing) and the practice as "fetiche," the 1705 English translation changed these terms to "poison" and the "Art of poisoning" (in the original Dutch, Bosman only used "vergift" to refer to poisoned arrows and venomous animals). Still, in comparing the practices on the Gold Coast to the "Italian Fetiche"—Italians being strongly connected to poison in the early modern period—Bosman made a connection to poison. Bosman, *Nauwkeurige Beschryving van de Guinese Goud-Tand-en Slavekust*, 137–138; Bosman, *New and Accurate Description*, 148.

63. Bosman, *New and Accurate Description*, 148.

64. Blier, *African Vodun*, 70; Hawthorne, *From Africa to Brazil*, 216–219; Chambers, *Murder at Montpelier*, 62; Sweet, *Domingos Álvares*, 124; Paton, "Witchcraft, Poison, Law," 243, 245.

65. Blier, *African Vodun*, 310. Witchcraft accusations were also often directed inwardly within communities of eighteenth-century Temne speakers in Sierra Leone. See Shaw, *Memories of the Slave Trade,* 221.

66. Blier, *African Vodun*, 117–118.

67. Blier, *African Vodun*, 113–114.

68. de Luna, "Sounding the African Atlantic," 609.

69. See Heywood and Thornton, *Central Africans, Atlantic Creoles*; Cecile Fromont, *The Art of Conversion: Christian Visual Culture in the Kingdom of Kongo* (Chapel Hill: University of North Carolina Press, 2014); Thornton, *Kongolese Saint Anthony*; John K. Thornton, "Afro-Christian Syncretism in the Kingdom of Kongo," *Journal of African History* 54 (2013): 53–77.

70. Heywood and Thornton, *Central Africans, Atlantic Creoles*, 64.

71. Bennett, *African Kings and Black Slaves*, 5–6, 53–54.

72. Heywood and Thornton, *Central Africans, Atlantic Creoles*, 215–216.

73. Gómez, "The Power of Unknowing," in Crawford and Gabriel, eds., *Drugs on the Page,* 268.

74. Breen, *Age of Intoxication*, 83–84, 131.

75. P. António da Silva Maia, *Lições de gramática de Quimbundo (Português e Banto), dialecto Omumbuim: Língua indígena de Gabela, Amboim, Quanza-Sul, Angola, Africa Ocidental Portuguesa* (Cucujães, Portugal: published by author, 1957), 159–160, 163, 170.

76. Francis Katamba, "Bantu Nominal Morphology," in *The Bantu Languages*, ed. Derek Nurse and Gérard Philippson (London: Routledge, 2003), 115–116.

77. José de Oliveira Ferreira Diniz, *Populações indígenas de Angola* (Coimbra, Portugal: Impresa da Universidade de Coimbra, 1918), 186.

78. Heywood and Thornton, *Central Africans, Atlantic Creoles*, 82–90, 99–102; Ferreira, *Cross-Cultural Exchange in the Atlantic World*, 180–181, 186–187, 201–202. For more on Ndongo history and the war with Portugal, see Thornton, *History of West Central Africa*, 89–122.

79. Ferreira, *Cross-Cultural Exchange in the Atlantic World*, 181; Heywood and Thornton, *Central Africans, Atlantic Creoles*, 103–105; Kalle Kananoja, "Healers, Idolaters, and Good Christians: A Case Study of Creolization and Popular Religion in Mid-Eighteenth-Century Angola," *International Journal of African Historical Studies* 43, no. 3 (2010): 444–445; Kananoja, *Healing Knowledge in Atlantic Africa*, 35–42.

80. Heywood and Thornton, *Central Africans, Atlantic Creoles*, 102.

81. ANTT IL Series 30, vol. 72, 74, 77, 86, 91–95; Ferreira, *Cross-Cultural Exchange in the Atlantic World*, 179, 182, 186–188; Kananoja, *Healing Knowledge in Atlantic Africa*, 45–49.

82. Confissão de Alexandre, 9 December 1698, ANTT IL Series 30, vol. 72, pp. 55–58. Kalle Kananoja also explores this case in *Healing Knowledge in Atlantic Africa*, 47–48.

83. Denúncia de Guiomar, 15 June 1720, ANTT IL Series 30, vol. 95, pp. 81–91.

84. Denúncia de Guiomar, p. 81; Confissão de Catherina Borges, 5 August 1698, ANTT IL Series 30, vol. 72, p. 39.

85. Kananoja, *Healing Knowledge in Atlantic Africa*, 48–49.

86. Denúncia de Pascoal Rodrigues, 4 August 1716, ANTT IL Series 30, vol. 86, pp. 42–46; Denúncia de Dom João Manoel, 14 January 1717, ANTT IL Series 30, vol. 95, pp. 59–65; Denúncia de Antonio Careque, Domingos a Ganga, Izabel Camuça Caganga, Pedro Quibuca Quiangolla, Fernão Lungariambamba, Manoel a Ganga, Antonio a Quilombo, Lourenço quituque, Domingos Aganga, 10 June 1717, ANTT IL Series 30, vol. 93, pp. 135–141. Kananoja also discusses the case of Lt. Pascoal Rodrigues in *Healing Knowledge in Atlantic Africa*, 66–67.

87. Denúncia de Antonio Caraque et al., p. 136.

88. Denúncia de Antonio Caraque et al., pp. 135v–136; Denúncia de Manoel da Costa, 15 June 1720, ANTT IL Series 30, vol. 95, pp. 93–99; Denúncia de João Alonzo Cabengue, c. 1719–1723, ANTT IL Series 30, vol. 91, pp. 43–62.

89. Denúncia de Manoel da Costa, pp. 93–99.

90. James Sweet has made extensive use of the *cadernos do promotor* in his work. See Sweet, *Recreating Africa*. See also Kananoja, *Healing Knowledge in Atlantic Africa*, 22.

91. Denúncia de Pascoal Rodrigues, p. 45; Confissão de Heitor Cardozo, 28 September 1720, ANTT IL Series 30, vol. 91, pp. 37–39; Denúncia de Joseph Carrea e Domingas João, 3 October 1720, ANTT IL Series 30, vol. 94, pp. 371–374; Denúncia de Guiomar, p. 81. The outlier was a fragment that did not go into much detail beyond mentioning "demons" and "superstitions": Termos dos juramentos de Capitão Mor Luisde Maya Carrea e. P. Joseph Camargo, April 1717, ANTT IL Series 30, vol. 86, p. 343.

92. Confissão de Heitor Cardozo, p. 37.

93. Confissão de Gregorio Pascoal, 30 September 1698, ANTT IL Series 30, vol. 72, pp. 36–38.

94. Bennett, *African Kings and Black Slaves*, 137.

95. Daniela Buono Calainho, *Metrópole das mandingas: Religiosidade negra e inquisição portuguesa no antigo regime* (Rio de Janeiro: Garamond, 2008), 54, 68.

96. After Portugal, the largest disembarkation region was Spain, where 3,273 captive Africans landed. England, France, and the Netherlands combined only accounted for 456 individuals brought directly from Africa. Of course, these numbers did not include enslaved people brought from colonies to Europe. *Slave Voyages Database* (accessed 25 May 2022), https://www.slavevoyages.org/voyages/dE23fFMg.

97. Fromont, *Art of Conversion*, 162–168; David Northrup, *Africa's Discovery of Europe: 1450–1850* (New York: Oxford University Press, 2002), 178.

98. ANTT IL Series 28, Processos de Fé.

99. Processo de António Correira de Aguiar, 1757–1761, ANTT IL Series 28, f. 6270; Processo de Sebastião, 1691, ANTT IL Series 28, f. 9498.

100. ANTT IL Series 28; Walker, *Doctors, Folk Medicine and the Inquisition*, 10, 22. I found only two of the total *feitiçaria* trials in the Lisbon Inquisition that ended in the defendant being "relaxed to the secular arm" for execution—one Guilherme Cardinall, born in Bristol, England, in 1552 for sacrilege and Lutheranism, and a sixty-eight-year-old Old Christian woman from southern Portugal named Mécia da Costa for a relapse into *feitiçaria* as a *curandeira*—a folk healer. See Processo de Guilliam Cardinall, 1552, ANTT IL Series 28, f. 591; Processo de Mécia da Costa, ANTT IL Series 28, f. 6973-1.

101. See Sweet, *Domingos Álvares*, 192, 194, 198–205.

102. For general statistics, I used the data from 1671 to 1802 taken from the index to the *cadernos*. The index is incomplete but contains more than 750 pages of basic information on cases entered into the *cadernos*. Indice Incompleto do Promotor, ANTT IL Series 30, vol. 328.

103. Walker, *Doctors, Folk Medicine and the Inquisition*, 84.

104. For more on the use of these power objects and their significance in Lisbon, see the entirety of Calainho, *Metrópole das mandingas*.

105. Indice Incompleto do Promotor, ANTT IL Series 30, vol. 328.

106. Walker, *Doctors, Folk Medicine and the Inquisition*, 39.

107. Cagle, *Assembling the Tropics*, 13, 64–65, 116–121.

108. In the last twenty years there has been a significant increase in work on the sixteenth- and seventeenth-century Iberian contributions to natural history and the history of science. See Cañizares-Esguerra, *Nature, Empire, and Nation*; Cagle, *Assembling the Tropics*; Crawford and Gabriel, eds., *Drugs on the Page*; Breen, *Age of Intoxication*; Mauro José Caraccioli, *Writing the New World: The Politics of Natural History in the Early Spanish Empire* (Gainesville: University of Florida Press, 2021). On the Dutch, see Harold J. Cook, *Matters of Exchange: Commerce, Medicine, and Science in the Dutch Golden Age* (New Haven: Yale University Press, 2007).

109. Breen, *Age of Intoxication*, 7. Breen revises and expands on Schiebinger's work on bioprospecting and botany by examining the range of early modern "drugs" of interest to bioprospectors beyond plants and by including the Portuguese empire as a crucial player in Atlantic bioprospecting. Compare Breen's "Chapter 1: Searching for Drugs: Inventing Quina in Seventeenth-Century Amazonia," with Londa Schiebinger, *Plants and Empire: Colonial Bioprospecting in the Atlantic World* (Cambridge, MA: Harvard University Press, 2004), "Chapter 2: Bioprospecting." For a discussion of European bioprospecting in Atlantic Africa, see Kananoja, *Healing Knowledge in Atlantic Africa*, 52, 54, 58–59.

110. MS 1017, British Library (BL) Sloane Manuscripts, Medicine Charms and Receipts, 1; MS 723, BL Sloane Manuscripts, Medicine Charms and Receipts, 16v. The anonymous 1609 manuscript is particularly fascinating as it was written in a unique system of runes—very helpfully decoded with a key by an archivist in 1829. For more on uses of plantains in the African Atlantic, see Judith Carney and Nicholas Rosomoff, *In the Shadow of Slavery: Africa's Botanical Legacy in the Atlantic World* (Berkeley: University of California Press, 2009), 36–37, 116.

111. Elaine Leong, *Recipes and Everyday Knowledge: Medicine, Science, and the Household in Early Modern England* (Chicago: University of Chicago Press, 2018), 57.

112. Parrish, *American Curiosity*, 314–315; Gómez, *Experiential Caribbean*, 5, 11.

113. Crawford and Gabriel, "Thinking with Pharmacopoeias," in Crawford and Gabriel, eds., *Drugs on the Page*, 6, 9.

114. Gómez, "Power of Unknowing," in Crawford and Gabriel, eds., *Drugs on the Page*, 264, 268.

115. For a recent collection of essays examining pharmacopoeias from many different angles (including textual traditions, the codification of knowledge, the construction of ideas

about new worlds, and emergent ideas about nations), see Crawford and Gabriel, eds., *Drugs on the Page*.

116. See D. Caetano de Santo António, *Pharmacopea Lusitana: Mathodo pratico de preparar & compor os medicamentos na forma Galenica com todas as receitas mais uzuais*, (facsimile of 1704 1st ed.), ed. João Rui Pita (Lisbon: Edições Minerva, 2000). Caetano's work, the first of its kind, was swiftly followed by Semedo's 1707 *Observaçoens medicas doutrinaes* and João Vigier's *Pharmacopea Ulyssiponense*; the first two respectively went into five and four editions in the first half of the eighteenth century.

117. Semedo, *Observacoens medicas*, 2, 8–9; Vigier, *Pharmacopea Ulyssiponense*, 48, 398–401; Breen, *Age of Intoxication*, 105–106.

118. Semedo, *Observaçoens medicas*, 22, 25; Vigier, *Pharmacopea Ulyssiponense*, 393, 402.

119. Semedo, *Observaçoens medicas*, 11; Vigier, *Pharmacopea Ulyssiponense*, 402–403, 433. Neither Semedo nor Vigier provided citations, but Semedo's description of snake eating in Angola is so close to that of Richard Mead's that it likely came from the same source cited in Duarte Lopes' *Report of the Kingdom of Congo* (translated from Italian to English in 1597). See Mead, *A Mechanical Account of Poisons in Several Essays* (London: Printed by R. J. for Ralph Smith, 1702), 32.

120. Porter, *Greatest Benefit to Mankind*, 245–247, 251–252, 259, 267, 270, 281–283; Kananoja, *Healing Knowledge in Atlantic Africa*, 3, 158, 166–173; Walker, *Doctors, Folk Medicine and the Inquisition*, 37, 45; Rankin, *Poison Trials*, 5–6; Suman Seth, *Difference and Disease: Medicine, Race, and the Eighteenth-Century British Empire* (Cambridge: Cambridge University Press, 2018), 51, 162.

121. Porter, *Greatest Benefit to Mankind,* 231, 302; Walker, *Doctors, Folk Medicine and the Inquisition*, 7–8, 11–12, 24, 395.

122. Walker, *Doctors, Folk Medicine and the Inquisition*, 37, 46, 50, 75–79; Porter, *Greatest Benefit to Mankind*, 282–283; Owen Davies, *Cunning-Folk: Popular Magic in English History* (London: Hambledon & London, 2003), xiii–xiv, 29, 70, 83; Willem de Blécourt, "'Evil People': A Late Eighteenth-Century Dutch Witch Doctor and His Clients," in *Beyond the Witch Trials: Witchcraft and Magic in Enlightenment Europe*, ed. Owen Davies and Willem de Blécourt (Manchester: University of Manchester Press, 2004), 149, 163.

123. Mead, *Mechanical Account of Poisons in Several Essays* (1702); Richard Mead, *A Mechanical Account of Poisons in Several Essays*, 3rd ed. (Dublin: Printed by S. Powell, for John Watson, 1729); Mead, *A Mechanical Account of Poisons in Several Essays*, 4th ed., corrected (London: Printed for J. Brindley, Bookseller to His Royal Highness the Prince of Wales, 1747).

124. Parrish, *American Curiosity*, 6–7, 314–315.

125. Seth, *Difference and Disease*, 14.

126. Hicks, "Blood and Hair," 71–74.

127. While ancient authorities had made up about one-third of Mead's citations in both the 1702 and 1747 editions of his work, for Felice Fontana's 1781 treatise, that number had dropped to 5 percent: the vast majority of the works Fontana did cite had been published in the eighteenth century, and about a quarter had been published in the six years previously. Mead, *Mechanical Account of Poisons in Several Essays* (1702), (1747); Felice Fontana, *Traité sur le vénin de la vipere, sur les poisons americains, sur le laurier-cerise et sur quelques autres poisons vegetaux* (Florence, 1781). About 75 percent of Fontana's citations were published in the eighteenth century, 45 percent were post-1750, and 24 percent were post-1775. By 1814 the percentage of ancient sources in the citations would drop to 1 percent in Mathieu Joseph Bonaventure Orfila's comprehensive work. See Orfila, *Traité des poisons: Tires des Régnes mineral, vegetal et animal, ou toxocologie générale, considérée sous les rapports de la physiologie, de la pathologie et de la medicine légale* (Paris: Chez Crochard, 1814). Fontana did cite Mead himself, but in the context of challenging his work on vipers.

128. Felice Fontana, *Treatise on the Venom of the Viper; on the American Poisons; and on the Cherry Laurel and Some Other Vegetable Poisons*, trans. Joseph Skinner (London: Printed for J. Murray, No. 32 Fleet Street, 1787), v. In one series of experiments, Fontana tested several of the "many boasted remedies" against viper venom, finding theriac, electricity, and sucking the poison out with the mouth each to be ineffective. He also attempted to resolve debates from earlier poison treatise authors Mead and Francesco Redi on subjects like the flavor of viper venom, noting that "these contradictions reduced me to the philosophical necessity of tasting the venom myself." See vol. 2, "Chapter 1: Examen des remedes pratiqués contre la morsure de la Vipere."

129. Fontana, *Treatise on the Venom of the Viper*, 181.

130. Fontana, *Traité sur le vénin de la vipere*, 2.84; Charles Marie de la Condamine, *Relation abrégée d'un voyage fait dans l'interieur de l'Amérique méridionale: Depuis la Côte de la Mer du Sud, jusqu'aux Côtes du Brésil & de la Guiane* (Paris: Chez la Veuve Pissot, 1745), 67–68. Fontana's earliest work on ticunas appeared in the *Philosophical Transactions*, vol. 68, 1778.

131. Fontana, *Traité sur le vénin de la vipere*, 2.86.

132. Seth, *Difference and Disease*, 55, 162; Parrish, *American Curiosity*, 6–7, 17, 280, 288–289. See also Christopher Iannini, *Fatal Revolutions: Natural History, West Indian Slavery, and the Routes of American Literature* (Chapel Hill: University of North Carolina Press, 2012).

133. Blier, *African Vodun*, 24, 27.

134. Chambers, *Murder at Montepelier*, 64.

135. Davis, "Judges, Masters, Diviners," 935–936.

136. Shaw, *Memories of the Slave Trade*, 211–216.

137. Edna Bay, *Wives of the Leopard: Gender, Politics, and Culture in the Kingdom of Dahomey* (Charlottesville: University of Virginia Press, 1998), 320; Sweet, *Domingos Álvares*, 22.

138. The history of the slave trade and the impact of African-European encounters on Africa is one of the largest and most debated in Atlantic history. For a recent reevaluation of this debate, particularly of the contributions of Walter Rodney and John Thornton, see Bennett, *African Kings and Black Slaves*, 22–26.

139. Achim von Oppen, *Terms of Trade and Terms of Trust: The History and Contexts of Pre-Colonial Market Production Around the Upper Zambezi and Kasai* (Münster: Lit Verlag, 1994), 47, 236–238; de Luna, *Collecting Food, Cultivating People*, "Chapter 5: Life on the Central Frontier"; Joseph C. Miller, *Way of Death: Merchant Capitalism and the Atlantic Slave Trade, 1730–1830* (Madison: University of Wisconsin Press, 1988), 146.

140. Miller, *Way of Death*, 105–106.

141. Miller, *Way of Death*, 141–146. For more recent scholarship, see Ferreira, *Cross-Cultural Exchange in the Atlantic World*, 52–55, 67–69; Candido, *An African Slaving Port and the Atlantic World*, 233–236.

142. Miller, *Way of Death*, 142; Janzen, *Lemba*, 44–45, 51, 299; Thornton, *Kongolese Saint Anthony*, 102, 206–207.

143. Janzen, *Lemba*, 3–6, 51, 326.

144. Janzen, *Lemba*, 3–4.

145. *lémba* (Kikongo: to calm, to speak to appease; to turn away the anger of a *nkisi*; to invoke or conjure a *nkisi* so that it will be obliged to turn away its anger); *lembika* (Kikongo, Kikongo-Fiote, Civili: to appease); *lémba* (Kikongo east variant: to neuter, to tame); *Lémbe* (Kikongo: *nkisi* that one carries in a basket and causes pain in the chest); *malémbe* (Kikongo, Civili: salutation of peace, health, prosperity). Bentley, *Dictionary and Grammar of the Kongo Language*, 322; Laman, *Dictionnaire Kikongo-Français*, 391; Mission de Lalanda, *Dictionnaire Français-Fiote* (Paris: Maison-Mère, 1890), 6; P. Marichelle, *Dictionnaire Vili-Français* (Loango: Imprimerie de la Mission, 1902), 93, 105.

146. Janzen, *Lemba*, 3–4, 29, 35; Kananoja, *Healing Knowledge in Atlantic Africa*, 19. Attested as *nlémbo* (Kikongo: palm oil); and *lembe* (Kikongo, Civili: cassava or manioc leaf). Laman, *Dictionnaire Kikongo-Français*; Marichelle, *Dictionnaire Vili-Français*. For more on the use of manioc in the Kingdom of Kongo, see Birgit Ricquier, "A Foodie's Guide to Kongo Language History," *Africana Linguistica* 22 (2016): 107–146.

147. Thornton, *Kongolese Saint Anthony*, 1–2, 42–43, 53–56, 100–111, 132, 138–139. See the entire book for a detailed analysis of the life of Dona Beatriz Kimpa Vita and the Antonian Movement. See also MacGaffey, *Kongo Political Culture*, 2.

148. MacJannet, *Chokwe-English English-Chokwe Dictionary*, 9, 42; Vansina, *How Societies Are Born*, 192–193; Miller, *Way of Death*, 38.

149. Matta, *Ensaio de Diccionario Kimbúndu-Portuguez*, 50, 149.

150. For more on Nyaneka and Nkhumbi speakers, see Vansina, *How Societies Are Born*, 132–157; Miller, *Way of Death*, 30.

151. Da Silva, *Dicionário Português-Nhaneca*, 145, 238, 339. Early twentieth-century ethnography also noted that a *vimbanda* among Nyaneka speakers would only speak to spirits at night when the fires had gone out, possibly in a nonpublic or clandestine way. See Diniz, *Populações indígenas de Angola*, 429.

152. This translation is my own, from the Portuguese in da Silva, *Dicionário Português-Nhaneca*, 336: "Aonde havemos de ir à água, sem que haja água turva? Onde havemos de construir casa, sem que ai haja feiticeiros?"

153. Baião, Lecomte, and Sutter, *Dicionário Ganguela-Português*, 61. Note the d>l sound change, regular for Southern Moxico.

154. Le Guennec and Valente, *Dicionário Português-Umbundu*, 199; Sanders and Fay, *Vocabulary of the Umbundu Language*, 54.

155. Le Guennec and Valente, *Dicionário Português-Umbundu*, 17, 87, 145, 276, 403; Sanders and Fay, *Vocabulary of the Umbundu Language*, 8, 50; Schadeberg, "Derivation," in *The Bantu Languages*, ed. Derek Nurse and Gérard Philippson, 78–82.

156. Sanders and Fay, *Vocabulary of the Umbundu Language*, 54.

157. Miller, *Way of Death*, xii–xiii.

158. Wilhelm J. H. Möhlig and Kari Peter Shiyaka-Mberema, *A Dictionary of the Rumanyo Language: Rymanyo-English/English-Rumanyo, Including a Grammatical Sketch* (Cologne: Rüduger Köppe, 2005), 123, 156, 255.

159. Attested in Lwena, Southern Moxico, and Dcrirku. Horton, *Dictionary of Luvale*; Baião, Lecomte, and Sutter, *Dicionário Ganguela-Português*; Möhlig and Shiyaka-Mberema, *Dictionary of the Rumanyo Language*.

160. Baião, Lecomte, and Sutter, *Dicionário Ganguela-Português*, 54.

161. Bentley, *Dictionary and Grammar of the Kongo Langauge*, 289; Laman, *Dictionnaire Kikongo-Français*, 213–215.

162. Ferreira, *Cross-Cultural Exchange in the Atlantic World*, 52, 67–69; Candido, *African Slaving Port and the Atlantic World*, 233, 235–236.

163. Kananoja, *Healing Knowledge in Atlantic Africa*, 202–205.

164. Buitrago, "Arvore da Vida," 8–16.

165. Voyages Database (accessed 5 May 2022); Schwartz, *Sugar Plantations in the Formation of Brazilian Society*, 348.

166. Buitrago, "Arvore da Vida," 63v. Buitrago explains in detail how he made an infusion from the bark by adding water drop by drop, resulting in rosy red water.

167. MacGaffey, "Dialogues of the Deaf."

Chapter 3

1. Trial of Eve, 23 January 1746, LVA Orange CCOB, vol. 4, 454–455. See also Morgan, *Slave Counterpoint*, 612; Schwarz, *Twice Condemned*, 92.

2. William Waller Hening, *The Statutes at Large: Being a Collection of All the Laws of Virginia, from the First Session of the Legislature, in the Year 1619*, 13 vols. (Richmond: Printed by and for Samuel Pleasants, junior, printer to the commonwealth, 1809), vol. 4, 104–112.

3. Trial of Tom, 9 June 1744, LVA Caroline CCOB, vol. 1741–46, 288–290. In his survey of alleged crimes committed by enslaved people in Virginia county court records, Stuart Schwarz discussed the cases of both Eve and Tom. See Schwarz, *Twice Condemned*, 92–96.

4. Abbé Raynal, *Histoire philosophic et politique, des établissemens & du commerce des Européens dans les deux Indes* (A. Amsterdam, 1770), vol. 4, 155.

5. For example, see Schwarz, *Twice Condemned*; Fick, *Making of Haiti*; Beeldsnijder, "*Om Werk Van Jullie te Hebben*"; Voeks, *Sacred Leaves of Candomblé*; Harding, *A Refuge in Thunder*; Moitt, *Women and Slavery in the French Antilles*; Chambers, *Murder at Montpelier*; Weaver, *Medical Revolutionaries*. Some other works on poison focus mainly or exclusively on the discourse and interpretations of poison by white slaveholders and the law. For example, John Savage, "'Black Magic' and White Terror: Slave Poisoning and Colonial Society in Early 19th Century Martinique," *Journal of Social History* 40, no. 3 (2007): 635–662; Handler and Bilby, *Enacting Power*; Oudin-Bastide, *L'effroi et la terreur*; Paton, *Cultural Politics of Obeah*. For works that address investigations led by the enslaved into poisonings in detail, see Fett, *Working Cures*; Sweet, *Recreating Africa*; Davis, "Judges, Masters, Diviners"; Randy Browne, "The 'Bad Business' of Obeah: Power, Authority, and the Politics of Slave Culture in the British Caribbean," *William and Mary Quarterly* 68, no. 3 (2011): 451–480; Bryson, "Art of Power."

6. For example, see Schwarz, *Twice Condemned*, 104.

7. Morgan, *Slave Counterpoint*, 614.

8. For the five accused healing practitioners who were not of African descent, see Denúncia de Mariana Pinheira, 8 July 1687, ANTT IL 30, vol. 59, pp. 235–236; Denúncia de Antonia da Costa, 5 August 1721, ANTT IL 30, vol. 113, pp. 254–255; Processo de António Rodrigues da Silva, 1725, ANTT IL 28, f. 11426; Denúncia de Joanna Florencia, 5 April 1753, ANTT IL 28, vol. 113, p. 184; Processo de Pedro Rodrigues, 1790, ANTT IL 28, f. 6881. For a breakdown of healing practitioners, I identified forty-two in cases from Bahia (1680–1849), fifty-six in the Dutch Guianas (1720–1829), sixty-one from Martinique (1730–1848), and thirty-one from Cumberland and Brunswick Counties in Virginia (1740–1849). Schwarz did not identify healing practitioners as a demographic category in his survey of surviving county court records, so I chose the two counties with the highest number of cases and conducted my own survey.

9. Schwarz, *Twice Condemned*, 100–101; Sweet, *Recreating Africa*, 130; Sweet, *Domingos Álvares*, 118; Fett, *Working Cures*, 50–55, 64, 159–162; Pierre Pluchon, *Vaudou, sorciers, empoisonneurs de Saint-Domingue à Haïti* (Paris: Éditions Karthala, 1987), 81–82. Europeans in Atlantic Africa also relied heavily on African health practitioners as both more available and more effective than European physicians. See Kananoja, *Healing Knowledge in Atlantic Africa*, 66–67, 88–90, 166–168.

10. Denúncia de Branca e Pedro de Sesqueira Barbosa, 14 August 1701, ANTT IL Series 30, vol. 81, pp. 239–248. James Sweet also discusses this case in *Recreating Africa*, 148–149. For more on Angolan *feitiçeiros/as* in Inquisition records from Angola, Bahia, and Minas Gerais, see Mott, "Feiticeiros de Angola."

11. "gàngà," Bantu Lexical Reconstructions, accessed 1 December 2017, http://www.africamuseum.be/collections/browsecollections/humansciences/blr/results_main.

12. Sweet, *Recreating Africa*, 139–142.

13. "Savant," *Dictionnaire de l'Académie française*, 4th ed. (Paris: Chex la Vve B. Brunet, 1762), 686.

14. Memoires de Pierre-Clément de Laussat, Archives Départmentales de la Martinique (ADM), Fonds Pierre-Clément de Laussat Série J24–1, vol. 1, p. 85.

15. "COMMITTED to the gaol of Charles City," 8 September 1774, *Virginia Gazette* (Clementina Rind, ed.), no. 435, p. 4; "COMMITTED to the jail of Isle of Wight county," 10 October 1777, *Virginia Gazette* (Alexander Purdie, ed.), no. 141, p. 3. Sharla Fett discusses "conjure doctors" and "root doctors" extensively: see Fett, *Working Cures*, 62–64, 85–106.

16. Davis, "Judges, Masters, Diviners," 956; John Gabriel Stedman, *Narrative of a Five Years' Expedition, Against the Revolted Negroes of Surinam, in Guiana, on the Wild Coast of South America, from the Year 1772, to 1777* (London: J. Johnson & J. Edwards, 1796), vol. 2, 266–267. Accusations of *wisi* as a practice among the Saramaka Maroons, as described by Moravian missionaries in the 1770s, also had multiple interpretations: missionaries identified the practices as "poison," while the Maroons termed it "sorcery." See Richard Price, *Alabi's World* (Baltimore: Johns Hopkins University Press, 1990), 159.

17. "lukkuman," in C. L. Schumann, "Neger-Englisch und Deutsches Woeterboek," 3rd ed., 1783, MS in the possession of the Moravians of Paramaribo, published online at "Languages of Suriname," created 26 February 2003, http://www.suriname-languages.sil.org/index.html. See also Davis, "Judges, Masters, Diviners," 951, 956, 958. *Obeah* and associated terms, e.g., *obeahman*, were mostly restricted to the British Caribbean, according to Handler and Bilby, *Enacting Power*, 5–6; Chambers, *Murder at Montpelier*, 62. In Suriname, some practitioners and practices were referred to using *obeah*, both by English-speaking observers like John Gabriel Stedman and modern Maroon oral histories. See Stedman, *Narrative of a Five Years' Expedition* (1796), vol. 2, 89, 138–139, 262, 347; Price, *Alabi's World*, 8, 27.

18. Proces van Kwamina, 24 August 1763, NADH RVP, vol. 808, n.p.

19. Stedman, *Narrative of a Five Year's Expedition* (1796), vol. 2, 262, 356.

20. Trials of African healers across the Americas sometimes noted payments for goods and services rendered. As a sampling, see Procès d'un negre, November 1755, ANOM Série F3, vol. 245, pp. 405–407; Denúncia de Mariana e Francisca, 18 July 1745, ANTT IL Series 30, vol. 106, p. 128; Proces van Schipio van Anka, Apollo, en Jasmijn, 17 July 1770, NADH RVP, vol. 818, pp. 51–59. As was often the case, the Virginia country court trial summaries were extremely limited on details such as payment: discussions of payments in Virginia more commonly appeared in personal plantation papers. Sharla Fett has found abundant evidence of payment in both coin and kind in nineteenth-century Virginian plantation papers. See Fett, *Working Cures*, 99.

21. James A. Bear and Lucia C. Stanton, eds., *Jefferson's Memorandum Books: Accounts, with Legal Records and Miscellany, 1767–1826*, vols. 1–2 (Princeton: Princeton University Press, 1997), vol. 2, 992, 1005; Robert Carter to William Berry, 31 July 1786, Bull Run Regional Library (BRRL), Robert Carter Letterbook VII, p. 62; William Berry to Robert Carter, 11 August 1786, Virginia Historical Society (VHS), Carter Family Papers 1651–1861, Robert Carter Correspondence, 1754–1804.

22. Proces van Scaramouche en anders, 14 May 1765, NADH RVP, vol. 810, n.p.

23. Proces van La Rocke, 1 February 1741, NADH RVP, vol. 694, n.p.; Denúncia de Branca e Pedro de Sesquira Barbosa, 243; Proces van André, 1 February 1741, NADH RVP, vol. 794, n.p.; Proces van Marquis en Akkra, 27 February 1771, NADH RVP, vol. 819, pp. 234–246. "Papa" was a variation of "Popo" and an ethnic term used in Suriname for people from the coast surrounding the city of Ouidah in the Bight of Benin and "gelt" was Yiddish for money. For more on the term "Papa," see Margot van den Berg, "Ningretongo and Bakratongo: Race/Ethnicity and Language Variation in 18th Century Suriname," *Revue belge de philologie et d'histoire* 91, no. 3 (2013): 742. For more on Ashkenazim and Sephardim Jewish communities in eighteenth-century Suriname, see Alex van Stipriaan, "An Unusual Parallel: Jews and Africans in Suriname in the 18th and 19th Centuries," *Studia Rosenthaliana* 31, no. 1/2 (1997): 80, 87 n.37, 88 n.39. Cowries became

currency in the Bight of Benin and the Yoruba-speaking interior region during the expansions of the Oyo, Benin, and Dahomey states: they were also powerful objects used in various divinatory rituals. The trial does not specifically state that the "papa gelt" was cowrie shells, but it is a plausible guess. For more on cowries and their use as currency and in rituals, see Akinwumi Ogundiran, "Cowries and Rituals of Self-Realization in the Yoruba Region, ca. 1600–1860," in Ogundiran and Saunders, eds., *Materialities of Ritual in the Black Atlantic*, 68–86. See also Price, *Alabi's World*, 308–309, n.5.

24. Denúncia de Paulo Gomes e Ignacia, 159v.

25. Sweet, *Recreating Africa*, 144–145; Luis Nicolau Parés, *The Formation of Candomblé: Vodun History and Ritual in Brazil*, trans. Richard Vernon (Chapel Hill: University of North Carolina Press, 2013), 79. For the wider use of the term *calundú* in the late eighteenth century, see João José Reis, "Magia Jeje na Bahia: A invasão do calundu do pasto de cachoeira, 1785," *Revista Brasileira de Historia* 8, no. 16 (1988): 57–81.

26. Procès de Jean Baptiste et outres, May 1766, ANOM Série F3, vol. 246, pp. 267–275.

27. Reis, "Magia Jeje na Bahia," 67–70.

28. Fett, *Working Cures*, 40–41; Sweet *Domingos Álvares*, 124, 196; Schwarz, *Twice Condemned*, 101–102; Oudin-Bastide, *L'effroi et le terreur*, 151–152. For more on the theory of medicine in Africa from the precolonial period to the present, see Feierman and Janzen, eds., *Social Basis of Health*.

29. Unfortunately for Jan, the Maroons returned him to Parimaribo. Proces van Jan, 20 October 1762, NADH RVP vol. 806, n.p.

30. Proces van Kwamina, 24 August 1763, NADH RVP, vol. 808, n.p.; Proces van Scaramouche en anders, 14 May 1765, NADH RVP, vol. 810, n.p.

31. Proces van Scaramouche, n.p.

32. Hening, *Statutes at Large*, vol. 4, 104–112.

33. Robert Carter to Bennett Neal, 15 September 1781, BRRL Carter Letterbook IV, 117–119; Robert Carter to William Berry, 31 July 1786, BRRL Carter Letterbook VII, 62; Robert Carter to William Berry, 26 February 1788, BRRL Carter Letterbook VIII, 88.

34. Robert Carter Pass to Sampson, 31 January 1788, Carter Letterbook VIII, 77.

35. Denúncia de Branca e Pedro de Sesqueira Barbosa, 14 August 1701, ANTT IL Series 30, vol. 81, pp. 239–248.

36. Davis, "Judges, Masters, Diviners," 959.

37. Davis, "Judges, Masters, Diviners," 971.

38. Processo de Simão, 1688, ANTT IL Series 28, f. 8464, pp. 10, 16v, 17v.

39. Proces van Mars, 19 January 1773, NADH RVP, vol. 823, 77.

40. Denúncia de Thereza e Luis, 494.

41. Proces van Mainbij en La Lande, 31 January 1732, NADH RVP, vol. 787, n.p. The upper right corners where the page numbers would be are torn for significant portions of this volume.

42. Schwarz, *Twice Condemned*, 101–102; Parrish, *American Curiosity*, 285.

43. "Déclaration du roi qui interdit aux nègres esclaves des îles de fabriquer ou de distribuer aucun remède," 1 February 1743, ANOM, Série A Acts du pouvoir souverain, vol. 25, f. 199; André de Melo e Castro to D. João V, 30 August 1743, AHU Conselho Ultramarino Brasil— Bahia, box 77, f. 6363; Hening, *Statutes at Large*, vol. 4, 104–112; J. A. Schiltkamp and J. th. de Smidt, *West Indisch Plakaatboek: Plakaten, Ordonnantiën en andere wetten, uitgevaardigd in Suriname*, 2 vols. (Amsterdam: S. Emmering, 1973), vol. 1, 550–551.

44. Pluchon, *Vaudou, sorciers, empoisonneurs*, 15–16.

45. Mott, *Bahia: Inquisição & Sociedade*, 40–62. For more on the Inquisition's policing of popular magic and healing practices, see Walker, *Doctors, Folk Medicine and the Inquisition*; Sweet, *Domingos Álvares*.

46. Parrish, *American Curiosity,* 259, 262; Paton, "Witchcraft, Poison, Law," 235; Sweet, *Recreating Africa,* 145; Sweet, *Domingos Álvares,* 69–70; Weaver, *Medical Revolutionaries,* 61–67; Bryson, "Art of Power," 73.

47. Landon Carter, *The Diary of Landon Carter of Sabine Hall, 1752–1778,* vol. 1–2, ed. Jack P. Greene (Charlottesville: University Press of Virginia, 1965); cases where L. Carter believed medicines had been improperly administered or that his assistants had been negligent: vol. 1, 201, 203, 411–412, 527; vol. 2, 768, 774. Cases where L. Carter had not been informed of an illness or its progress: vol. 1, 217–218, 219, 297, 377, 520; vol. 2, 665, 776. Cases with a clear difference in medical treatment: vol. 2. 774, 793. For more on Landon Carter and Nassau's relationship, see Isaac, *Landon Carter's Uneasy Kingdom,* 315–322.

48. Jefferson hired "Perkins's Sam" to come to Monticello on two occasions to treat the strange declines of George Jr. and Sr. Since his semiretirement to Monticello in 1794, Jefferson had occasionally paid white practitioners for medicine, but in only two instances did he pay for the services of an enslaved practitioner: both were for Sam to treat the Georges. Bear and Stanton, eds., *Jefferson's Memorandum Books,* vol. 2, 31 February 1796, 936–937; 27 June 1798, 986; 27 July 1798, 998; 18 March 1799, 1000. Since George, George Jr., and Ursula apparently had similar symptoms, with Ursula lingering for four months and George Jr. ill for nearly a year and a half, it is reasonable to conclude that Jefferson's second payment to Sam in August 1799 was to treat George in the months before his death in November. Sam therefore was very likely the practitioner involved in each of the four unusual Monticello deaths. For Jefferson's two payments to "Perkins's Sam," see Bear and Stanton, eds., *Jefferson's Memorandum Books,* vol. 2, 25 November 1798, 992; 24 August 1799, 1005. See Martha Jefferson Randolph to Thomas Jefferson, 30 January 1800, vol. 31, 347–348 (see the footnote by Barbara Oberg); Thomas Mann Randolph to Thomas Jefferson, c. 19 April 1800, vol. 31, 522–524. See also Robert Carter to Dr. Thomas Thompson, 4 August 1786, BRRL Carter Letterbook VII, 138; Robert Carter to Dr. Timothy Harrington, 30 October 1787, BRRL Carter Letterbook VIII, 23; Robert Carter to Dr. Timothy Harrington, 30 July 1788, BRRL Carter Letterbook VIII, 155; Robert Carter to Bennett Neal, 15 September 1781, BRRL Carter Letterbook IV, 117–119; Robert Carter to William Berry, 31 July 1786, BRRL Carter Letterbook VII, 62; Robert Carter to William Berry, 26 February 1788, BRRL Carter Letterbook VIII, 88.

49. Pluchon, *Vaudou, sorciers, empoisonneurs,* 19; Weaver, *Medical Revolutionaries,* 1, 31–35, 50; Savage, "'Black Magic' and White Terror," 645.

50. van Stipriaan, *Surinaams contrast,* 362–368; Beeldsnijder, *"Om Werk Van Jullie te Hebben,"* 86, 150, 206–208; Davis, "Judges, Masters, Diviners," 951.

51. Denúncia de Jacome Rodrigues e Pedro Nunes, 27 April 1708, ANTT IL Series 30, vol. 76, p. 407.

52. Manoel de Magalhães to P. Francisco da Guerra, 18 May 1745, ANTT Amário Jesuitico e Cartório dos Jesuitas (AJCJ), box 70, f. 120.

53. Denúncia de Pedro Coelho Pimentel, 28 March 1686, ANTT IL Series 30, vol. 59, p. 135; Denúncia de Branca e Pedro de Sesqueira Barbosa, 14 August 1701, ANTT IL Series 30, vol. 81, pp. 239–248; Denúncia de Manoel Lopes e Barbara da Silva, 9 January 1743, ANTT IL Series 30, vol. 113, p. 188.

54. See Sweet, *Domingos Álvares,* 76–94 for more discussion of hiring out practices and medicine in urban Brazil.

55. Raymond de Laborde, "Effet dangereux de l'erreur et de la superstition dans les colonies françaises de l'Amérique," 1775, ANOM Série C8b, box 14, f. 4.

56. Procès d'un negre, January 1755, ANOM Série F3, vol. 245, p. 300. Pierre Pluchon also discusses this case in *Vaudou, sorciers, empoisonneurs,* 159–160.

57. Procès de Jacques (1767), 407–414.

58. *Jatropha curcas*, Kew Science, Plants of the World Online, accessed 4 December 2018, http://plantsoftheworldonline.org/taxon/urn:lsid:ipni.org:names:131462-2. According to the National Institutes of Health, cases of poisoning by *Jatropha curcas* are only from ingestion of the plant, especially the seeds. R. K. Singh, D. Singh, and A. G. Mahendrakar, "Jatropha Poisoning in Children," *Medical Journal of the Armed Forces India* 66 (January 2010): 80–81. In contrast, see the *manceniller* or *manchineel* tree (*Hippomane mancinella*), a tree still common today in Martinique mangrove swamps, which was well known for causing severe rashes on contact as early as Cosomo Bruni's 1660 report on the island. See "Description des îles d'Amerique en l'estat qu'elles estoient l'année 1660," 6 April 1660, ANOM Série C8b, box 1, f. 3. One of Thomas Walduck's letters from 1712 also mentions this tree and treatments for the inflammation caused by contact. See Thomas Walduck to James Petiver, Letter 8, n.d. (1712), BL Sloane Manuscripts, vol. 2302.

59. Mémoires de Pierre-Clément de Laussat, 13 September 1807, pp. 87–88.

60. Jean Baptiste Labat, *Nouveau voyage aux ils de l'Amerique, contenant l'histoire naturelle de ce pays* (Paris: Chez Guillaume Cavalier, 1722), vol. 4, 191.

61. Labat, *Nouveau voyage aux ils de l'Amerique*, vol. 4, 192–193.

62. Labat, *Nouveau voyage aux ils de l'Amerique*, vol. 1, 495.

63. Labat, *Nouveau voyage aux ils de l'Amerique*, vol. 1, 495–499.

64. André de Melo e Castro to D. João V, 8 July 1741, AHU, Administração Central Bahia, box 71, f. 5959, reel 73; André de Melo e Castro to D. João V, 30 September 1743, AHU, Administração Central Bahia, box 78, f. 6444, reel 79. In the 1743 report, Galveas expressed alarm as apparently over five thousand had sickened and died in recent years, throwing the colony into an "unfortunate, and terrible" situation. For a growing sense of crisis following illnesses in the 1730s, see Jesuit records, João Dias to P. Provintial, 28 July 1731, ANTT, Armário Jesuitico e Cartório dos Jesuitas, box 70, f. 380; Mattheus de Souza to P. Luis Valhozo, 13 January 1732, ANTT, Armário Jesuitico e Cartório dos Jesuitas, box 70, f. 166. On the 1743 ordinance, see André de Melo e Castro to D. João V, 30 August 1743, AHU, Administração Central Bahia, box 77, f. 6363, reel 78.

65. ANTT IL Series 30, vol. 55–131.

66. ANTT IL Series 30, vol. 55–131. See, for example, Denúncia de Paulo Gomes e Ignacia, 21 October 1749; Denúncia de Miguel e Maria Monjola, 25 July 1746, ANTT IL Series 30, vol. 118, pp. 90-94. This case is also interesting as it offers a rare glimpse of local judicial proceedings regarding feitiçaria. At the time of the denunciation of Maria Monjola and Miguel, local authorities already held them in the Jacobina jail.

67. Denúncia de Lucrecia Vieira, 6 May 1708, ANTT IL Series 30, vol. 76, p. 416; Denúncia de Lourença e outros, 1 April 1713, ANTT IL Series 30, vol. 80, p. 32; Denúncia de Cristina Lopes, 31 January 1732, ANTT IL Series 30, vol. 113, p. 259; Denúncia de Manoel do Valle Pontes, 23 March 1737, ANTT IL Series 30, vol. 113, p. 263; Processo de António Rodrigues da Silva, 1725, ANTT IL Series 28, f. 11426; Denúncia de Jacome Rodrigues e Pedro Nunes, 27 April 1708, ANTT IL Series 30, vol. 76, p. 407. Some local priests began to engage with and sometimes even incorporate African ideas into their practices, even if the church's laws did not. Often this syncretism was part of a deliberate and explicit effort to draw patients away from unsanctioned practitioners. Mott, *Bahia: Inquisição & Sociedade*, 34; Sweet, *Recreating Africa*, 222–223.

68. For example, see Proces van Apollo, 4 August 1742, NADH RVP, vol. 795; Proces van Osirus, Amanthea, en Macenissa, 25 August 1769, NADH RVP, vol. 816, pp. 29–31v.

69. 11 March 1749, NADH Sociëteit van Suriname (SVS), Resoluties van Gouverneur en Raden, vol. 141. Beeldsnijder also discusses this case in *"Om Werk Van Jullie te Hebben,"* 225.

70. Dinsdag den 12 Augustus 1766, NADH SVS, Resoluties van Gouverneur en Raden, vol. 158. This detail appears in the SVS resolutions; it is unclear how long Bettie's execution was delayed or if it was suspended. For her trial, where she and two others were sentenced to burn for

allegedly poisoning other enslaved people, see Proces van Sara, Januarij, en Bettie, 4 August 1766, NADH RVP, vol. 812.

71. Hening, *Statutes at Large*, vol. 4, 105.

72. For example, see Trial of Isaac and Quash, 29 May 1759, LVA Cumberland CCOB, vol. 1758–62, pp. 56–57, reel 23.

73. LVA CCOB from Brunswick and Cumberland Counties.

74. "Miscellaneous Documents, Colonial and State: From the Originals in the Virginia State Archives," *Virginia Magazine of History and Biography* 18 (October 1910): 395–396.

75. Marquis de Champigny de Noroy and César Marie de La Croix to Compte de Maurepas, 8 October 1741, ANOM Série C8a, box 53, f. 207. For more on earlier concerns about deaths of livestock and enslaved people—framed as disastrous economic losses for slaveholders—see Marquis de Feuquières to Comte de Maurepas, 30 October 1725, ANOM Série C8a, box 34, f. 113. For a broader French Caribbean context on livestock die-offs, see Garrigus, "'Like an Epidemic.'"

76. Since the 1682 Affair of the Poisons, the legal definition of *maléfice* had been "pretended magic," but in the French Caribbean colonies the term was used almost synonymously and frequently in conjunction with "poison." Oudin-Bastide, *L'effroi et la terreur*, 23–27; Paton, "Witchcraft, Poison, Law," 255–256.

77. ANOM Série F3, vol. 244–246; Pluchon, *Vaudou, sorciers, empoisonneurs*, 156–158. Strikingly, given courts' concerns in the late eighteenth and early nineteenth centuries, few of these mid-century cases involved specifically identified mineral poisons, such as arsenic. Only three cases, one from 1747 and two from 1755, mentioned arsenic at all, and one was ruled an accident (a young enslaved boy had unknowingly transported drugs that had been carelessly mixed with arsenic by his owner). Oudin-Bastide, *L'effroi et la terreur*, 31; Procès d'un petit negre, March 1755, ANOM Série F3, vol. 245, pp. 312–314 (accident); Procès de Confident, May 1755, ANOM Série F3, vol. 245, pp. 346–350; Procès d'une negresse, November 1747, ANOM Série F3, vol. 244, pp. 613–614.

78. He was convicted "d'avoir porté sur luy des poudres et Drogues suspectes et inconnues, et dont les usages et consequences ne pouvoient etre que très prejudiciable." Procès de Pierre dit Cartouche, January 1753, ANOM Série F3, vol. 245, pp. 111–112. Sometimes captured Maroons were found carrying such "suspicious drugs," which they claimed were for curing snakebites, protection from gunshots, or what the court vaguely termed "superstitious practices." Procès de trois negres marons, November 1755, ANOM Série F3, vol. 245, pp. 400–401; Procès de deux negres, January 1755, ANOM Série F3, vol. 245, pp. 297–299; Procès d'un negre, November 1755, ANOM Série F3, vol. 245, pp. 405–407.

79. Procès de Jean François, January 1742; Déclaration du roi qui interdit aux nègres esclaves des îles de fabriquer ou de distribuer aucun remède, et qui ordonne l'exécution de l'édit de février 1724 sur les empoisonneurs, 1 February 1743, ANOM Série A, vol. 25, f. 199.

80. Governeur Mauicius to Sociëteit van Suriname, 8 May 1745, NADH SVS, vol. 275, pp. 766–775, reel 3102.

81. Proces van Baron, 10 May 1742, NADH RVP, vol. 795, n.p.; Proces van Sambo, 10 May 1742, NADH RVP, vol. 795, n.p.; Proces van Abraham, 10 May 1742, NADH RVP, vol. 795, n.p.; Proces van Emanuiel, 4 August 1742, NADH RVP, vol. 795, n.p..

82. Fuentes, *Dispossessed Lives*, 8, 37–40.

83. Governeur Mauicius to Sociëteit van Suriname, 8 May 1745.

84. No. 449 Notifikatie: Bestraffing van slaven die mensen of beesten vergiftigen, 22 December 1745, in Schiltkamp and Smidt, *West Indisch Plakaatboek*, vol. 1, 550; Davis, "Judges, Masters, Diviners," 963–964.

85. For a discussion of a similar temporary decision following an alleged poisoning in 1768 Barbados to bury bodies of the convicted at sea to prevent funerals among the enslaved, see

Fuentes, *Dispossessed Lives*, 101, 103, 117–119. For more on the importance of funeral practices within enslaved communities more generally, see Vincent Brown, *The Reaper's Garden: Death and Power in the World of Atlantic Slavery* (Cambridge, MA: Harvard University Press, 2008), 61–62.

86. Proces van Goliath, 18 December 1745, NADH RVP, vol. 798; Proces van Philip, 18 December 1745, NADH RVP, vol. 798; Proces van Bossoe, 18 December 1745, NADH RVP, vol. 798.

87. Hening, *Statutes at Large*, vol. 4, 105; Schwarz, *Twice Condemned*, 97.

88. William Blackstone, ed., *Commentaries on the Laws of England* (Oxford: Clarendon, 1765), book 4, 193, 196.

89. Sweet, *Domingos Álvares*, 149. For more on how the Lisbon Inquisition operated in Bahia, see Mott, *Bahia: Inquisição & Sociedade*.

90. Mott, *Bahia: Inquisição & Sociedade*, 44, 49–50, 52.

91. Denúncia de Thereza e Luis, 17 January 1778, ANTT IL Series 30, vol. 129, pp. 490–494.

92. Davis, "Judges, Masters, Diviners," 971.

93. Oudin-Bastide, *L'effroi et la terreur*, 109.

94. Maxim de Bompar and Charles Marin Hurson to Antoine Louis Rouillé, 16 June 1753, ANOM Série C8a, box 60, f. 7.

95. André de Melo e Castro to D. João V, 30 September 1743, AHU, Administração Central Bahia, box 78, f. 6444.

96. Davis, "Judges, Masters, Diviners," 967–968; Beeldsnijder, *"Om Werk Van Jullie te Hebben,"* 244–247.

97. Davis, "Judges, Masters, Diviners," 971.

98. *Le Code Noir ou Edit du Roy, 1685* (Paris: Chez Claude Girard, 1735); Nicolas François Arnoul de Vaucresson to Comte de Pontchartrain, 20 May 1713, ANOM Série C8a, box 19, f. 341.

99. Proces van Kees, 5 May 1735, NADH RVP, vol. 789, pp. 47–48v, 58–60v. Beeldsnijder also discusses Kees's case: see Beeldsnijder, *"Om Werk Van Jullie te Hebben,"* 227, n.66.

100. Proces van Sambo, 10 May 1742, NADH RVP, vol. 795, n.p.

101. Procès de Jean Baptiste et outres, May 1766, ANOM Série F3, vol. 246, pp. 267–275; Procès de Jacques, September 1767, ANOM Série F3, vol. 246, pp. 407–414.

102. de Laborde, "Effet dangereux de l'erreur."

103. From his file, it appears the Kees was not punished by the court, but his fate is unclear.

104. Proces van Kees, pp. 47–48v; Proces van Sambo, n.p.

105. Procès de Jacques, pp. 410–411.

106. Mémoires de Pierre-Clément de Laussat, 18 February 1808, pp. 94, 97–98.

107. Trial of Tom, 9 June 1744, LVA Caroline CCOB, vol. 2, pp. 288–290; Hening, *Statutes at Large*, vol. 4, 104–106.

108. Mémoires de Pierre-Clément de Laussat, 18 February 1808, p. 100.

109. *Dictionnaire de l'Académie française*, 1st ed. (Paris: Chez la Veuve de Jean Baptiste Coignard, Imprimeur ordinaire du Roy, & de l'Académie Françoise, 1694), vol. 2, 270; *Dictionnaire de l'Académie française*, 4th ed. (Paris: Chez la Veuve b. Brunet, 1762), vol. 1, 389, vol. 2, 412; *Dictionnaire de l'Académie française*, 6th ed. (Paris: Imprimerie et Librarie de Firmin Didot frères, Imprimeurs de l'Institut de France, 1835), vol. 1, 400; Orfila, *Traité des poisons*, vol. 1.1, 146, 183–184; vol. 1.2, 12, 227; vol. 2.1, 104.

110. *Dictionnaire de l'Académie française* (1835), 1:629. For more on changing discourses on suicide and poison in nineteenth-century Bahia, see Jackson André da Silva Ferreira, "Loucos e pecadores: Suicide na Bahia do século XIX" (PhD diss., Universidade Federal da Bahia, 2004)

111. *Dictionnaire de l'Académie française* (1694) 2:621, (1762) 2:913, (1835) 2:915; "venefice," *Trésor de la langue Française informatisé (TLFi)* (accessed 23 July 2016); Émile Littré, *Dictionnaire de la langue française*, 4 vols. (Paris: L. Hachette, 1873–74), 4:2438.

112. Samuel Farr, "Elements of Medical Jurisprudence," originally published 1788, in Thomas Cooper, *Tracts on Medical Jurisprudence* (Philadelphia: James Webster, 1819), 47–54; William Dease, "Remarks on Medical Jurisprudence; Intended for the General Information of Juries and Young Surgeons," originally published 1793, in Thomas Cooper, *Tracts on Medical Jurisprudence* (Philadelphia: James Webster, 1819), 89, 98–100.

113. "toxicology, n.," *OED Online* (accessed 21 July 2016); "toxicology," *TFLi*, accessed 8 July 2016. Orfila based his classification system on the work of François-Emmanuel Fodéré: see *Traité de médecine légale et d'hygiène publique, ou de police de santé*, 2nd ed. (Paris: L'imprmerie de Mame, 1813).

114. Orfila, *Traité des poisons*, vii–viii.

115. Littré, *Dictionnaire de la langue française*, vol. 4, 2290.

116. Orfila, *Traité des poisons*, vol. 2.2, 4–7, 180–183, 225–227. On the poisoned arrows, Orfila corresponded with Alexander von Humboldt.

117. Orfila, *Traité des poisons*, 1.1 Poisons mercuriels, 1.2 Poisons arsénicaux, 1.3 Poisons antimoniaux.

118. Examples included a toddler eating rat poison containing mercury sublimate, a tormented young woman putting arsenic in her soup, and a young man accidentally overdosing on opium. Orfila, *Traité des poisons*, vol. 1.1, 67, 143; vol. 2.1, 143. Mead mentioned opium as a poison if taken in too large a dose as early as 1702. See Mead, *Mechanical Account of Poisons in Several Essays*, "Essay the Fourth: Of Opium," 131–148.

119. Orfila, *Traité des poisons*, vol. 2.2, 294.

120. John Garrigus describes the construction of narratives about poison as a collaborative form of myth-making in the case of Makandal in 1750s Saint Domingue. See Garrigus, "'Like an Epidemic,'" 651.

Chapter 4

1. An earlier version of part of this chapter appeared in *Medicine and Healing in the Age of Slavery*, ed. Sean Morey Smith and Christopher D. E. Willoughby, Copyright 2021 by Louisiana State University Press. Reproduced by permission of LSU Press.

2. "Swart Jan" (Black John) was how this man referred to himself when asked by the court to state his name during his examination. Accordingly, I will refer to him as such. For information on the plantation and its geographic location, see Alexander de Lavaux, "Algemeene kaart van de Colonie of Provintie van Suriname," 1737, Bijzondere Collecties van de Universiteit van Amsterdam. The term "Coromanti/Coromantee" in English referred generally to Akan peoples from the Gold Coast of West Africa. See Gwendolyn Midlo Hall, "African Ethnicities and the Meaning of 'Mina,'" in Lovejoy and Trotman, eds., *Trans-Atlantic Dimensions of Ethnicity*, 70.

3. On *wissimen*, see Davis, "Judges, Masters, Diviners," 956; Stedman, *Narrative of a Five Years' Expedition*, vol. 2, 266–267; Price, *Alabi's World*, 159.

4. On *wiriwiri*, see Beeldsnijder, "*Om Werk Van Jullie te Hebben*," 228. For an analysis on the relationships between plants and magical power in Suriname, see Tinde van Andel, Rofie Ruysschaert, Kobeke Van de Putte, and Sara Groenendijk, "What Makes a Plant Magical? Symbolism and Sacred Herbs in Afro-Surinamese *Winti* Rituals," in *African Ethnobotany in the Americas*, ed. Robert Voeks and John Rashford (New York: Springer, 2013), 247–284.

5. Interestingly, in his testimony Swart Jan noted in explaining his wife's death by suicide that she was a Coromantee (Akan). People from the Gold Coast had a reputation on slave ships and in the slave societies of the Atlantic for suicide. For more, see Terri L. Snyder, *The Power to Die: Slavery and Suicide in British North America* (Chicago: University of Chicago Press, 2015), 10.

6. Proces van Swart Jan, 10 December 1744, NADH RVP, vol. 797, n.p. The upper corners of this and several other volumes in the collection have been damaged by water, eliminating page numbers.

7. MacGaffey, *Kongo Political Culture*, 2. The literature on this subject is vast. As a brief sampling, see E. E. Evans-Pritchard, *Witchcraft, Oracles, and Magic Among the Azande* (Oxford: Clarendon, 1976); Robert M. Baum, "Crimes of the Dream World: French Trials of Diola Witches in Colonial Senegal," *International Journal of African Historical Studies* 37, no. 2 (2004): 201–228; Thornton, "Cannibals, Witches, and Slave Traders."

8. Gordon, *Invisible Agents*, 28–34; Kathryn M. de Luna, "Affect and Society in Precolonial Africa," *International Journal of African Historical Studies* 46, no. 1 (2013): 124–133; David Schoenbrun, "A Mask of Calm: Emotion and Founding the Kingdom of Bunyoro in the Sixteenth Century," *Comparative Studies in Society and History* 55, no. 3 (2013): 638–639; Nancy Rose Hunt, "The Affective, the Intellectual, and Gender History," *Journal of African History* 55, no. 3 (2014): 335–338. Hunt's article is also useful as a state of the field on dozens of affective African histories, with articles accelerating in the past twenty years, for further reading. For a slightly more critical take on methods relating to emotion, affect, and performance, see Tom McCaskie, "Unspeakable Words, Unmasterable Feelings: Calamity and the Making of History in Asante," *Journal of African History* 59, no. 1 (2018): 4, 19–20. For an introduction to the field of the history of emotions more broadly, see William M. Reddy, *The Navigation of Feeling: A Framework for the History of Emotions* (Cambridge: Cambridge University Press, 2001); Barbara H. Rosenwein, "Worrying About Emotions in History," *American Historical Review* 107, no. 3 (2002): 821–845; Nicole Eustace et al., "AHR Conversation: The Historical Study of Emotions," *American Historical Review* 117, no. 5 (2012): 1487–1531.

9. McCaskie, "Unspeakable Words, Unmasterable Feelings," 20. McCaskie's article focuses on Asante storytelling relating to the reigns of two eighteenth-century rulers.

10. Denúncia de Thereza e Luis, 17 January 1778, ANTT IL Series 30, vol. 129, pp. 490–494.

11. Proces van Mainbij en La Lande, 31 January 1732, NADH RVP, vol. 787, n.p.

12. De Laborde, "Effet dangereux de l'erreur"; Pierre Dessalles, *La vie d'un colon à la Martinique au XIXème Siècle: Correspondance 1808-1834*, ed. Fenri de Fremont (La Haye du Puits: Imprimerie Cauchard, 1980), 85, 181; Étienne Rufz de Lavison, *Recherches sur les empoisonnements pratiqués par les nègres à la Martinique* (Paris: Chez J. B. Ballière, 1844), 5. Laborde and Rufz de Lavison were both skeptics of poisoning claims, arguing for other possible causes of *mal d'estomac* than poisoning. Rana Hogarth explores *mal d'estomac*, defined as a "slave disease" called Cachezia Africana, or dirt eating, in the nineteenth-century British Caribbean. See Hogarth, *Medicalizing Blackness*, 81–103.

13. de Laborde, "Effet dangereux de l'erreur."

14. Proces van Swart Jan, n.p.

15. Notably, convulsions and swelling were also frequently noted symptoms of the bite of greatly feared venomous snakes in the Caribbean, particularly the fer-de-lance (a name used to refer to at least two species of viper, including *Bothrops asper* on the mainland Caribbean and *Bothrops lanceolatus* endemic specifically to the island of Martinique). Both species were extremely dangerous, as they lived in lowland areas and came into frequent contact with humans—especially in the cane fields. However, there is no indication from my sources that either enslaved people or enslavers identified these convulsions and fits that had such a direct and obvious cause with deliberate human-caused poisoning, despite the overlap in symptoms. Mémoires de Pierre-Clément de Laussat, vol. 1, pp. 61–62; Stedman, *Narrative of a Five Years' Expedition* (1796), vol. 2, 133–134.

16. Proces van Swart Jan, n.p.

17. Proces van Coffie, 20 April 1739, NADH RVP, vol. 793, pp. 56–56v.

18. Processo de Gracia, 1699, ANTT IL Series 28, f. 12658.

19. Dessalles, *La vie d'un colon à la Martinique*, 68; Martha Jefferson Randolph to Thomas Jefferson, 30 January 1800, in *The Papers of Thomas Jefferson*, ed. Barbara B. Oberg (Princeton: Princeton University Press, 2004), vol. 31, 347–348.

20. Beeldsnijder, *"Om Werk Van Jullie te Hebben,"* 227.

21. For the significance of the belly in Africa and examples in West African languages, see Blier, *African Vodun*, 32–33, 145, 295, 309–310; Christaller, *Dictionary of the Asante and Fante Languages*, 556; Williamson, *Dictionary of Ònìchà Igbo*, 5.

22. Blier, *African Vodun*, 144.

23. Blier, *African Vodun*, 142.

24. Christaller, *Dictionary of the Asante and Fante Languages*, 556.

25. Williamson, *Dictionary of Ònìchà Igbo*, 5.

26. Blier, *African Vodun*, 145, 295, 309.

27. Blier, *African Vodun*, 310.

28. Blier, *African Vodun*, 32–33.

29. MacGaffey, "Dialogues of the Deaf," 249–267. For more on how such convergences facilitated cross-cultural medical interactions in Atlantic Africa, see Kananoja, *Healing Knowledge in Atlantic Africa*, 32–33, 158–160.

30. Proces van Banielje, Spadelje en Diekje, 16 May 1766, NADH RVP, vol. 812, p. 484; Proces van Seba, Roselina, Quassiba, en Margo, 11 May 1769, NADH RVP, vol. 815, n.p.

31. Copie d'un jugement rendu par le tribunal special de la Martinique condemmant à être brûlée vive la négresse Émilie, 9 June 1806, ANOM Série C8a, box 112, f. 210; Louis Thomas Villaret de Joyeuse to Denis Decrès, 15 June 1806, ANOM Série C8a, box 112, f. 219. This case is well known to scholars of the French Caribbean. For more details, see Oudin-Bastide, *L'effroi et la terreur*, 87.

32. Villaret to Decrès, 15 June 1806; Mémoires de Pierre-Clément de Laussat, vol. 1, pp. 76–77.

33. Mémoires de Pierre-Clément de Laussat, vol. 1, p. 76.

34. Mémoires de Pierre-Clément de Laussat, vol. 1, p. 77.

35. Clark, *Thinking with Demons*, 111, 133.

36. Levack, *Witch-Hunt in Early Modern Europe*, 9, 13, 16–17.

37. For more on the "Medea myth" and the trope of vengeful wife as poisoner, see Mollenauer, *Strange Revelations*, 53–56.

38. Jean Nicot, *Thresor de la langue françoyse, tant ancienne que modern* (Paris: David Douceve, 1606), vol. 1, 225; for the connection between sorcery and poison, see vol. 2, 601.

39. Thomas Elyot, "The Dictionary of Syr Thomas Eliot Knyght (1538)," *Lexicons of Early Modern English*, University of Toronto, https://leme.library.utoronto.ca.

40. Games, *Witchcraft in Early North America*, 52.

41. Levack, *Witch-Hunt in Early Modern Europe*, 1, 19–21, 214–215, 227–228; Bengt Ankarloo and Stuart Clark, "Introduction," in *Witchcraft and Magic in Europe: The Eighteenth and Nineteenth Centuries*, ed. Ankarloo and Clark (London: Athlone, 1999), ix.

42. Raphael Bluteau, *Vocabulario Portuguez & Latino* (Coimbra: No Collegio das Artes da Companhia de Jesus, 1728), vol. 4, 63–66.

43. Semedo, *Observaçoens medicas doutrinaes*, 566–567. For more on the uses of menstrual blood in love magic and as a poison, see Mollenauer, *Strange Revelations*, 57, 86; von Germeten, *Violent Delights, Violent Ends*, 110.

44. Mollenauer, *Strange Revelations*, 53, 61–65, 74–77, 84–86, 95.

45. Randa Helfield, "Poisonous Plots: Women Sensation Novelists and Murderesses of the Victorian Period," *Victorian Review* 21, no. 2 (Winter 1995): 161–188.

46. For more on fingernails as an ingredient in conjure packets in the US South, see Fett, *Working Cures*, 102.

47. Proces van Picard, 4 August 1742, NADH RVP, vol. 795, n.p.

48. Governor the Earl of Bellomont to the Council of Trade and Plantations, 26 July 1700, Colonial State Papers Online, accessed 2 August 2017, https://search.proquest.com/csp/.

49. For more on eighteenth-century anti-Catholic sentiment and conflict between the British and French in North America, see Linda Colley, *Britons: Forging the Nation, 1707–1837* (New Haven: Yale University Press, 1992).

50. Labat, *Nouveau voyage aux isles de l'Amerique*, vol. 4, 198.

51. Edward Long, *The History of Jamaica: or, General Survey of the Ancient and Modern State of the Island*, 3 vols. (London: Printed for T. Lowndes, 1774), vol. 3, 779.

52. Anthony Blom, *Verhandeling over den Landbouw, in de Colonie Suriname, volgens eene negentien-jarrige ondervinding zamen gbsteld* (Haarlem, Netherlands: Cornelis van de Aa., 1786), 387–388.

53. Stedman, *Narrative of a Five Years' Expedition*, vol. 1, 404; vol. 2, 266–267.

54. NADH RVP, vols. 823–829.

55. de Laborde, "Effet dangereux de l'erreur"; Mémoires de Pierre-Clément de Laussat, 13 September 1807, vol. 1, pp. 86–87.

56. Collard, *Crime of Poison in the Middle Ages*, 50.

57. Robert Boyle, "The Notion of Specific Remedies Prov'd Agreeable to Mechanical Philosophy" (1686), in *The Philosophical Works of the Honourable Robert Boyle*, ed. Peter Shaw (London: Printed for W. and J. Innys, J. Osborn, and T. Longman, 1725), vol. 3, 550. See also Benjamin Patrick Breen, "Tropical Transplantations: Drugs, Nature, and Globalization in the Portuguese and British Empires, 1640–1755" (PhD diss., University of Texas, Austin, 2015), 144, 157, for a discussion of European ideas about Africa as a "poisoned landscape."

58. Carter, *Diary of Landon Carter*, vol. 2, 994.

59. Robert Carter to Bennett Neal, 15 September 1781, BRRL Carter Letterbook IV, 117–119; Robert Carter to William Berry, 31 July 1786, BRRL Carter Letterbook VII, 62.

60. For example, see Denúncia de Pedro Coelho Pimentel, 28 March 1686, ANTT IL Series 30, vol. 59, p. 135.

61. Denúncia de Mai Catherina, 12 May 1704, ANTT IL Series 30, vol. 76, pp. 11–12.

62. The numbers for total cases, total cases with a target, and total cases with an enslaved target that I have seen are as follows: Bahia (1680–1839), 99, 27, 12; Suriname (1722–1825), 128, 102, 71; Virginia (1706–1784), 179, 136, 46; Martinique (1730–1848), 117, 100, 56. ANTT IL Series 28 and Series 30, vol. 55–131; NADH RVP vol. 783–915; Schwarz, *Twice Condemned*, Table 10, p. 96; LVA, Brunswick CCOB, vol. 1–36; LVA, Cumberland CCOB, vol. 1749–51 to 1844–51; ANOM Série F3, Collection Moreau de Saint-Méry, Annales du Conseil souverain de la Martinique, vol. 244–246; ANOM Dépôt des papiers des colonies, greffes Martinique, Cour d'assises de Fort-de-France and Saint-Pierre; ANOM Série C8, Correspondance à l'arrivée en provenance de la Martinique (for cases from Villaret's tribunal, 1806–1808); ADM Série U7, Cour Prévôtale. Schwarz's analysis of Virginia trials of enslaved people runs from 1706 to 1784, but the first poison cases did not appear until 1730.

63. For examples of the former, see Denúncia de Macaco, 1 July 1698, ANTT IL Series 30, vol. 71, p. 430; Denúncia de Thereza e Francisco, 19 November 1754, ANTT IL Series 30, vol. 113, pp. 318–319; Mémoires de Pierre-Clément de Laussat, vol. 1, pp. 71–72; Pierre Dessalles to Albis de Gissac, 26 July 1823, in Dessalles, *La vie d'un colon à la Martinique*, 94. For examples of the latter, see Proces van Adoja, 21 May 1736, NADH RVP, vol. 790, pp. 89–90; Denúncia de Paulo Gomes e Ignacia, 21 October 1749, ANTT IL Series 30, vol. 109, pp. 153–160; Procès de Thelemaque, July 1754, ANOM Série F3, vol. 245, p. 250; Procès de Toiny, July 1754, ANOM Série F3, vol. 245, p. 250; Procès d'un negre, January 1755, ANOM Série F3, vol. 245, p. 300. Eighteenth-century Virginia county court trial summaries are so sparse—often listing little more than basic information on the accused, the crime, and the outcome of the case—that it is difficult to pull motives

from this data. However, the trope of conjure men causing afflictions among women did appear frequently in nineteenth-century conjure narratives. See Fett, *Working Cures*, 91.

64. Proces van Isaac, 10 May 1731, NADH RVP, vol. 787, n.p.; Proces van Dirk, 13 May 1732, NADH RVP, vol. 787, n.p.; Proces van Askaan, 1 June 1742, NADH RVP, vol. 795, n.p. For more on the fraught position of drivers within enslaved communities, see Browne, *Surviving Slavery*, 73–74.

65. Proces van Swart Jan, n.p.

66. Gómez, *Experiential Caribbean*, 130.

67. Feierman and Janzen, "Introduction," in Feierman and Janzen, eds., *Social Basis of Health*, 14; Janzen, *Lemba*, 299. For examples of health practices and complex social politics within communities of African descent in the Americas, see Sweet, *Domingos Álvares*, 126–143; Browne, *Surviving Slavery*, 134–135; Fett, *Working Cures*, 6, 37, 87, 101.

68. Proces van Swart Jan, n.p.; Proces van Daniel, 2 April 1761, NADH RVP, vol. 805, n.p.; Proces van Chocolaat, 20 February 1762, NADH RVP, vol. 806, n.p.; Proces van Andries, 8 September 1768, NADH RVP, vol. 814, n.p.; Proces van Corolaad, 8 February 1770, NADH RVP, vol. 817, p. 96; Proces van Paay, 28 February 1776, NADH RVP, vol. 829, p. 156.

69. Proces van Swart Jan, n.p.

70. Souza, *The Devil and the Land of the Holy Cross*, 169; Reis, "Candomblé and Slave Resistance in Nineteenth-Century Brazil," in Luis Nicolau Parés and Roger Sansi, eds., *Sorcery in the Black Atlantic*, (Chicago: University of Chicago Press, 2011), 69–70; Burnard and Garrigus, *Plantation Machine*, 106–107; João José Reis, *Divining Slavery and Freedom: The Story of Domingos Sodré, an African Priest in Nineteenth-Century Brazil*, trans. H. Sabrina Gledhill (Cambridge: Cambridge University Press, 2015), 132–135. For an example of taming used by Indigenous Barbacoans in early eighteenth-century Columbia, see Lane, "Taming the Master."

71. Mollenauer, *Strange Revelations*, 84–85.

72. Walker, *Doctors, Folk Medicine and the Inquisition*, 68; Ruth Behar, "Sex and Sin, Witchcraft and the Devil in Late-Colonial Mexico," *American Ethnologist* 14, no. 1 (1987), 40; von Germeten, *Violent Delights, Violent Ends*, 107, 110.

73. Procès de Jupiter et Gouan, May 1754, ANOM Série F3, vol. 245, pp. 235–237.

74. Procès de Jupiter et Gouan, July 1754, 251.

75. Procès de Jupiter et Gouan, July 1754, 252.

76. Gómez, *Experiential Caribbean*, 48–49, 58–60. For an example of the intensity of this competition, see the story of Diego López and Paula de Eguiluz in seventeenth-century Cartagena. Gómez, *Experiential Caribbean*, 73–78; von Germeten, *Violent Delights, Violent Ends*, 103, 119, 123.

77. For example, see Walker, *Doctors, Folk Medicine and the Inquisition*; Cagle, *Assembling the Tropics*; Breen, *Age of Intoxication*; Kananoja, *Healing Knowledge in Atlantic Africa*.

78. Sweet, *Recreating Africa*, 164–167; Reis, *Divining Slavery and Freedom*, 132–144, 154.

79. Gómez, *Experiential Caribbean*, 71.

80. Reis, "Candomblé and Slave Resistance," 69–70.

81. Blier, *African Vodun*, 5, 24, 62, 118, 310.

82. Blier, *African Vodun*, 113–114. James Sweet also explores similar ideas in *Domingos Álvares*, 70–71.

83. Blier, *African Vodun*, 73, 142. On twentieth-century Yoruba practices using herbs defensively to "cool" aggression, see Reis, *Divining Slavery and Freedom*, 73, 142.

84. See the analysis of the word root *-dèmb-* in Chapters 1 and 2. For more on the *lemba* institution specifically and its relationship to the transatlantic slave trade, see Janzen, *Lemba*, 3–6, 21.

85. D. Fernando José de Portugal to Martinho de Melo e Castro, 24 December 1789, Arquivo Historical Ultramarino (AHU) Administração Central Bahia, box 70, f. 13366..

86. Proces van Clarinda en Nero, 7 August 1733, NADH RVP, vol. 188, n.p. For a similar case involving an enslaved woan trying to "soften" her master through "powders," see Beeldsnijder, *"Om Werk Van Jullie te Hebben,"* 225.

87. Procès d'un negre et une negresse, November 1756, ANOM Série F3, vol. 245, p. 531.

88. Procès de Gabriel, Roze, et Sarra, May 1754, ANOM Série F3, vol. 245, p. 228.

89. João Joaquim da Silva to João José de Moura Magalhães, 28 March 1848, APEB Colônia e Província, Polícia, assuntos diversos, box 3113, f. 14. João Reis discusses this case and others in a wave of poison cases in the second half of the nineteenth century. See Reis, *Divining Slavery and Freedom,* 135.

90. Proces van Clarinda en Nero, n.p.

91. Garrigus, "'Like an Epidemic,'" 639. For an earlier, though still recent, interpretation that focused instead on spoiled food in the context of the blockade during the Seven Years' War, see Burnard and Garrigus, *Plantation Machine,* 106–107. Documents on Médor's confession, the interrogation of several enslaved women, and reports on the wider Makandal case were organized together by M. L. E. Moreau de Saint-Méry and can be found in the same box at the French colonial archives. See ANOM, Série F3, box 88. Burnard and Garrigus's arguments challenge the predominant interpretation of the Makandal case as an example of resistance and attempted revolt. See Fick, *Making of Haiti*; Weaver, *Medical Revolutionaries.*

92. de Luna, "Sounding the African Atlantic," 597–599.

93. de Luna, "Sounding the African Atlantic," 599–601.

94. Clark, "Inversion, Misrule, and the Meaning of Witchcraft"; Clark, *Thinking with Demons,* 129–133.

95. Souza, *The Devil and the Land of the Holy Cross,* 169; Reis, "Candomblé and Slave Resistance in Nineteenth-Century Brazil," 69–70; Beeldsnijder, *"Om Werk Van Jullie te Hebben,"* 225.

96. Proces van Bolletrie en André, 29 May 1745, NADH RVP, vol. 798, n.p.

97. Procès d'un negre et une negresse (1756), 531–532.

98. For more on conjure packets and their uses, see Fett, *Working Cures,* 102.

99. Yvonne Chireau, *Black Magic: Religion and the African American Conjuring Tradition* (Berkeley: University of California Press, 2003), 17.

100. Morgan, *Slave Counterpoint,* 287–288.

101. Sylvia R. Frey and Betty Wood, *Come Shouting to Zion: African American Protestantism in the American South and British Caribbean to 1830* (Chapel Hill: University of North Carolina Press, 1998) 119.

102. Chireau, *Black Magic,* 6–8.

103. McCaskie, "Unspeakable Words, Unmasterable Feelings," 20.

104. Proces van Swart Jan, n.p.

Chapter 5

1. An earlier version of parts of this chapter appeared in Victoria Barnett-Woods, ed., *Cultural Economies of the Atlantic World,* Copyright 2020 by Routledge. Reproduced by permission of the Taylor & Francis Group.

2. Denúncia de Paulo Gomes e Ignacia, 21 October 1749, ANTT IL Series 30, vol. 109, pp. 153–160.

3. Denúncia de Paulo Gomes e Ignacia, pp. 156, 158v, 160.

4. Denúncia de Paulo Gomes e Ignacia, pp. 153–154, 158. For another complex tale of a practitioner of African descent navigating the competitive medical marketplace of seventeenth-century Cartagena, see the story of surgeon Diego Lopez and Paula de Eguiluz. Von Germeten, *Violent Delights, Violent Ends,* 103–107, 119–123; Gómez, *Experiential Caribbean,* 72–78.

5. I borrow this turn of phrase from Neil Kodesh, "Networks of Knowledge: Clanship and Collective Well-Being in Buganda," *Journal of African History* 49 (2008): 208.

6. See, for example (in chronological order), Fett, *Working Cures*; Stephan Palmié, *Wizards and Scientists: Explorations in Afro-Cuban Modernity & Tradition* (Durham, NC: Duke University Press, 2002); Sweet, *Recreating Africa*; Juanita de Barros, "'Setting Things Right': Medicine and Magic in British Guiana, 1803–38," *Slavery & Abolition* 25, no. 1 (2004): 28–50; Walker, *Doctors, Folk Medicine and the Inquisition*; Weaver, *Medical Revolutionaries*; Parrish, *American Curiosity*; Santos, "As bolsas de mandinga "; Calainho, *Metrópole das mandingas*; Parés and Sansi, eds., *Sorcery in the Black Atlantic*; Sweet, *Domingos Álvares*; Voeks and Rashford, eds., *African Ethnobotany in the Americas*; Ogundiran and Saunders, eds., *Materialities of Ritual in the Black Atlantic*; Gómez, *Experiential Caribbean*; Schiebinger, *Secret Cures of Slaves*; Cagle, *Assembling the Tropics*; Breen, *Age of Intoxication*; Kananoja, *Healing Knowledge in Atlantic Africa*.

7. Gómez, *Experiential Caribbean*, 132; Schiebinger, *Secret Cures of Slaves*, 45–64; Ogundiran and Saunders, "On the Materiality of Black Atlantic Rituals," in Ogundiran and Saunders, eds., *Materialities of Ritual in the Black Atlantic*, 4, 16–21.

8. Gómez, *Experiential Caribbean*, 48–51, 58–59, 67.

9. For example, see Hogarth, *Medicalizing Blackness*, 83–84, 87, 94, 96.

10. Hicks, "Blood and Hair," 71–74; Parés, *Formation of Candomblé*, 79–81, 84, 89–93; Reis, "Magia Jeje na Bahia," 78.

11. Guyer and Belinga, "Wealth in People as Wealth in Knowledge," 110–113, 119.

12. For example, see Kodesh, "Networks of Knowledge," 199, 208; de Luna, "Affect and Society in Precolonial Africa," 129; Hunt, "The Affective, the Intellectual, and Gender History," 332; Cameron Gokee and Amanda L. Logan, "Comparing Craft and Culinary Practice in Africa: Themes and Perspectives," *African Archaeological Review* 31, no. 2 (2014): 96; Ann B. Stahl, "Africa in the World: (Re)Centering African History Through Archaeology," *Journal of Anthropological Research* 70, no. 1 (2014): 18. For an extension of Guyer and Belinga's key insight to the African diaspora, see James H. Sweet, "Defying Social Death: The Multiple Configurations of African Slave Family in the Atlantic World," *William and Mary Quarterly* 70, no. 2 (2013): 256.

13. Procès d'un negre, January 1755, pp. 295–297.

14. Santos, "As bolsas de mandinga," 205; Sweet, *Recreating Africa*, 148; Denúncia de Branca e Pedro de Sesueira Barbosa, 242v; Denúncia de Vitoria e outros, 28 June 1757, ANTT IL 30, vol. 120, p. 182.

15. Denúncia de Paulo Gomes e Ignacia, 157v.

16. Ogundiran and Saunders, "On the Materiality of Black Atlantic Rituals," in Ogundiran and Saunders, eds., *Materialities of Ritual in the Black Atlantic*, 2–4.

17. There are many examples of these objects in poison cases. As a selection of such cases involving the makers of these objects, see Denúncia de João e Manoel, 2 March 1758, ANTT IL Series 30, vol. 121, pp. 6–7; Procès de Jupiter et Gouan, 250–253; Proces van Titus en Dafina, 30 November 1763, NADH RVP, vol. 808, n.p.

18. Procès de Toiny, July 1754, ANOM Série F3, vol. 245, pp. 249–250.

19. Proces van Samsam, 11 May 1736, NADH RVP, vol. 790, n.p.; Procès de deux negres, January 1755, ANOM Série F3, vol. 245, pp. 297–299; Complaint against the negro Hans, 17 June 1819, NA-Kew CO 116 British Guiana, Fiscal's Reports (1819-1832), vol. 138, p. 63; Gómez, *Experiential Caribbean*, 82. For more on cupping practices in Atlantic Africa, see Kananoja, *Healing Knowledge in Atlantic Africa*, 30, 32, 66.

20. Gómez, *Experiential Caribbean*, 140–142.

21. de Laborde, "Effet dangereux de l'erreur."

22. Surviving records are even more fragmental for other colonies in the British Atlantic, such as Barbados. See Fuentes, *Dispossessed Lives*, 2.

23. Fett, *Working Cures*, 94, 102–103.

24. Jugement rendu par le tribunal spécial contre des esclaves appartenant aux sieurs Eyma, de Leyritz, Pécoul, Chalvet, Fortier, Gradis, Lavener, Serrand, Ducoudray et Valmont accusés d'empoisonnements et de complot d'assassinat contre les économes du quartier, 2 November 1807, ANOM Série C8a, box 115, f. 51. See also similar accusation from the 1820s Cour Prévôtale: Procés de Catherine Rosane et outres, 29 August 1822, ADM Série U7, vol. 1, n.p.; Procés de Raimond et outres, 27 November 1823, ADM Série U7, vol. 1, n.p.

25. Proces van Goliath en Prins.

26. Breen, "Tropical Transplantations," 178; Mott, *Bahia: Inquisição e Sociadade*, 106; Calainho, *Metropole das mandingas*, 95, 98.

27. Processo de António Rodrigues da Silva, 1725, ANTT IL Series 28, f. 11246; Denúncia de Miguel e Maria Monjola, 92v–93; Processo de Mateus Pereira Machado, 1750–1756, ANTT IL Series 28, f. 1131; Processo de Luis Pereira de Almeida, 1750–1756, ANTT IL Series 28, f. 1134; Processo de João da Silva, 1750–1756, ANTT IL Series 28, f. 502; Processo de José Martins, 1750–1756, ANTT IL Series 28, f. 508. See also Mott, *Bahia: Inquisição e Sociedade*, 101–117.

28. The documentation for the case is in a series of letters, reports, and transcripts of interrogations from 1757 to 1759 compiled by Moreau de Saint-Méry. See ANOM Série F3, box 88, f. 212–252. For a recent interpretation of the case and the particular significance of this bundle, see Burnard and Garrigus, *Plantation Machine*, 109; Garrigus, "'Like an Epidemic,'" 639–640.

29. Denúncia de Miguel e Maria Monjola, 92v–93. Today, the worship of Caboclos is a major subset of Candomblé practices in Bahia. See Parés, *Formation of Candomblé*, 68; Voeks, *Sacred Leaves of Candomblé*, 88, 106.

30. **-gàngà* (expert, healer-diviner) regularly takes noun class 1/2 (with NC 2 being the regular plural of NC 1) or 9/10; **-gàngà* (medicine) regularly takes noun class 14.

31. For an example of *ganga* in Lisbon Inquisition cases, see Denúncia de Branca e Pedro de Sesqueira Barbosa, p. 241v. For a rare example of a preserved *bolsa* in Inquisition records, see Matthew Francis Rarey, "Assemblage, Occlusion, and the Art of Survival in the Black Atlantic," *African Arts* 51, no. 4 (2018): 21. In Baudry's work, derivatives from this root appear in a serious of efforts at one-to-one translation as follows: *amarrer* (to tie to)=*kanga*; *chirurgien* (surgeon)=*gangan kizi*; *serrer* (to grip, to tighten)=*kanga*. Louis-Narcisse Baudry des Lozières, *Second voyage à la louisiane, faisant suite au premier de l'auteur de 1794 a 1798* (Paris: Chez Charles, Imprimeur, 1803), vol. 1, 109, 117, 142. **-kàng-* is an established variant of the Proto-Bantu root **-gàng-*. For more on the making of Baudry's dictionary and the layers of insight it offers on the ideas and expressions of Kikongo speakers enslaved on his plantation, see de Luna, "Sounding the African Atlantic," 582–583. For an example of *wanga* in North America, see Michael Gomez, *Exchanging Our Country Marks: The Transformation of African Identities in the Colonial and Antebellum South* (Chapel Hill: University of North Carolina Press, 1998), 50–51.

32. Tiana Andrade Lima, Marcos André Torres de Souza, and Glaucia Malerba Sene, "Weaving the Second Skin: Protection Against Evil Among the Valong Slaves in Nineteenth-Century Rio de Janeiro," *Journal of African Diaspora Archaeology & Heritage* 3 (2014): 117–119.

33. Denúncia de Thereza e Francisco, 19 November 1754, ANTT IL Series 30, vol. 113, pp. 318–319; Proces van April, 4 August 1742, NADH RVP, vol. 795, n.p.

34. Proces van Isaac, 10 May 1731, NADH RVP, vol. 787, n.p.

35. Blier, *African Vodun*, 117–118.

36. Fett, *Working Cures*, 102; Mark P. Leone, Jocelyn E. Knauf, and Amanda Tang, "Ritual Bundle in Colonial Annapolis," in Ogundiran and Saunders, eds., *Materialities of Ritual in the Black Atlantic*, 198–211.

37. For more on social tensions and *minkisi*, see MacGaffey, *Kongo Political Culture*, 93–95.

38. Paton, "Witchcraft, Poison, Law," 256–257; Burnard and Garrigus, *Plantation Machine*, 102; João José Reis, *Slave Rebellion in Brazil: The Muslim Uprising of 1835 in Bahia*, trans. Arthur

Brakel (Baltimore: Johns Hopkins University Press, 1993), 93; Stedman, *Narrative of a Five Years' Expedition* (1796), vol. 2, 89, 138–139, 347.

39. Andrade Lima, Torres de Souza, and Sene, "Weaving the Second Skin," 103–136.

40. Suzanne Blier compiled a similar list of goals for empowerment objects in the Bight of Benin recorded by Olyme Bhêly-Quénum, Julien Alapini, Melville Herskovits, and Albert de Surgy. See Blier, *African Vodun*, 117–118.

41. Proces van Fortuijn en Africaan, 15 February 1735, NADH RVP, vol. 789, p. 24; Proces van La Rocke, 1 February 1741, NADH RVP, vol. 794, n.p.; Procès d'un negre et une negresse, November 1756, ANOM Série F3, vol. 245, p. 531; Procès de Zéphir, September 1768, ANOM Série F3, vol. 246, p. 516; Proces van Coffij en La Rose, 16 August 1779, NADH RVP, vol. 836, p. 216; Proces van Sergeant, 25 May 1798, NADH RVP, vol. 858, n.p.; Procès de Gustave et outres, 13 December 1824, ADM Série U7, vol. 1, n.p.

42. Denúncia de Rafael Margues, 11 December 1707, ANTT IL Series 30, vol. 76, p. 59; Processo de dois soldados, 1781, ANTT IL Series 28, f. 12970.

43. de Laborde, "Effet dangereux de l'erreur"; Procès de deux negres, January 1755, ANOM Série F3, vol. 245, p. 297.

44. Processo de António Rodrigues da Silva, 1725, ANTT Series 28, f. 11426.

45. Processo de António Rodrigues da Silva; Procès de deux negres.

46. de Laborde, "Effet dangereux de l'erreur."

47. Denúncia de Bento José, 8 October 1748, ANTT IL Series 30, vol. 109, p. 14; Denúncia de Antonio Veira, 14 October 1748, ANTT IL Series 30, vol. 109, p. 223; Processo de José Fernandes, 1760, ANTT IL Series 28, f. 8909; Procès de Zéphir, p. 516; de Laborde, "Effet dangereux de l'erreur"; Proces van Sergeant, n.p.

48. Proces van La Rocke, n.p.; Proces van Titus en Dafina, 30 November 1763, NADH RVP, vol. 808, n.p.; Proces van Fiulo, 17 January 1774, NADH RVP, vol. 825, p. 73; de Laborde, "Effet dangereux de l'erreur."

49. de Laborde, "Effet dangereux de l'erreur."

50. Proces van Baron, 10 May 1742, NADH RVP, vol. 795, n.p.; Processo de João da Silva, 1750, ANTT IL Series 28, f. 502; Procès d'un negre et une negresse, p. 531; de Laborde, "Effet dangereux de l'erreur."

51. Processo de Luis Pereira de Almeida, 1750, ANTT IL Series 28, f. 1134; Procès de deux negres, p. 297.

52. Denúncia de Manoel da Silva, 15 October 1703, ANTT IL Series 30, vol. 75, p. 225; Proces van Clarinda en Nero, 7 August 1733, NADH RVP, vol. 788, n.p.; Proces van Fortuijn en Africaan, p. 24; Proces van Baron, n.p.; Proces van Abraham, 10 May 1742, NADH RVP, vol. 795, n.p.; Proces van Apollo, 4 August 1742, NADH RVP, vol. 795, n.p.; Denúncia de Paulo Gomes e Ignacia, p. 153; "Dinsdag den 11 Maart 1749," NADH Sociëteit van Suriname, Resoluties van Gouverneur en Raden, vol. 141, n.p.; Procès de Jupiter et Gouan, July 1754, p. 250; Procès d'un negre, November 1755, p. 405; Procès d'un negre et une negresse, p. 531; Proces van Hendrik, 31 March 1790, NADH RVP, vol. 835, p. 20.

53. Procès de Gabriel, Roze, et Sarra, May 1754, ANOM Série F3, vol. 245, p. 228; D. Fernando José de Portugal to Martinho de Melo e Castro, 24 December 1789, AHU Administração Central Bahia, Series Bahia-CA, box 70, f. 13366; João Joaquim da Silva to João José de Moura Magalhães, 28 March 1848, APEB Colônia e Província, Polícia assuntos diversos, maço 3113, f. 14.

54. Bosman, *New and Accurate Description*, 147, 153–154. For more on *feitiçaria* accusations in Angola, see Ferreira, *Cross-Cultural Exchange in the Atlantic World*, 166–179, 201.

55. The idiom of binding someone with power was not unique to Atlantic Africa; overlap on the significance of tying/untying from multiple ontologies in the creole societies of the Americas opened spaces for convergences. For example, in eighteenth-century Mexico—a colony with centuries of convergence and interaction between Indigenous, African, and Spanish cultures,

mestiza women confessed to procuring from Indigenous practitioners means to sexually "tie up" their husbands and render them "tamed" or impotent. Behar, "Sex and Sin," 34, 40–43.

56. Proces van Marquis en Akkra, 27 February 1771, NADH RVP, vol. 819, p. 234; Proces van Present en Abraham, 8 September 1798, NADH RVP, vol. 859, l.

57. Rufz de Lavison, *Recherches sur les empoisonnements*, 26.

58. Davis, "Judges, Masters, Diviners," 935–936. For more detail on West Central African tribunals, see Ferreira, *Cross-Cultural Exchange in the Atlantic World*, 69; Candido, *African Slaving Port and the Atlantic World*, 235. For changes in West Africa, see Shaw, *Memories of the Slave Trade*, 211–216; Bay, *Wives of the Leopard*, 320; Sweet, *Domingos Álvares*, 19–20, 22.

59. Westermann, *Evefiala*, vol. 1, 26, 28; Segurola, *Dictionnaire Fon-Franççais*, 286; Christaller, *Dictionary of the Asante and Fante Language*, 214, 498. See also Blier, *African Vodun*, 26, 78.

60. Denúncia de Paulo Gomes e Ignacia, pp. 155, 156v–157. See also Sweet, *Domingos Álvares*, 7; for a more detailed exploration of the formation of "Mina" identity, see 33–34.

61. Proces van Bienvenue, 13 May 1743, NADH, Oud Archief Suriname: RVP, vol. 796. Many of the volumes in this collection are missing page numbers due to damage on the edges.

62. Procès d'un negre et une negresse, pp. 531–532.

63. Sweet, *Domingos Álvares*, 56; Denúncia de Pedro Coelho Pimentel, 28 March 1686, ANTT IL Series 30, vol. 59, p. 135; Processo de Simão, 1688, ANTT IL Series 28, Processos, f. 8464. Sweet also discusses these two cases in *Recreating Africa*, 165, 120–122.

64. Sweet, *Recreating Africa*, 145, 156–157, 218, 222–223; Chireau, *Black Magic*, 53; Davis, "Judges, Masters, Diviners," 956; Morgan, *Slave Counterpoint*, 623.

65. Gómez, *Experiential Caribbean*, 3; Voeks, *Sacred Leaves of Candomblé*, 2–4.

66. Gómez, *Experiential Caribbean*, 3.

67. Denúncia de Paulo Gomes e Ignacia, p. 159v.

68. Rarey, "Assemblage, Occlusion," 24–26. See also Santos, "As bolsas de mandinga."

69. Sweet, *Recreating Africa*, 127–128. For an example in the Inquisition records originating in Bahia, see Denúncia de Rosa Maria Berreira, 29 October 1757, ANTT IL Series 30, vol. 120, pp. 161–162.

70. Denúncia de Paulo Gomes e Ignacia, pp. 156v, 158v–159.

71. Gómez, *Experiential Caribbean*, 77; Sweet, *Domingos Álvares*, 77, 195, 207.

72. See Chapter 3 in this book for more details regarding the demographic data.

73. Lewis, *Hall of Mirrors*, 149, 156.

74. Parrish, *American Curiosity*, 280. Virginian snakeroot also became an important part of European pharmacopoeias in the Atlantic. See Vigier, *Pharmacopea Ulyssiponese*, 445–446; Breen, *Tropical Transplantations*, 264; A. M. G. Rutten, *Dutch Transatlantic Medicine Trade in the Eighteenth Century Under the Cover of the West India Company* (Rotterdam: Erasmus, 2000) appendix V.

75. Thomas Walduck to James Petiver, 24 November 1710, BL Sloane Manuscripts, vol. 2302; Proces van Quashie, 28 July 1731, NADH RVP, vol. 787, n.p.; Proces van Jacob, 3 May 1734, NADH RVP, vol. 788, pp. 202–202v; Proces van Samson, 9 May 1741, NADH RVP, vol. 794, n.p.

76. For an example, see Gordon's analysis of the oral tradition as origin story of the Crocodile Clan in Gordon, *Invisible Agents*, 33. For a comparative analysis of the concept of autochthony across a deep time scale in Cameroon and the Netherlands, see Peter Geschiere, *The Perils of Belonging: Autochthony, Citizenship, and Exclusion in Africa and Europe* (Chicago: University of Chicago Press, 2009).

77. Procès de Zéphir, 517; de Laborde, "Effet dangereux de l'erreur"; Rufz de Lavison, *Recherches sur les empoisonnements*, 25; Oudin-Bastide, *L'effroi et la terreur*, 188.

78. Rufz de Lavison, *Recherches sur les empoisonnements*, 25–26.

79. Gordon, *Invisible Agents*, 1–5, 9–10.

80. Fett, *Working Cures*, 56; Sweet, *Recreating Africa*, 120, 123, 127–128, 130, 135, 139, 142–146, 151–157; Handler and Bilby, *Enacting Power*, 26. For works on the specific context of practices for communicating with spirits in Africa, see Feierman and Janzen, eds., *Social Basis of Health*; Gordon, *Invisible Agents*.

81. Sweet, *Recreating Africa*, 156–157. See the practices of Domingos Álvares at his *terreiro* (healing house) in Rio de Janeiro in the late 1730s and early 1740s, in Sweet, *Domingos Álvares*, 104–105, 126-130.

82. Denúncia de Mariana e Francisca, 18 July 1745, ANTT IL Series 30, vol. 106, p. 128. For similar accusations of healers of African descent speaking in the voices of specific deceased individuals, see Denúncia de Pedro Coelho Pimentel, 28 March 1686, ANTT IL Series 30, vol. 59, p. 135; Denúncia de Branca e Pedro de Sesueira Barbosa, pp. 239–248.

83. Proces van April, n.p.; Complaint against the negro Hans, pp. 60–63. As Randy Browne notes in his article on *watermama* and *obeah* in early nineteenth-century Berbice, "minje" was an Ijo word for "water." Browne, "'Bad Business' of Obeah," 463. Browne also discusses the case of Hans in detail on pp. 463–468.

84. Stedman, *Narrative of a Five Years' Expedition* (1796), vol. 2, 177–179.

85. Proces van April, n.p.

86. Fett, *Working Cures*, 101–102; Chireau, *Black Magic*, 50. By 1800, African-born individuals were a statistically insignificant portion of the Virginian enslaved population. Morgan, *Slave Counterpoint*, 61.

87. Complaint against the negro Hans, pp. 60, 63; Procès de Jacques, September 1767, ANOM Série F3, vol. 246, pp. 408–409.

88. David, "Judges, Masters, Diviners," 951; Price, *Alabi's World*, 32.

89. Stedman, *Narrative of a Five Years' Expedition* (2010), 426, 551–552, 582.

90. Price, *Alabi's World*, 32.

91. Proces van Coffij en La Rose, p. 216.

92. Parrish, *American Curiosity*, 287; Morgan, *Slave Counterpoint*, 625–626.

93. Hening, *Statutes at Large*, vol. 4, 105; Schwarz, *Twice Condemned*, 97.

94. Denúncia de Paulo Gomes e Ignacia, pp. 156–157, 159–159v.

95. "RAN AWAY, about the First Day of June last," 21 November 1745, *Virginia Gazette* (W. Parks ed.), no. 486, p. 4; "RUN AWAY from the Subscriber," 4 November 1763, *Virginia Gazette* (J. Royle, ed.), no. 668, p. 4; "COMMITTED to the gaol of Charles City," 8 September 1774, *Virginia Gazette* (Clementina Rind, ed.), no. 435, p. 4; "COMMITTED to the jail of Isle of Wight county," 10 October 1777, *Virginia Gazette* (Alexander Purdie, ed.), no. 141, p. 3.

96. For examples of the mobility of Virginian healers of African descent in county court trials, see Trial of Webster, Sarah, and Jenny, 25 July 1758, LVA Brunswick CCOB, vol. 7, pp. 233–234; Trial of Tom, Judy, Margery, and Abraham, 20 June 1764, LVA Goochland CCOB, vol. 9, pp. 384–385. Cases of "exhibiting" poisons, medicines, of "poisonous medicines" were numerous. See Trial of Isaac and Quash, 29 May 1759, LVA Cumberland CCOB, vol. 1758–62, pp. 56–57; Trial of Toby, 17 March 1764, LVA Cumberland CCOB, vol. 1762–64, pp. 394–395; Trial of Harry, 5 November 1764, LVA Amelia CCOB, vol. 8, pp. 247–248; Trial of Will and York, 9 February 1765, LVA Goochland CCOB, vol. 9, pp. 451–452; Trial of Peter, 23 May 1765, LVA Cumberland CCOB, vol. 1764–67, pp. 124–125; Trial of Dick and Peg, 4 June 1765, LVA Goochland CCOB, vol. 10, pp. 126–127; Trial of Caesar, 21 October 1773, LVA Cumberland CCOB, vol. 1772–74, pp. 452–453; Trial of Obee, Dick, and Mary, 29 July 1778, LVA Spotsylvania CCMB, vol. 1774–82, p. 94.

97. Robert Carter to Bennett Neal, 15 September 1781, BRRL, RCC, Letterbook 4, pp. 117–119; Robert Carter to William Berry, 31 July 1786, BRRL RCC, Letterbook 7, p. 62; Robert Carter to William Berry, 26 February 1788, BRRL RCC, Letterbook 8, p. 88; Robert Carter Pass to

Sampson, 31 January 1788, BRRL RCC, Letterbook 8, p. 77. For a Brazilian example of similar practices, see Sweet *Domingos Álvares*, 76.

98. ANTT IL Series 30, vol. 55–131; ANTT IL Series 28; NADH RVP, vol. 787–915; ANOM Série F3, vol. 244–246; Archives Départementales de la Martinique, Série U7 Cour Prévôtale. I have examined 154 cases with practitioners of African descent in total; in 32 of these cases the individual's reputation was explicitly discussed by the court.

99. Proces van La Rocke, 1 February 1741, NADH RVP, vol. 794, n.p.; Proces van André, 1 February 1741, NADH RVP, vol. 794, n.p.

100. Proces van La Rocke, n.p.

101. Proces van André, n.p.

102. Proces van Tromp en Manuel, 29 April 1741, NADH RVP, vol. 794, n.p.

103. Proces van La Rocke, n.p.; Proces van André, n.p.; Proces van Samson, 9 May 1741, NADH RVP, vol. 794, n.p.

104. See, for example, Proces van Tromp en Manuel, n.p.; Proces van Coffij, 1 June 1742, NADH RVP, vol. 795, n.p.

105. Parés, *Formation of Candomblé*, 75–76. For a selection of works on the debates about Afro-Caribbean and Afro-Brazilian religions, see Roger Bastide, *The African Religions of Brazil: Toward a Sociology of the Interpenetration of Civilizations*, trans. Helen Sebba (Baltimore: Johns Hopkins University Press, 1978); Pluchon, *Vaudou, sorciers, empoisonneurs de Saint-Domingue*; Harding, *Refuge in Thunder*; Palmié, *Wizards and Scientists*; Reis, *Divining Slavery and Freedom*.

106. Reis, "Magia Jeje na Bahia," 78.

107. Reis, "Magia Jeje na Bahia," 67–79; Parés, *Formation of Candomblé*, 82–83.

108. Capitão-mor of São Francisco to Governador Conde da Ponte, 1807, Arquivo Publico do Estado da Bahia (Salvador) (APEB) Series Colônia e Província, Correspondência Recebida dos Capitães-Mores, box 417-1, f. São Francisco 1807–1809, p. 10; Manoel de Cezeda Rodrigues de Sa to Capitão-Mor of São Francisco, 23 Jun 1807, APEB Series Colônia e Província, Correspondência Recebida dos Capitães-Mores, box 417-1, f. São Francisco 1807–1809, p. 44; To the Capitão-mor of São Francisco, 19 June 1807, APEB Series Colônia e Província, Correspondência Recebida dos Capitães-Mores, box 417-1, f. São Francisco 1807–1809, p. 85; Joquim Ignacio de Sequeira Bulção to Governador Conde da Ponte, 23 Jun 1807, APEB Series Colônia e Província, Correspondência Recebida dos Capitães-Mores, box 417-1, f. São Francisco 1807–1809, pp. 99–104. This case has been frequently discussed in studies on the formation of Candomblé. See Parés, *Formation of Candomblé*, 88; Harding, *Refuge in Thunder*, 80. The police in another 1830 raid accused the leader of a Candomblé house of being partially responsible for four hundred runaways in his district. Antonio Gomes de Abreu Guimares to Luiz Paulo Araejo Basto, 10 December 1830, APEB Series Colônia e Província, Correspondência Recebida de Juizes, box 2681, f. 1.

109. The use of amulets for this purpose had also been prominent in eighteenth-century revolts, such as Tackey's Revolt in 1760 Jamaica and the war on the Cottica River described by John Gabriel Stedman in 1796. See Burnard and Garrigus, *Plantation Machine*, 122–131; Paton, "Witchcraft, Poison, Law," 257–258; Stedman, *Narrative of a Five Years' Expedition (1796)*, vol. 2, 107, 347.

110. Reis, *Slave Rebellion in Brazil*, 203.

111. Parés, *Formation of Candomblé*, 91–93. Historians and anthropologists who study Candomblé make clear that these affiliations, Nagô, Jeje, Angola, among others, that continue in Candomblé houses today, were spiritual and not necessarily determined by the ethnic background of participants, who were multiethnic. See Parés, *Formation of Candomblé*, 68–69, 84; João José Reis, "Candomblé in Nineteenth-Century Bahia: Priests, Followers, Clients," in *Rethinking the African Diaspora: The Making of a Black Atlantic World in the Bight of Benin and*

Brazil, ed. Kristen Mann and Edna G. Bay (Portland, OR: F. Cass, 2001), 132. This is also the case for Richard Price on the ritual practices among the Saramaka maroons and Stephen Palmié on Cuban Santeria. See Price, *Alabi's World*, 308–309; Palmié, *Wizards and Scientists*, 159–160, 196–197.

112. Padre Marianno de Santa Roza de Lima, "A Feiticeria entre nós: Ella não pode ser extirpada senão pela acção poderosa e não interrompida da policia, Artigo 5," *O noticiador Catholico*, vol. 2, no. 89 (1850): 365; Reis, *Divining Slavery and Freedom*, 6, 166–169.

113. Reis, *Divining Slavery and Freedom*, 172.

114. *Collecção das leis do Imperio do Brazil de 1830*, vol. 1 (Rio de Janeiro: Typographia Nacional, 1876); Reis, *Divining Slavery and Freedom*, 127.

115. Reis, *Divining Slavery and Freedom*, 129–130. For an example of a raid for "disturbing the peace," see João Joaquim da Silva to Francisco José de Sousa Soares d'Andrea, 28 December 1846, APEB Series Colônia e Província, Polícia assuntos diversos, box 3114, f. 7.

116. For more on the Cour Prévôtale, see Oudin-Bastide, *L'effroi et la terreur*; and Savage, "'Black Magic' and White Terror."

117. Procès de Jean Baptiste et outres, 267–275.

118. Mémoires de Pierre-Clément de Laussat, 13 September 1807, vol. 1, 83; "Jugement rendu par le tribunal spécial contre des esclaves appartenant aux sieurs Eyma, de Leyritz, Pécoul, Chalvet, Fortier, Gradis, Lavener, Serrand, Ducoudray et Valmont accusés d'empoisonnements et de complot d'assassinat contre les économes du quartier," 2 November 1807, ANOM Série C8a, box 115, f. 51; Louis Thomas Villared de Joyeuse to Denis Decrès, 1 December 1807, ANOM Série C8a, box 115, f. 47.

119. Gouverneur Donzelot to Marquis de Clermont-Tonnerre, 28 September 1822, ANOM Série Géographiques (SG) Martinique, box 52, f. 430.

120. Savage, "'Black Magic' and White Terror," 639; Oudin-Bastide, *L'effroi et la terreur*, 138.

121. Ada Ferrer, *Freedom's Mirror: Cuba and Haiti in the Age of Revolutions* (New York: Cambridge University Press, 2014), 271–328.

122. A. J. R. Russell Wood, "Ports of Brazil," in *Atlantic Port Cities: Economy, Culture, and Society in the Atlantic World*, ed. Franklin W. Knight and Peggy K. Liss (Knoxville: University of Tennessee Press, 1991), 199.

123. Denúncia de Miguel e Maria Monjola, 94.

Chapter 6

1. Lucia Stanton, *"Those Who Labor for My Happiness": Slavery at Thomas Jefferson's Monticello* (Charlottesville: University of Virginia Press, 2012), 108–113.

2. Martha Jefferson Randolph to Thomas Jefferson, 30 January 1800, in Oberg, ed., *Papers of Thomas Jefferson*, vol. 31, 347–348.

3. Martha Jefferson Randolph to Thomas Jefferson, 347–348.

4. Thomas Mann Randolph to Thomas Jefferson, 19 April 1800, Oberg, ed., *Papers of Thomas Jefferson*, vol. 31, 522–524.

5. Willem de Blécourt and Cornelie Usborne, eds., *Cultural Approaches to the History of Medicine: Mediating Medicine in Early Modern and Modern Europe* (New York: Palgrave Macmillan, 2004), 4, 8–9.

6. John Garrigus explores this idea of shared myth creation in the specific context of Saint-Domingue and the famous 1758 Makandal case. See Garrigus, "'Like an Epidemic,'" 651. For an example of a way that people of European and African descent could have very different origins for their ideas that converged into similar practices (in this case with the practice of bloodletting), see Hicks, "Blood and Hair," 62.

7. While I did not find this theme of drawing physical evidence from the bodies of the afflicted in the trials I have examined from Martinique and the Dutch Guianas, anecdotal evidence from British colonies and cases from Bahia suggest that there was a widely shared idea of what Sharla Fett describes as the porous body, "permeable to graveyard dirt, snakeskin powder, and the spiritual forces they contained." Fett, *Working Cures*, 94.

8. Thomas Walduck to James Petiver, n.d. 1712, BL Sloane Manuscripts, vol. 2302, p. 28v.

9. Carter, *Diary of Landon Carter*, vol. 2, 610 (10 August 1771), 742 (19 October 1772); Fett, *Working Cures*, 93–94; Chireau, *Black Magic*, 104–106.

10. Denúncia de Miguel e Maria Monjola, p. 90.

11. Denúncia de Joanna Maria, 11 June 1752, ANTT IL Series 30, vol. 113, p. 66; Denúncia de Sebastião, 30 April 1698, ANTT IL Series 30, vol. 72, p. 324.

12. Gómez, *Experiential Caribbean*, 145–147, 158–159.

13. Buitrago, "Arvore da Vida," 61v, 64.

14. Denúncia de Paulo Gomes e Ignacia, pp. 157v–159.

15. Gómez, *Experiential Caribbean*, 130–131; Fett, *Working Cures*, 6, 101.

16. Fett, *Working Cures*, 101–106.

17. Complaint against the negro Hans, pp. 60–63. Pablo Gómez discusses similar "[discoveries] of incriminating evidence" in cases from the seventeenth-century Spanish Caribbean. See Gómez, *Experiential Caribbean*, 132.

18. Denúncia de Paulo Gomes e Ignacia, p. 158v; Fett, *Working Cures*, 106; Games, *Witchcraft in Early North America*, 39; Brian Hoggard, "The Archaeology of Counter-Witchcraft and Popular Magic," in Davies and de Blécourt, eds., *Beyond the Witch Trials*, 168–169, 170–173.

19. Caroline Oudin-Bastide also examines these letters in detail in *L'effroi et la terreur*, 104–108, 183–184.

20. Pierre Dessalles to Albis de Gissac, 2 August 1824, in Dessalles, *La vie d'un colon à la Martinique*, 125.

21. Pierre Dessalles to Albis de Gissac, 28 July 1824, in Dessalles, *La vie d'un colon à la Martinique*, 123–124. For the trial, see Procès de Barbe et outres, 16 August 1824, ADM Série U7, vol. 1, n.p.

22. Pierre Dessalles to Albis de Gissac, 4 July 1824, in Dessalles, *La vie d'un colon à la Martinique*, 114.

23. Pierre Dessalles to Albis de Gissac, 12 July 1824, in Dessalles, *La vie d'un colon à la Martinique*, 116–118.

24. Copy of a letter from M. Lasalle to Pierre Dessalles, 18 July 1824, 121; and copy of a letter from Pierre Dessalles to M. Lasalle, 18 July 1824, both in Dessalles, *La vie d'un colon à la Martinique*, 122–123.

25. Pierre Dessalles to Albis de Gissac, 22 January 1825, in Dessalles, *La vie d'un colon à la Martinique*, 139–140.

26. Pierre Dessalles to Albis de Gissac, 18 February 1825, in Dessalles, *La vie d'un colon à la Martinique*, 143. See Procès de Charlotte et outres, 6 May 1825, ADM Série U7, vol. 1, n.p.

27. Pierre Dessalles to Albis de Gissac, 18 July 1824, in Dessalles, *La vie d'un colon à la Martinique*, 122. For more on the contemporary argument attributing "poison" to anthrax, see Garrigus, "'Like an Epidemic.'"

28. Richard H. Grove, *Green Imperialism: Colonial Expansion, Tropical Island Edens and the Origins of Environmentalism, 1600–1860* (Cambridge: Cambridge University Press, 1995); Schiebinger, *Plants and Empire*; Parrish, *American Curiosity*; Cañizares-Esguerra, *Nature, Empire, and Nation*; Breen, *Age of Intoxication*; Elizabeth Polcha, "Voyeur in the Torrid Zone: John Gabriel Stedman's *Narrative of a Five Years Expedition Against the Revolted Negroes of Surinam, 1773–1838*," *Early American Literature* 54, no. 3 (2019): 673–710; Crawford and Gabriel, "Introduction: Thinking with Pharmacopoeias," in *Drugs on the Page*, 6.

29. André João Antonil, *Cultura e opulencia do Brasil por suas drogas e minas, com varias noticias curiosas do modo de fazer o assucar; plantar & beneficiar o tabaco; tirar ouro das minas; & descubrir as da prata* (Lisbon: Na Officina Real Deslandesiana, 1711), 24, 28. See also Sweet, *Recreating Africa*, 41.

30. For more on Labat's time in Martinique, see Pluchon, *Vaudou, sorciers, empoisonneurs*, 19–26.

31. Maarit Forde and Diana Paton, "Introduction," in Paton and Forde, eds., *Obeah and Other Powers*, 14. See Labat, *Nouveau voyage aux isles de l'Amerique*, vol. 1, 488–501; Long, *History of Jamaica*, vol. 2, 387, and vol. 3, 807; Bryan Edwards, *The History, Civil and Commercial, of the British Colonies in the West Indies* (London: Printed for John Stockdale, 1801), vol. 1, 32–33, 40, 44, 92, and vol. 2, 93, 207–209.

32. Breen, *Age of Intoxication*, 70–74.

33. Parrish, *American Curiosity*, 273–274.

34. Antonil, *Cultura e opulencia*, 24.

35. Labat, *Nouveau voyage aux isles de l'Amerique*, vol. 4, 137.

36. M. L. E. Moreau de Saint-Méry, *Description topographique, physique, civile, politique, et historique de la partie française de l'isle Saint-Domingue*, 2nd ed. (Paris: T. Morgand, 1875), vol. 1, 36.

37. de Laborde, "Effet dangereux de l'erreur."

38. Governor Charles Wales to Lord Bathurst, 14 February 1814, NA-Kew WO 1 West Indies and South America, box 47. Thank you to Alix Rivière for sharing this letter with me.

39. Wales's letter stands in interesting contrast to the difference between British conceptions of *obeah* and French conceptions of *poison* explored by Diana Paton. See Paton, "Witchcraft, Poison, Law."

40. For more on the Brinvilliers case, see Mollenauer, *Strange Revelations*, 53. Pierre-Clément de Laussat included *brinvilliers* in his list of poisons allegedly used by enslaved poisoners, claiming that it caused instant and atrocious convulsions in animals. *Brinvilliers* also appeared in a list of poisons in an 1827 letter from the prosecutor A. Rivière to the governor as part of his campaign to reinstate the Cour Prévôtale. Mémoires de Pierre-Clément de Laussat, 13 September 1807, vol. 1, 89; Procureur du Roi Riviere to Governeur le Comte de Chabrol, 27 July 1827, ANOM Série Géographique: Martinique, box 52, f. 431.

41. Jean-Baptiste Ricord-Madianna, *Recherches et experiences sur les poisons d'Amérique tires des trois règnes de la nature* (Bordeaux: Charles Lawalle, 1826), 33, 42–43, 50. Ricord-Madianna put his own work in direct conversation with European works like Orfila's 1814 *Traité des poisons*. Ricord-Madianna at one point corrects Orfila for one of his anecdotes on the *mancenillier* (manchineel) tree (*Hippomane mancinella*). See Ricord-Madianna, *Recherches et experiences sur les poisons d'Amérique*, 91; Orfila, *Traité des poisons*, vol. 2.2, 76. The copy of Ricord-Madianna's book I read was signed and sent to the Directeur du Jardin des Plantes de Marseilles, illustrating the circles Ricord-Madianna was trying to enter with this botanical work.

42. For a description of cassava preparation in Barbados in the early eighteenth century, see Thomas Walduck to James Petiver, n.d. (1710), BL Sloane Manuscripts, vol. 2302.

43. Long, *History of Jamaica*, vol. 3, 777–779. However, not all works in this period pointed to cassava as a tool for deliberate poisoning. Stedman described cassava use, preparation, and poisonous qualities in detail without making claims to its use to intentionally poison—despite discussions elsewhere in his work on the "art of poisoning" practiced by both enslaved Africans and Indigenous Americans. Stedman, *Narrative of a Five Years' Expedition*, vol. 1, 389–390, and vol. 2, 266–267.

44. Mémoires de Pierre-Clément de Laussat, 13 September 1807, vol. 1, 88.

45. Rufz de Lavison, *Recherches sur les empoisonnements*, 144–145.

46. Thomas Jefferson to Thomas Mann Randolph, 13 January 1800, Oberg, ed., *Papers of Thomas Jefferson*, vol. 31, 304–307; Thomas Jefferson to Thomas Mann Randolph, 4 February 1800, *Papers of Thomas Jefferson*, vol. 31, 359–361. According to Oberg, Richardson's letter informing Jefferson of Jupiter's death has not been found. See Thomas Jefferson to Richard Richardson, 10 February 1800, *Papers of Thomas Jefferson*, vol. 31, 363–364.

47. For more on Thomas Mann Randolph's theory on how the "poison" physically worked, see Thomas Mann Randolph to Thomas Jefferson, 19 April 1800, Oberg, ed., *Papers of Thomas Jefferson*, vol. 31, 522–524. On the language of biological materialism in eighteenth-century Europe, see Porter, *Greatest Benefit to Mankind*, 251–252.

48. Thomas Mann Randolph to Thomas Jefferson, 19 April 1800, Oberg, ed., *Papers of Thomas Jefferson*, vol. 31, 522–524.

49. Stanton, *"Those Who Labor for My Happiness,"* 24.

50. Bryson, "Art of Power," 65–66; Savage, "'Black Magic' and White Terror," 645; Boaz, "'Instruments of Obeah': The Significance of Ritual Objects in the Jamaican Legal System, 1760 to the Present," in Ogundiran and Saunders, eds., *Materialities of Ritual in the Black Atlantic* 147; Weaver, *Medical Revolutionaries*, 117–118.

51. Martha Jefferson Randolph to Thomas Jefferson, 347–348.

52. Ogundiran and Saunders, "On the Materiality of Black Atlantic Rituals,", 4–8, 18; Leone, Knauf, and Tang, "Ritual Bundle in Colonial Annapolis," 200.

53. Davis, "Judges, Masters, Diviners," 933.

54. Procès de Marie Therese et Thélémaque, May 1773, ANOM Série F3, vol. 246, pp. 699–700.

55. Proces van Masongoe, 11 December 1781, NADH RVP, vol. 839, pp. 278–282v.

56. Ordonnance concernant les nègres empoisonneurs, 5 November 1749, ADM Série B, vol. 8, pp. 130–131; Marquis de Caylus to Antoine Louis Rouillé, 4 October 1749, ANOM Série C8a, box 58, f. 258.

57. Ordonnance concernant les nègres empoisonneurs, 5 November 1749, ADM Série B Conseil Souverain, vol. 8, pp. 130–131.

58. Ordonnance concernant les nègres empoisonneurs, 5 November 1749; Ordonnance concernant les nègres et autre personnes empoisonnés, 12 November 1758, ADM Série B, vol. 9, pp. 91–92. The 1758 update also mandated that surgeons perform this service for free to further encourage slaveholders to use them for autopsies.

59. Ordonnance concernant les nègres et autre personnes empoisonnés.

60. de Laborde, "Effet dangereux de l'erreur."

61. Pierre Dessalles to Albis de Gissac, 12 July 1824, in *La vie d'un colon à la Martinique,* 118; Pierre Dessalles to Albis de Gissac, 6 December 1824, in *La vie d'un colon à la Martinique,* 134.

62. Proces van Masongoe, 278–282v; Proces van Mustapha, 29 May 1787, NADH RVP, vol. 850, pp. 28–29.

63. Trial of Tom (1744), 288.

64. Procès de Jean Baptiste et outres, 267.

65. Proces van Coffij en La Rose, 16 August 1779, NADH RVP, vol. 836, p. 216.

66. Processo de Simão, 1688, ANTT IL Series 28 Processos, no. 8464, 6v–7, 15, 22v–24.

67. See, for example, Proces van Goliath en Prins; Proces van Bienvenue; Mémoires de Pierre-Clément de Laussat, vol. 1, pp. 71–72.

68. Denúncia de Paulo Gomes e Ignacia, pp. 154v, 160.

69. Proces van Coffij. Coffij's claim is similar to that of Hans in 1819 Berbice, who told the court that he could "smell" poison where it was hidden. See Browne, "'Bad Business' of Obeah," 478.

70. Proces van Quashie, 28 July 1731, NADH RVP, vol. 787, n.p.

71. Procès de Jean Baptiste et outres, p. 269.

72. Proces van Karel, Datra, en Avans, 22 August 1798, NADH RVP, vol. 859, pp. 24–30v.

73. Fett, *Working Cures*, 90.

74. António Brásio, *Monumenta missionaria Africana: Africa occidental*, 2nd series (Lisbon: Agência Geral do Ultramar, 1958), vol. 1, 703.

75. Davis, "Judges, Masters, Diviners," 932; Bosman, *New and Accurate Description*, 226–228; Barbot, *Barbot on Guinea*, 590; Olaudah Equiano, *The Interesting Narrative of the Life of Olaudah Equiano, or Gustavus Vassa, the African: Written by Himself* (London: Printed for and sold by the author, 1789), vol. 1, 34–36; Matthews, *Voyage to the River Sierra-Leone*, 121–124.

76. Bosman, *New and Accurate Description*, 226–228.

77. Davis, "Judges, Masters, Diviners," 933.

78. Bosman, *New and Accurate Description*, 149–150. Barbot and Atkins also reported belief in terrible agony resulting from perjury, see Barbot, *Barbot on Guinea*, 2: 572; Atkins, *Voyage to Guinea*, 103–104.

79. A word used in late nineteenth-century Twi, *aká-bó* (to undergo the ordeal by water), made a connection between *bo* empowerment objects with this ordeal, specifically the "bitter water." Christaller, *Dictionary of the Asante and Fante Languages*, 214. On the root *bo* among Gbe-speakers, see Blier, *African Vodun*, 4. In the vocabulary Barbot compiled, he noted among Ewe speakers the word *bodou-houy* [vodunnunu] (to drink fetish, possibly to seal a pact). See Jean Barbot, *Barbot's West African Vocabularies of c. 1680*, ed. P. E. H. Hair (Liverpool: Centre of African Studies, University of Liverpool, 1992), 22.

80. For Sierra Leone "red water," see Atkins, *Voyage to Guinea*, 52–53; Matthews, *Voyage to the River Sierra-Leone*, 124–125. For Gold Coast "bitter water," see Barbot, *Barbot on Guinea*, 2: 572. For Gold Coast "oath-draught" and Gold Coast "edible fetish," see Atkins, *Voyage to Guinea*, 103–104.

81. Its bark has been used for many purposes, including as an emetic, a fishing poison, and an antidote. H. M. Burkhill, *The Useful Plants of West Tropical Africa* (Kew: Royal Botanic Gardens, 1985), vol. 3, 116–120; Ficalho, *Plantas uteis da Africa Portuguza*, 168–171.

82. Brown, *Reaper's Garden*, 66–69; Davis, "Judges, Masters, Diviners," 956–957; Price, *Alabi's World*, 87, n.13, 312–313. For a particularly detailed and fascinating case from Suriname that involved a coffin ritual, see Proces van Quacoe en anders, 21 February 1775, NADH RVP, vol. 827, pp. 72–77.

83. Such practices were even more widespread, appearing in accounts from Sierra-Leone to the Gold Coast to the Kingdom of Kongo. Atkins, *Voyage to Guinea*, 52–53; Matthews, *Voyage to the River Sierra-Leone*, 124–127; Bosman, *New and Accurate Description*, 150. See also Davis, "Judges, Masters, Diviners," 933; Heywood and Thornton, *Central Africans, Atlantic Creoles*, 106.

84. Sweet, *Recreating Africa*, 121–123. For the full case, see Processo de Simão.

85. Davis, "Judges, Masters, Diviners," 965; Browne, "'Bad Business' of Obeah," 459.

86. Proces van Quacoe en anders.

87. Davis, "Judges, Masters, Diviners," 967–968; Beeldsnijder, *"Om Werk Van Jullie te Hebben,"* 244–247; Pierre Dessalles to Albis de Gissac, 12 July 1824, 28 July 1824, 15 September 1824, 6 November 1824, 6 December 1824, 1 February 1825, in Dessalles, *La vie d'un colon à la Martinique*, 119–121, 123–125, 127–128, 132, 134–135, 140.

88. Davis, "Judges, Masters, Diviners," 953, 971.

89. To further break down these cases, Virginia had seven, Bahia eight, Suriname seventeen, and Martinique zero. The number of Virginia cases with enslaved witnesses may be artificially low, as the majority of case summaries did not list the names of those testifying at all beyond "sundry" or "divers" witnesses, which may have included enslaved people. As the surviving eighteenth-century Martinique cases are also summaries from the Conseil Supérieur as the automatic court of appeal, it is unclear whether there were witnesses in individual cases or what their status was.

90. For more on the way chains of cases could rapidly escalate, see Levack, *Witch Hunt in Early Modern Europe.*

91. Proces van Francies, 16 August 1738, NADH RVP, vol. 792, p. 131.

92. Denúncia de Simão.

93. Denúncia de Paulo Gomes e Ignacia, p. 153.

94. Proces van Samsam, 11 May 1736, NADH RVP, vol. 790, n.p. For an example of a detailed examination of a witness without a confrontation, see Proces van Coffie, 20 April 1739, NADH RVP, vol. 793, p. 56.

95. Proces van Coffie; Proces van Assurant, 27 May 1737, NADH RVP, vol. 791, pp. 72–75.

96. Trial of Boatswain, 27 December 1764, LVA Amelia CCOB, vol. 8, p. 327.

97. ANTT Inquisição Lisboa, Series 30 Cadernos do Promotor and Series 28 Processos; APEB Seção Judiciário, Devassas; Schwarz, *Twice Condemned*, Table 10, p. 96 (for the Virginia data); NADH Raad van Politie en Criminele Justitie; NA-Kew CO 116 British Guiana, Berbice Records of the Court of Policy and Criminal Justice; ANOM Série F3 Collection Moreau de Saint-Méry, Annales du Conseil souverain de la Martinique; ANOM Dépôt des papiers des colonies, greffes Martinique, Cour d'assises de Fort-de-France and Saint-Pierre; ANOM Série C8 Correspondance à l'arrivée en provenance de la Martinique (for cases from Villaret's tribunal, 1806–1808); ADM Série U7 Cour Prévôtale.

98. Randy Browne has examined these two cases in detail in his work on the Berbice fiscal records. See Browne, "'Bad Business' of Obeah"; Browne, *Surviving Slavery*, 132–156.

99. Complaint against the negro Hans, pp. 60–63; Browne, "'Bad Business' of Obeah"; Paton, *Cultural Politics of Obeah*, 84–85.

100. Paton, *Cultural Politics of Obeah*, 83. See also Handler and Bilby, *Enacting Power.*

101. Boaz, "'Instruments of Obeah,'" 149.

102. NADH RVP, vol. 787–858.

103. Procès d'un negre (1756), ADM Série U7.

104. Pluchon, *Vaudou, sorciers, empoisonneurs*, 153–154; Oudin-Bastide, *L'effroi et la terreur*, 161.

105. Maxim de Bompar and Charles Marin Hurson to Antoine Louis Rouillé, 16 June 1753, ANOM Série C8a, box 60, f. 7; Oudin-Bastide, *L'effroi et la terreur*, 60–68, 71–72, 128–130.

106. ANOM, Série F3, vol. 244–246.

107. Arrêté de Villaret-Joyeuse portant création d'un tribunal spécial qui sera chargé de juger les crimes d'empoisonnements, incendies et enlèvements de canots et pirogues commis par les esclaves, 17 October 1803, ANOM Série C8a, box 107, f. 188; Arrêté relatif à l'établissement d'un tribunal spécial, 21 October 1803, ADM Série B, vol. 24, pp. 57–60. Villaret-Joyeuse attached a copy of this act in a letter to the Ministère de la Marine. For the cover letter, see Louis Thomas Villaret de Joyeuse to Denis Decrès, 28 November 1803, ANOM Série C8a, box 107, f. 112.

108. Louis Thomas Villaret de Joyeuse to Pierre Clément de Laussat, 9 June 1805, ANOM Série C8a, box 111, f. 111.

109. Mémoires de Pierre-Clément de Laussat, 16 September 1807 to 8 November 1807, vol. 1, pp. 83–94. This manuscript was part of Laussat's preparation for writing his memoir of his time in Martinique, published in 1831. The entries are the original text from his journals and have their original dates, copied out and rearranged into Laussat's planned chapters. Some entries were repeated when information from them appeared in multiple sections. For the published memoir, see Pierre-Clément de Laussat, *Mémoires sur ma vie à mon fils: Pendant les années 1803 et suivants* (Pau: É. Vignancour, imprimeur, 1831).

110. Louis Thomas Villaret de Joyeuse to Denis Decrès, 2 April 1808, ANOM Série C8a, box 116, f. 17.

111. From April 1809 to October 1811 alone, the tribunal tried 203 enslaved people and free people of color, mainly for poisoning, resulting in 66 executions; from 1809 to 1815 the tribunal sentenced 127 people to die. Oudin-Bastide, *L'effroi et la terreur*, 63–64.

112. Extrait du Registre des Delibérations du Conseil de Gouvernement & d'Administration, 9 August 1822, ANOM SG Martinique, box 52, f. 430. See also A la suite d'une lettre du Gouverneur Donzelot pour enquêter sur les empoisonnements, 9 September 1818, ADM Série B, vol. 26, p. 200.

113. ADM Série U7 Cour Prévôtale.

114. ADM Série U7; ANOM Série F3, vol. 244–246.

115. Governeur Donzelot to Marquis de Clermont-Tonnerre; Savage, "'Black Magic' and White Terror," 637; Oudin-Bastide, *L'effroi et la terreur*, 159.

116. Oudin-Bastide, *L'effroi et la terreur*, 31.

117. Extrait d'une letter de la Martinique de 14 7bre 1823, 14 September 1823, ANOM SG Martinique, box 52, f. 430.

118. Extrait d'une letter de la Martinique de 14 7bre 1823.

119. Directeur Général de l'intérieur to Gouverneur François Marie Michel de Bouillé, March 1827, ANOM SG, box 52, f. 431.

120. Oudin-Bastide, *L'effroi et la terreur*, 66.

121. Baron Delamardelle to Duc de Clermont-Tonnerre, 25 January 1823, ANOM SG Martinique, box 52, f. 431.

122. Gouverneur François Marie Michel de Bouillé to Comte de Chabrol, 9 February 1827, ANOM SG Martinique, box 52, f. 430; Procureur du Roi Riviere to Gouverneur le Comte de Chabrol, 27 July 1827, ANOM SG Martinique, box 52, f. 431; Oudin-Bastide, *L'effroi et la terreur*, 67.

123. Garrigus, "'Like an Epidemic,'" 651. For a classic discussion of this idea, see Marc Bloch, *The Historian's Craft* (New York: Vintage Books, 1953), 107.

124. Parrish, *American Curiosity*, 259. I'd also like to thank Mike Zuckerman for sharing this insight with me as feedback following a presentation of an earlier version of this chapter at the McNeil Center for Early American Studies in October 2020.

Conclusion

1. See, for example, the case of Benjamin Pousset in Davis, "Judges, Masters, Diviners," 968. For discussion of the 1788 Lejeune affair, a similar case in Saint-Domingue, see Pluchon, *Vaudou, sorciers, empoisonneurs*, 200–202; Garrigus, "'Like an Epidemic,'" 648–649.

2. Procureur Général to Gouverneur Pierre Louis Aimé Mathieu, 12 April 1847, ANOM SG Martinique, box 33, f. 284. This folder contains a flurry of official correspondence regarding the case. I want to thank Alix Rivière for noticing the file and calling me over to her desk in the ANOM in a serendipitous archival moment. Caroline Oudin-Bastide briefly mentions this case in *L'effroi et la terreur*, 106–107.

3. Procureur Général to Gouverneur Pierre Louis Aimé Mathieu.

4. The phrase "terreur salutaire" was from a speech by Governor Donzelot to the Conseil du Gouvernement et Administration establishing the Cour Prévôtale in 1822. See Extrait du Registre des Delibérations du Conseil de Gouvernement & d'Administration, 9 August 1822, box 52, f. 430.

5. Pierre Dessalles to Albis de Gissac, 8 September 1822, *La vie d'un colon à la Martinique*, 69. This letter was attached to Dessalles's letter from 1 September 1822.

6. Procureur du Roi Riviere to Gouverneur le Comte de Chabrol (1827); Procureur du Roi Riviere to Gouverneur Louis Henri de Saulces de Freycinet, 15 October 1829, ANOM SG Martinique, box 52, f. 431. Caroline Oudin-Bastide also talks about Rivière's letters in *L'effroi et la terreur*, 81–82.

7. Procureur Général to Gouverneur Pierre Louis Aimé Mathieu.

8. Procureur Général to Gouverneur Pierre Louis Aimé Mathieu.

9. For an earlier precedent of skepticism in the Martinique context, see de Laborde, "Effet dangereux de l'erreur" from 1775. Garrigus discusses this history of skepticism in a wider French Caribbean context, including de Laborde's report, in Garrigus, "'Like an Epidemic,'" 640–643, 647, 649–651.

10. Rufz de Lavison, *Recherches sur les empoisonnements*, 6.

11. Rufz de Lavison, *Recherches sur les empoisonnements*, 33–34.

12. Procureur Général to Gouverneur Pierre Louis Aimé Mathieu. See also Burnard and Garrigus, *Plantation Machine*, 106–107; Garrigus, "'Like an Epidemic,'" 637–640.

13. Procureur Général to Gouverneur Pierre Louis Aimé Mathieu.

14. Procureur Général to Gouverneur Pierre Louis Aimé Mathieu, 9 April 1847, ANOM SG Martinique, box 33, f. 284.

15. Procureur Général to Gouverneur Claude Rostoland, 21 February 1848, ANOM SG Martinique, box 33, f. 284.

16. de Luna, "Sounding the African Atlantic," 585.

17. Isaac, *Transformation of Virginia*, 5.

Appendix A

1. Ehret, *History and the Testimony of Language*, 3.

2. de Luna and Fleisher, *Speaking with Substance*, 18–20.

3. de Luna and Fleisher, *Speaking with Substance*, 5.

4. Ehret, *History and the Testimony of Language*, 22–23.

5. de Luna, *Collecting Food, Cultivating People*, 41–42; de Luna and Fleisher, *Speaking with Substance*, 4.

6. Schoenbrun, *Green Place, Good Place*, 28. Changes in vocabulary related to crops or technologies, for example, can reveal changes and adaptations in agricultural practice. See Fields-Black, *Deep Roots*, 12–13. For examples of classic works, see Jan Vansina, *Paths in the Rainforest: Toward a History of Political Tradition in Equatorial Africa* (Madison: University of Wisconsin Press, 1990); Christopher Ehret, *An African Classical Age: Eastern and Southern Africa in World History, 1000 BC to AD 400* (Charlottesville: University Press of Virginia, 1998). For examples of more recent works, see Rhiannon Stephens, *A History of African Motherhood: The Case of Uganda, 700–1900* (Cambridge: Cambridge University Press, 2013); de Luna, "Affect and Society in Precolonial Africa"; de Luna, *Collecting Food, Cultivating People*. For an example that focuses on the African Atlantic, see Almeida, "African Voices from the Congo Coast."

7. Ehret, *History and the Testimony of Language*, 13.

8. de Luna and Fleisher, *Speaking with Substance*, 14–15.

9. For example, see Vansina, *How Societies Are Born*; de Luna, *Collecting Food, Cultivating People*. For an example of the new phylogenetic classification, see de Schryver et al., "Introducing a State-of-the-Art Phylogenetic Classification of the Kikongo Language Cluster." This team's work was part of the Kongo King interdisciplinary research project that included historians, linguists, and archaeologists. For historical linguistic works that have come out of the new classification in this project, see Jaspar De Kind, Gilles-Maurice de Schryver, and Koen Bostoen, "Pushing Back the Origin of Bantu Lexicography: The 'Vocabularium Congense' of 1652, 1928, 2012," *Lexicos* 22 (2012): 159–194; Bostoen et al., "On the Origin of the Royal Kongo Title *Ngangula*"; Koen Bostoen and Gilles-Maurice de Schryver, "Linguistic Innovation, Political Centralization and Economic Integration in the Kongo Kingdom: Reconstructing the Spread of Prefix Reduction," *Diachronica* 32, no. 2 (2015): 139–185.

10. Ehret, *History and the Testimony of Language*, 28–29. An asterisk (*) is the standard way to show that a word has been reconstructed.

11. For more on tones, and particularly tone shifts and tone spreading phenomena in Bantu languages, see Michael R. Marlo and David Odden, "Tone," in *The Bantu Languages*, ed. Mark Van de Veld, Koean Bostoen, Derek Nurse, and Gérard Philippson, 2nd ed. (New York: Routledge, 2019), 150–171.

12. Fields-Black, *Deep Roots*, 17–18; de Luna and Fleisher, *Speaking with Substance*, 4, 12; Ehret, *History and the Testimony of Language*, 82–104; Bostoen and de Schryver, "Linguistic Innovation, Political Centralization," 173; de Schryver et al., "Introducing a State-of-the-Art Phylogenetic Classification of the Kikongo Language Cluster," 143. On prestige borrowing, see Ehret, *History and the Testimony of Language*, 52.

13. Schoenbrun, "Mixing, Moving, Making, Meaning," 302.

14. de Luna and Fleisher, *Speaking with Substance*, 15; Vansina, *How Societies Are Born*, 5; Ehret, *History and the Testimony of Language*, 13. For more on the history, uses, and some of the pitfalls of "words and things," see Koen Bostoen, "Pots, Words and the Bantu Problem: On Lexical Reconstruction and Early African History," *Journal of African History* 48, no. 2 (2007): 175.

15. Grollemund et al., "Bantu Expansion Shows"; Vansina, *Paths in the Rainforests*, "Appendix of Comparative Lexical Data"; Schoenbrun, *Historical Reconstruction of Great Lakes Bantu Cultural Vocabulary*; P. Dahin, *Vocabulaire Français-Adouma* (Kempten: Jos. Kösel, 1893); A. Sims, *A Vocabulary of the Kiteke as Spoken by the Bateke (Batio) and Kindred Tribes on the Upper Congo* (London: Hodder and Stoughton, 1886).

16. Schoenbrun, "Mixing, Moving, Making, Meaning," 296, 312; Bostoen, "Pots, Words and the Bantu Problem," 174–177.

17. de Luna and Fleisher, *Speaking with Substance*, 15–16, 19; Schoenbrun, "Mixing, Moving, Making, Meaning," 295–296. For a creative look at a very specific context of elicitation—that of a Brazilian clerk and several West Central African translators interviewing enslaved people taken from an illegal slaving voyage in 1850, see Almeida, "African Voices from the Congo Coast," 172–175, 177, 187.

18. de Luna and Fleisher, *Speaking with Substance*, 17.

19. Bostoen, "Pots, Words, and the Bantu Problem," 183.

20. de Luna and Fleisher, *Speaking with Substance*, 18.

21. Schoenbrun, "Mixing, Moving, Making, Meaning," 308.

Appendix C

1. David Schoenbrun examines this same root in the context of spirit consecration in the Great Lakes region of East Africa. See Schoenbrun, *Historical Reconstruction of Great Lakes Bantu Cultural Vocabulary*, 178; Schoenbrun, "Conjuring the Modern in Africa," 1421.

2. On the connection between *-kìtì nature spirits specifically, see Vansina, *Paths in the Rainforests*, 297; Vansina, *How Societies Are Born*, 51; Schoenbrun, *Historical Reconstruction of Great Lakes Bantu Cultural Vocabulary*, 187–188.

Appendix D

1. Sweet, *Domingos Álvares*, 149, 152–153. Of the approximately forty thousand cases from the Portuguese empire that went to full trial, Sweet counts only forty-six involving Africans accused of *feitiçaria*. For a history of the Inquisition's activities in Brazil from the sixteenth to the nineteenth century, see the entirety of Mott, *Bahia: Inquisição & Sociedade*. There was a jurisdictional divide, where cases of "feitiçarias, spells, and superstitions" were to be reported to the

Inquisition only when they were "manifest heresy or apostasy." Several Inquisitorial trials hint at the existence of trials for *feitiçaria* crimes under the secular judicial system; unfortunately, their records for the bulk of the eighteenth century have not survived.

2. Davis, "Judges, Masters, Diviners," 941, 959; van Stipriaan, *Surinaams contrast*, 38; Beeldsnijder, *"Om Werk Van Jullie te Hebben,"* 30.

3. Davis, "Judges, Masters, Diviners," 941, 959; van Stipriaan, *Surinaams contrast*, 38; Beeldsnijder, *"Om Werk Van Jullie te Hebben,"* 30. The role of the fiscal would take on new dimensions under British rule and nineteenth-century British policies of amelioration. See Browne, *Surviving Slavery*, 5.

4. Davis, "Judges, Masters, Diviners," 960, 976–978; Beeldsnijder, *"Om Werk Van Jullie te Hebben,"* 236–237.

5. Appendix B: *Constitutio Criminalis Carolina* (1532), translated into English, in John H. Langbein, *Prosecuting Crime in the Renaissance: England, Germany, France* (Cambridge, MA: Harvard University Press, 1974), 280–282; Levack, *Witch-Hunt in Early Modern Europe*, 212–213. For more on the application of the Carolina in witchcraft trials, see "Chapter 7: The Chronology and Geography of Witch-Hunting."

6. Isaac, *Transformation of Virginia*, 92. Trial of Dido, 3 May 1756, vol. 1752–58, pp. 388–389; Trial of Isaac and Quash, 29 May 1759, vol. 1758–62, pp. 56–57; Trial of Peter and Mingo, 24 January 1763, vol. 1762–64, pp. 129–130; Trial of Frank and Dick, 4 September 1769, vol. 1767–70, p. 428; Trial of Caesar, 21 October 1773, vol. 1772–74, pp. 452–453, all from LVA Cumberland CCOB.

7. Friedman, *History of American Law*, 51; Thomas D. Morris, *Southern Slavery and the Law, 1619–1860* (Chapel Hill: University of North Carolina Press, 1996), 214; Hugh F. Rankin, *Criminal Trial Proceedings in the General Court of Virginia* (Charlottesville: University Press of Virginia, 1956), 212; Isaac, *Transformation of Virginia*, 113; Annette Gordon-Reed, *The Hemingses of Monticello: An American Family* (New York: W. W. Norton, 2008), 45.

8. Oudin-Bastide, *L'effroi et la terreur*, 57.

9. Nicolas François Arnoul de Vaucresson to Comte de Pontchartrain, 22 May 1712, ANOM Série C8, box 18, f. 410; Nicolas François Arnoul de Vaucresson to Comte de Pontchartrain, 20 May 1713, ANOM Série C8, box 19, f. 341; Charles Bernard to Joseph Jean Baptiste Fleuriau d'Armenonville, 2 September 1720, ANOM Série C8a, box 27, f. 351.

10. For Bahia, see D. Sebastião Monteiro Vide, *Constituições primeiras do Arcebispado da Bahia (1707)* (São Paulo: Tipografia 2 de Dezembro, 1853), 313–317. The Dutch colonies in the Guianas lacked a slave code comparable to the French Code Noir. Instead, laws regarding enslaved Africans in the colonies came in the form of ad hoc ordinances issued by the local governments—in the case of Suriname, by the eponymous Society. Ordinances pre-1764 for Berbice have not survived, as they were destroyed in the 1763–1764 slave uprising. For Suriname, see Appendix B: *Constitutio Criminalis Carolina* (1532), translated into English, in Langbein, *Prosecuting Crime in the Renaissance*, 280–282; Davis, "Judges, Masters, Diviners," 941, 960, 976–978; Beeldsnijder, *"Om Werk Van Jullie te Hebben,"* 236–237.[1] No. 134 Reglement voor plantagebedienden, 9–24 May 1686, in Schiltkamp and Smidt, *West Indisch Plakaatboek*, vol. 1, 166–169. There *were* several ordinances regarding poison in the late seventeenth century, but of a very particular kind: its use as a fishing practice. The existence of four separate bans on the practice, as well John Gabriel Stedman's description of its widespread use from his time in the colony in the 1770s, indicates a lack of success in enforcement. None of the bans gave any indication of a concern about people intentionally using this technique to poison others. No. 94 Plakaat: Verontreiniging van kreeken, 17 July 1681, in Schiltkamp and Smidt, *West Indisch Plakaatboek*, vol. 1, 112–113; No. 131 Plakaat: verontreininging van kreeken; vrij cisserij in de kreeken; schoonhouden van grensafbakeningen tussen plantagies, 22 September 1685, in Schiltkamp and Smidt, *West Indisch Plakaatboek*, vol. 1, 162–164; No. 141 Plakaat: verbod om wild te schieten

in de Paramaribo-Divisie; verontreiniging van sloten op societeitsplantages; verbod om hout te kappen op societeitsplantages, 7 September 1687, in Schiltkamp and Smidt, *West Indisch Plakaatboek*, vol. 1, 175–176; No. 296 Bekendmaking: aanvulling van het verbod om kreken te verontreiningen, September 1722, in Schiltkamp and Smidt, *West Indisch Plakaatboek*, vol. 1, 347; Stedman, *Narrative of a Five Years' Expedition* (1796), vol. 1, 402. For Virginia, see Hening, *Statutes at Large*, vol. 3, 102–103. For Martinique, see *Le Code Noir ou Edit du Roy, 1685* (Paris: Chez Claude Girard, 1735); *Edit du Roy Pour la punition de differents crimes: Registé en Parlement le 31 aoust 1682* (Paris: Chez François Muguet, Imprimeur du Roy & de son Parlement, 1682); Mollenauer, *Strange Revelations*, 130; Paton, "Witchcraft, Poison, Law," 241–242; Oudin-Bastide, *L'effroi et la terreur*, 25. The 1724 application of the edict to Martinique and the other Isles du Vent kept most of the language from the original law, with some significant exceptions. The preface of the 1682 law was rooted in the circumstances of the case, emphasizing pretended "Diviners, Magicians & Enchanters," who added *maléfices* (evil spells), *vénéfice* (poison by magical means) and "poison" to their sacrilege, and the dangers of their seduction of the gullible. In the Martinique law, the preface reflected different circumstances and a different perceived threat: the "enormous Crimes" of "malicious" enslaved Africans, serving "Venefices and poisons to the detriment of the lives of our subjects." Édit pour la punition et la prevention des crimes par empoisonnement, dans les îles du Vent, February 1724, ANOM, Série A, Acts du pouvoir souverain, vol. 25, f. 81.

11. For an example of how the interaction between guiding concepts from different parts of the Atlantic world could combine in the drastically unequal power relationships of western Atlantic societies to create new guiding interpretations of events, see Sharples, "Discovering Slave Conspiracies," 829–839.

12. "Déclaration du roi qui interdit aux nègres esclaves des îles de fabriquer ou de distribuer aucun remède," 1 February 1743, ANOM, Série A, Acts du pouvoir souverain, vol. 25, f. 199; André de Melo e Castro to D. João V, 30 August 1743, AHU Conselho Ultramarino Brasil—Bahia, box 77, f. 6363; Hening, *Statutes at Large*, vol. 4, 104–112; Schiltkamp and Smidt, *West Indisch Plakaatboek*, vol. 1, 550–551.

13. ANTT IL, Series 28; ANTT IL, Series 30, vol. 55–131. The four full trials from 1750, all of people of African descent, were interconnected cases involving *bolsas de mandinga* made with pieces of consecrated host in the backcountry town of Jacobina. Luiz Mott discusses these cases in detail in *Bahia: Inquisição & Sociedade*, 99–117.

14. ANTT IL, Series 30, vol. 55–131. The volume numbers do not always correspond with chronological order.

15. NA-Kew, CO 116 British Guiana, Berbice Records of the Court of Policy and Criminal Justice, vol. 106–117.

16. Schwarz, *Twice Condemned*, 39, 92. In his sampling of county court records, Philip Morgan counted 175 poison trials from the eighteenth-century. Morgan, *Slave Counterpoint*, 613–614.

17. ANOM, Série F3, vol. 244–246.

18. From 1735 to 1739, poison cases had made up 10 percent of all trials and 19 percent of all trials involving enslaved people, but another five-year sample from 1761 to 1765 shows a drop to 5 percent of total cases, and 6 percent of those involving enslaved people. NADH RVP, vol. 789–793, 805–811.

19. NADH RVP, vol. 829–836.

20. Schwarz, *Twice Condemned*, 92.

21. ANTT IL, Series 30, vol. 55–131; Mott, *Bahia: Inquisição & Sociedade*, 11; Schwartz, *Sugar Plantations in the Formation of Brazilian Society*, 473–488; Reis, *Slave Rebellion in Brazil*, 141–142. See the entirety of Reis's book for an analysis of the 1835 Malê rebellion as the culmination and largest expression of a series of revolts in the late eighteenth and early nineteenth

centuries. For more on this period in the Portuguese Atlantic more broadly, see Gabriel Paquette, *Imperial Portugal in the Age of Atlantic Revolutions: The Luso-Brazilian World, c. 1770-
1850* (New York: Cambridge University Press, 2013); Matthew Brown and Gabriel Paquette, eds.,
Connections After Colonialism: Europe and Latin America in the 1820s (Tuscaloosa: University of
Alabama Press, 2013). For more on the suppression of the Cour Prévôtale in 1826 and protests
by slaveholders against the suppression, see Oudin-Bastide, *L'effroi et la terreur*, 66, 67; Gouverneur François Marie Michel de Bouillé to Comte de Chabrol, 9 February 1827, ANOM SG
Martinique, box 52, f. 430; Procureur du Roi Riviere to Gouverneur le Comte de Chabrol, 27
July 1827, ANOM SG Martinique, box 52, f. 431.

22. For a similar shift involving discussion of the efficacy of the work of African bloodletting practitioners in Bahia, see Hicks, "Blood and Hair," 71–74.

23. *Collecção das leis do Imperio do Brazil de 1830* (Rio de Janeiro: Typographia Nacional,
1876) vol. 1, 144, 174; Browne, *Surviving Slavery*, 5–8; Paton, *Cultural Politics of Obeah*, 9–10;
Danielle N. Boaz, "'Instruments of Obeah': The Significance of Ritual Objects in the Jamaican
Legal System, 1760 to the Present," in Ogundiran and Saunders, eds., *Materialities of Ritual in
the Black Atlantic*, 147–150; Handler and Bilby, *Enacting Power*, 21; Morris, *Southern Slavery and
the Law*, 271; Friedman, *History of American Law*, 281–282; Isaac, *Transformation of Virginia*,
318; Oudin-Bastide, *L'effroi et la terreur*, 27; Projet de Code Pénal pour les esclaves, January 1831,
ANOM Séries Généralités, box 189, f. 1455, Art 170, 174, 177–178, 204–206, 218–220, 235.

Appendix E

1. Voyages Database.

2. Voyages Database.

3. Recensement des îles Amérique, 12 April 1683, ANOM Série C8b, box 17, f. 9; Recensement
general de l'isle Martinique fait à la fin de l'année mil sept cent vingt six, 16 February 1727, ANOM
Série C8a, box 37, f. 14; Alison Games, "Cohabitation, Suriname-Style: English Inhabitants in
Dutch Suriname After 1667," *William and Mary Quarterly* 72, no. 2 (2015): 217, 233; Davis, "Judges,
Masters, Diviners," 929–930; van Stipriaan, *Surinaams contrast*, 311, 314; Berlin, *Generations of
Captivity*, 272; Schwartz, *Sugar Plantations in the Formation of Brazilian Society*, 86–88.

BIBLIOGRAPHY

Manuscript

Brazil

Arquivo Publico do Estado da Bahia (Salvador)
Seção Colônia
417 Correspondência Recebida dos Capitães-Mores e Sargento Mor: Maragojipe, Sergipe d'El Rei (1809–1820)
Seção Judiciário
Processos Crime, Devassas
Seção Colônia—Provincia
Correspondência Recebida de Juízes
Correspondência Recebida da Polícia, diversos assuntos
Correspondência Recebida da Secretaria da Polícia

France

Archives Départementales de la Martinique (Fort-de-France, Martinique)
B: Conseil Souverain (1712–1820)
U2: Cour Royal & Cour d'appel
U7: Cour Prévôtale (1822–1826)
J24: Fonds Pierre-Clément de Laussat (1804–1809)
Archives Nationales d'Outre-Mer (Aix-en-Provence)
C8: Correspondance à l'arrivée en provenance de la Martinique
DPPC: Dépôt des papiers des colonies, greffes Martinique
Cour d'assises de Fort-de-France (1830–1907)
Cour d'assises de Saint-Pierre (1830–1907)
F3: Collection Moreau de Saint-Méry
Annales du Conseil souverain de la Martinique (1726–1778)
Généralités (1829–1831), Box 189
Séries Géographiques (SG): Martinique (1793–1931)

The Netherlands

Nationaal Archief (The Hague)
Sociëteit van Suriname (1650, 1682–1796)

C2: Ingekomen Stukken uit de Kolonie
    Resoluties van Gouverneur en Raden (1695–1795)
    Bekendmakingen en plakkaten van het Hof van Politie en Criminele Justitie (27 December 1759–11 February 1762)
    Ingekomen brieven en papieren van de Gouverneur en andere overheidspersonen (1683–1794)
Raad van Politie en Criminele Justitie en voorgangers, in Suriname (1699–1828)
Processtukken betreffende criminele zaken (1705–1828)

Portugal

Arquivo Histórico Ultramarino (Lisbon)
    Conselho Ultramarinho: no. 5 Brasil-Bahia (1604–1828)
Arquivo Nacional Torre do Tombo (Lisbon)
    AJCJ: Amário Jesuitico e Cartório dos Jesuitas
    IL: Inquisição Lisboa (1536–1821)
    IL 28 Processos
    IL 30 Cadernos do Promotor
Biblioteca Nacional de Portugal (Lisbon)
    Manuscritos reservados
        Buytrago, Francisco de. *Arvore da Vida, e Thezouro Descuberto da Avore Irmãa da que se Fez a Cruz da Nossa Redempção: Para Livrar dos Malefícios do Demonio, P.A. Vida e Saude dos Enfeitiçados ou Vexados do Mesmo Demonio, e Outras Mtas.* 1731.

United Kingdom

British Library (London)
    Sloane Manuscripts
National Archives (Kew)
    CO: Records of the Colonial Office
        CO 111 British Guiana, formerly Berbice, Demerara, and Essequibo, Original Correspondence (1781–1951)
        CO 116 British Guiana, formerly Berbice, Demerara, and Essequibo, Miscellanea including Papers of the Dutch West India Company (1681–1943)
            68–72 Berbice Ordinances & Instructions (1681–1794)
            106–117 Berbice Records of the Court of Policy and Criminal Justice (1764–1793)
            138–142 Berbice Fiscal's Reports (1819–1832)
            156–163 Demerara and Essequibo Reports of Protectors (1826–1834)
        CO 137/248 Jamaica Despatches (1840)
        CO 166 Secretary of State for the Colonies and War and Colonial Department: Martinique, Original Correspondence, Entry Books and Shipping Returns (1693–1815)
    WO: Records of the War Office
        WO 1 War Office, In-letters and Miscellaneous Papers; Of the French Wars, West Indies and South America: Martinique (1791–1815)

United States

Bull Run Regional Library (Manassas, VA)
Robert Carter Letterbooks, I–IX (1772–1794) (microfilm)
Library of Virginia (Richmond, VA)
County Court Order Books and County Court Minute Books (microfilm)
Amelia County, Vol. 3 (1751–1755), Vol. 8 (1764–1765); Reels 40–41
Brunswick County, Vol. 1–21 (1732–1844); Reels 29–43
Cumberland County, Vol. 1749–1751 to 1844–1851; Reels 1–35
Goochland County, Vol. 7 (1750–1757), Vol. 9–10 (1761–1766), Reels 23, 24
Orange County, Vol. 4–6 (1743–1763); Reels 31, 32
Powhatan County, Vol. 1 (1777–1784); Reel 22
Spotsylvania County, Vol. 1774–1782; Reel 45
University of Virginia, Small Special Collections Library (Charlottesville, VA)
Account Book of Phebe Jackson (1843–1846)
Atcheson L. Hench Papers (1776–1939)
Charles Beale Medical Notes and Daybook (1815–1819)
Cocke Family Papers (1725–1939)
Correspondence Between Nathanial H. Hooe and William A. Harrison (1832–1836)
Henkel Family Papers (1800–1846)
Papers of Dr. James Carmichael (1816–1834)
Virginia Historical Society (Richmond, VA)
Carter Family Papers (1651–1861)

Published Primary

Dictionaries

Baião, Domingos Viera, Ernesto Lecomte, and José Sutter. *Dictionário Ganguela-Português: Língua falada nas regiões do Cubango, Nhemba e Luchaze, Província de Angola.* Lisbon: Centro de Estudos Filológicos, 1940.

Barbot, Jean. *Barbot's West African Vocabularies of c. 1680.* Edited by P. E. H. Hair. Liverpool: Centre of African Studies, University of Liverpool, 1992.

Bentley, W. Holman. *Dictionary and Grammar of the Kongo Language, as Spoken at San Salvador.* London: Baptist Missionary Society and Trübner, 1887–1895.

Blom, Anthony. *Verhandeling over den Landbouw, in de Colonie Suriname, volgens eene negentien-jarrige ondervinding zamen gbsteld.* Haarlem: Cornelis van den A., 1786.

Bluteau, Raphael. *Vocabulario Portuguez & Latino.* 8 volumes. Coimbra: No Collegio das Artes da Companhia de Jesus, 1728.

Christaller, J. G. *Dictionary of the Asante and Fante Language Called Tshi (Twi).* 2nd ed. Basel: Printed for the Basel Evangelical Missionary Society, 1933.

Clarke, Mary Lane. *A Limba-English Dictionary: or Tampen Ta Ka Talun To Ka Hulimba Ha In Huinkilisi Ha.* Westmead, UK: Gregg International Publishers, 1971.

Daeleman, Jan. *Ko-Holo (notes provisoires).* Paris: Heverlee & Leuven, 1961.

Dahin, P. *Vocabulaire Français-Adouma.* Kempten: Jos. Kösel, 1893.

da Matta, J. D. Cordeiro. *Ensaio de Diccionario Kimbúndu-Portuguez.* Lisbon: Da Casa Editoria Antonio Maria Pereira, 1893.

da Silva, António Joaquim. *Dicionário Portugûes-Nhaneca*. Lisbon: Instituto de Investigação Científica de Angola, 1966.

da Silva Maia, António. *Lições de gramática de Quimbundo (Portugûes e Banto), dialecto Omumbuim: Língua indígena de Gabela, Amboim, Quanza-Sul, Angola, Africa Ocidental Portuguesa*. Cucujães, Portugal: published by the author, 1957.

de Moraes Silva, Antonio. *Diccionario da lingua Portugueza: Composto pelo Padre D. Rafael Bluteau, reformado, e accrescentado por Antonio de Moraes Silva, natural do Rio de Janeiro*. Lisbon: Na Officinia de Simão Thaddeo Ferreira, 1789.

Deutsches Wörterbuch von Jacob Grimm und Wilhelm Grimm auf CD-ROM und im Internet. Universitëit Trier. 2019. http://dwb.uni-trier.de/de/ (accessed 27 January 2019).

Dictionnaire de l'Académie Française. 1st ed. Paris: Chez la Veuve de Jean Baptiste Coignard, Imprimeur ordinaire du Roy, & de l'Académie Françoise, 1694.

Dictionnaire de l'Académie Française. 4th ed. Paris: Chez la Veuve de Brunet, 1762.

Dictionnaire de l'Académie Française. 6th ed. Paris: Imprimerie et Librairie de Firmin Didot frères, Imprimeurs de l'Institut de France, 1835.

Diouf, Jean-Léopold. *Dictionnaire Wolof-Français et Français-Wolof*. Paris: Éditions Karthala, 2003.

do Nascimento, J. Pereira. *Diccionario Portuguez-Kimbundu*. Huilla, Angola: Typographia da Missão, 1903.

Etymologiebank.nl. 2010. http://www.etymologiebank.nl (accessed 27 January 2019).

Féraud, Jean François. *Dictionnaire critique de la langue française*. Marseille: J. Mossy, 1787.

Glare, P. G. W. *Oxford Latin Dictionary*. 4 volumes. Oxford: Clarendon, 1973.

Gusimana, Barthelemy. *Dictionnaire Pende-Français*. Bandundu, Democratic Republic of Congo: Publications Ceeba, 1972.

Horton, Albert E. *A Dictionary of Luvale*. El Monte, CA: Rahn Brothers Printing & Lithographic, 1953.

———. *A Grammar of Luvale*. Johannesburg: Witwatersrand University Press, 1949.

Innes, Gordon. *A Mende-English Dictionary*. Cambridge: Cambridge University Press, 1969.

Johnston, Harry. *A Comparative Study of the Bantu and Semi-Bantu Languages*. Oxford: Clarendon, 1919.

Kloppers, J. K. *Bukenkango: Rukwangali-English, English-Rukwangali Dictionary*. Edited by A. W. Bredell. Windhoek, Namibia: Gamsberg Macmillan, 1995.

Kluge, Friedrich. *Etymological Dictionary of the German Language*. 4th ed., translated from the German. London: Bell, 1891.

Koelle, S. W. *Polyglotta Africana, or a Comparative Vocabulary of Nearly Three Hundred Words and Phrases in More Than One Hundred Distinct African Languages*. 2nd ed. Graz, Austria: Akademische Druck U. Verlagsanstalt, 1963.

Kolbe, F. W. *An English-Herero Dictionary with an Introduction to the Study of Herero and Bantu in General*. Cape Town: J. C. Juta, 1883.

Laman, K. E. *Dictionnaire Kikongo-Français: Avec une etude phonetique décrivent les dialects les plus importants de la langue dite Kikongo*. Originally published 1936. Ridgewood, NJ:Gregg Press, 1964.

Le Guennec, Grégoire, and José Francisco Valente. *Dicionário Português-Umbundu*. Luanda, Angola: Instituto d'Investigação Cientifica d'Angola, 1972.

Lexicons of Early Modern English. University of Toronto. https://leme.library.utoronto.ca (accessed 17 February 2019).

Littré, Émile. *Dictionnaire de la langue française.* 4 volumes. Paris: L. Hachette, 1873–74.

Machado, José Pedro. *Dicionário etimológico da língua Portuguesa: Com a mais antiga documentação escrita e conhecida de muitos dos vocábulos estudados.* Lisbon: Editorial Confluência, 1952.

MacJannet, Malcom Brooks. *Chokwe-English English-Chokwe Dictionary and Grammar Lessons.* Missão da Biula, Angola, 1949.

Maes, J. "Vocabulaire des populations de la region du Kasai-Lulua-Sankuru." *Journal de la Société des Africanistes* 4, no. 2 (1934): 209–268.

Marichelle, P. *Dictionnaire Vili-Français.* Loango: Imprimerie de la Mission, 1902.

Mission de Landana. *Dictionnaire Français-Fiote.* Paris: Maison-Mère, 1890.

Möhlig, Wilhelm J. G., and Kari Peter Shiyaka-Mberema. *A Dictionary of the Rumanyo Language: Rumanyo-English/English-Rumanyo, Including a Grammatical Sketch.* Cologne: Rüdiger Köppe Verlag, 2005.

Mudinaambi, Lumbwe. *Dictionnaire Mbala-Français.* Bandundu, Democratic Republic of Congo: Ceeba Publications, 1974.

Nash, Jay. "Ruund 1996." *Comparative Bantu Online Dictionary.* University of California, Berkeley. Accessed 21 April 2016.

Nicot, Jean. *Thresor de la langue françoyse, tant ancienne que modern.* Paris: David Douceve, 1606.

Oxford English Dictionary Online. March 2015. Oxford University Press. www.oed.com (accessed 30 June 2016).

Oxford Portuguese Dictionary. Oxford: Oxford University Press, 2015.

Raynal, Abbé. *Histoire philosophic et politique, des établissemens & du commerce des Européens dans les deux Indes.* A. Amsterdam, 1770.

Sanders, W. H., and W. E. Fay. *Vocabulary of the Umbundu Language, Comprising Umbundu-English and English-Umbundu.* Boston: Beacon, 1885.

Segurola, P. B. *Dictionnaire Fon-Français.* Paris: Cotonou, 1963.

Sewel, William. *A Large Dictionary English and Dutch, in Two Parts: Wherein Each Language Is Set Forth in Its Proper Form; The Various Significations of the Words Being Exactly Noted, and Abundance of Choice Phrases and Proverbs Intermixt.* 2nd ed. Amsterdam: Weduwe van Steven Swart, 1708.

Sims, A. *A Vocabulary of the Kiteke, as Spoken by the Bateke (Batio) and Kindred Tribes on the Upper Congo.* London: Hodder and Stoughton, 1886.

Trésor de la langue Française informatisé (TLFi). Université de Lorraine. http://atilf.atilf.fr (accessed 8 July 2016).

Tobias, G. W. R., and B. H. C. Turvey. *English-Kwanyama Dictionary.* Johannesburg: Witwatersrand University Press, 1965.

Westermann, D. H. *Evefiala: Ewe-English Dictionary.* Berlin: Reimer, 1928.

———. *Gbesela Yeye: English-Ewe Dictionary.* Berlin: Reimer, 1930.

———. *Evefiala or Ewe-English Dictionary: Gbesela Yeye or English-Ewe Dictionary,* 2nd ed. Nendeln, Liechtenstein: Kraus Reprint, 1973.

Williamson, Kay. *Dictionary of Ọ̀nịchà Igbo.* Prepared and edited by Roger Blench. Benin: Ethiope Press, 1972.

Other

Acts of the General Assembly of Virginia. Richmond: Samuel Shepherd, Printer to the Commonwealth, 1843.

Antonil, André João. Cultura e opulencia do Brasil por suas drogas e minas, com varias noticias curiosas do modo de fazer o assucar; plantar & beneficiar o tabaco; tirar ouro das minas; & descubrir as da prata. Lisbon: Na Officina Real Deslandesiana, 1711.

Atkins, John. A Voyage to Guinea, Brasil, and the West Indies. London: Printed for Cesar Ward and Richard Chandler, 1735.

Barbot, Jean. Barbot on Guinea: The Writings of Jean Barbot on West Africa, 1687–1712. Edited by P. E. H. Hair, Adam Jones, and Robin Law. 2 volumes. London: Hakluyt Society, 1992.

Baudry des Lozières, Louis-Narcisse. Second voyage à la louisiane, faisant suite au premier de l'auteur de 1794 a 1798. Paris: Chez Charles, Imprimeur, 1803.

Bear, James A., and Lucia C. Stanton, eds. Jefferson's Memorandum Books: Accounts, with Legal Records and Miscellany, 1767–1826. Vol. 1–2. Princeton: Princeton University Press, 1997.

Blackstone, William. Commentaries on the Laws of England. 4 volumes. Oxford: Clarendon, 1765–1769.

Bosman, Willem. A New and Accurate Description of the Coast of Guinea, Divided into the Gold, the Slave, and the Ivory Coasts. London: Printed for James Knapton at the Crown, 1705.

———. Nauwkeurige Beschryving van de Guinese Goud-Tand-en Slavekust:Nevens alle desselfs landen, koningryken, en gemenebesten. 2nd edition. Calvinus, Netherlands: Isaak Stokmans, 1709.

Boyle, Robert. "The Notion of Specific Remedies Prov'd Agreeable to Mechanical Philosophy: With the Advantages of Simple Medicines Consider'd: And Their Use Recommended (1686)," in The Philosophical Works of the Honourable Robert Boyle. Edited by Peter Shaw. Vol. 3. London: Printed for W. and J. Innys, J. Osborn, and T. Longman, 1725.

Brasio, António, ed. Monumenta missionaria Africana: Africa occidental. Second series. 6 volumes. Lisbon: Agência Geral do Ultramar, 1958–1991.

Caetano de Santo António, D. Pharmacopea Lusitana: Methodo pratico de preparar & compor os medicamentos na forma Galenica com todas as receitas mais uzuais. Edited by João Rui Pita. Facsimile of 1st ed. (1704). Lisbon: Edições Minerva, 2000.

Carter, Landon. The Diary of Landon Carter of Sabine Hall, 1752–1778. Vol. 1–2. Edited by Jack P. Greene. Charlottesville: University Press of Virginia, 1965.

Cavazzi, Giovanni Antonio. Istorica descrittione de tre regni Congo, Matamba, et Angola. Milan: Nella stampe del l'Agnelli, 1690.

Le Code Noir ou Edit du Roy, 1685. Paris: Chez Claude Girard, 1735.

Collecção das leis do Imperio do Brazil de 1830. Volume 1. Rio de Janeiro: Typographia Nacional, 1876.

Condamine, Charles Marie de la. Relation abrégée d'un voyage fait dans l'interieur de l'Amérique méridionale: Depuis la Côte de la Mer du Sud, jusqu'aux Côtes du Brésil & de la Guiane. Paris: Chez la Veuve Pissot, 1745.

Cooper, Thomas, ed. Tracts on Medical Jurisprudence: Including Farr's Elements of Medical Jurisprudence, Dease's Remarks on Medical Jurisprudence, Male's Epitome of Juridical or Forensic Medicine, and Haslam's Treatise on Insanity. Philadelphia: James Webster, 1819.

de Laussat, Pierre-Clément. Mémoires sur ma vie à mon fils: Pendant les années 1803 et suivants. 3 volumes. Pau, France: É. Vignancour, imprimeur, 1831.

Dessalles, Pierre. *La vie d'un colon à la Martinique au XIXème siècle: Correspondance 1808–1834.* Edited by Fenri de Fremont. La Haye du Puits, France: Imprimerie Cauchard, 1980.

Edit du Roy Pour la punition de differents crimes: Registré en Parlement le 31 aoust 1682. Paris: Chez François Muguet, Imprimeur du Roy & de son Parlement, 1682.

Edwards, Bryan. *History, Civil and Comercial, of the British Colonies in the West Indies.* London: Printed for John Stockdale, 1801.

Equiano, Olaudah. *The Interesting Narrative of the Life of Olaudah Equiano, or Gustavus Vassa, the African: Written by Himself.* London: Printed for and sold by the author, 1789.

Ficalho, Conde de. *Plantas uteis da Africa Portugueza.* Lisbon: Imprensa Nacional, 1884.

Fontana, Felice. *Traité sur le venin de la vipere, sur les poisons americains, sur le laurier-cerise et sur quelques autres poisons vegetaux.* Florence, 1781.

———. *Treatise on the Venom of the Viper; on the American Poisons; and on the Cherry Laurel and Some Other Vegetable Poisons.* Translated from the original French by Joseph Skinner. London: Printed for J. Murray, No. 32 Fleet Street, 1787.

Hening, William Waller. *The Statutes at Large: Being a Collection of All the Laws of Virginia, from the First Session of the Legislature, in the Year 1619.* 13 volumes. Richmond: Printed by and for Samuel Pleasants, junior, printer to the commonwealth, 1809.

Labat, Jean Baptiste. *Nouveau voyage aux isles de l'Amerique, contenant l'histoire naturelle de ces pays.* 6 volumes. Paris: Chez Guillaume Cavalier, 1722.

Long, Edward. *The History of Jamaica: or, General Survey of the Ancient and Modern State of the Island.* 3 volumes. London: Printed for T. Lowndes, 1774.

Looney, J. Jefferson. *The Papers of Thomas Jefferson: Retirement Series.* Vol. 4, 6, 8. Princeton: Princeton University Press, 2007–2012.

Matthews, John. *A Voyage to the River Sierra-Leone on the Coast of Africa.* London: Printed for B. White and Son, at Horace's Head Fleet Street, and J. Sewell, Cornhill, 1788.

Mead, Richard. *A Mechanical Account of Poisons in Several Essays.* London: Printed by R. J. for Ralph Smith, 1702.

———. *A Mechanical Account of Poisons in Several Essays.* 3rd ed. Dublin: Printed by S. Powell, for John Watson, 1729.

———. *A Mechanical Account of Poisons in Several Essays.* 4th ed., corrected. London: Printed for J. Brindley, Bookseller to His Royal Highness the Prince of Wales, 1747.

"Miscellaneous Documents, Colonial and State: From the Originals in the Virginia State Archives." *Virginia Magazine of History and Biography* 18 (October 1910): 394–407.

Moreau de Saint-Méry, M. L. E. *Description topographique, physique, civile, politique, et historique de la partie française de l'isle Saint-Domingue.* 2nd ed. Paris: T. Morgand, 1875.

Oberg, Barbara, ed. *The Papers of Thomas Jefferson.* Vol. 30–31. Princeton: Princeton University Press, 2003–2004.

O Noticiador Catholico. Salvador, 1850.

Orfila, Mathieu Joseph Bonaventure. *Traité des poisons: Tirés des régnes minéral, végétal et animal, ou toxocologie générale, considérée sous les rapports de la physiologie, de la pathologie et de la médicine légale.* 2 volumes. Paris: Chez Crochard, 1814.

Park, Mungo. *Travels in the Interior Districts of Africa.* Edited by Kate Ferguson Marsters. Durham, NC: Duke University Press, 2000.

Ricord-Madianna, Jean-Baptiste. *Recherches et experiences sur les poisons d'Amérique tires des trois règnes de la nature.* Bordeaux: Charles Lawalle, 1826.

Rufz de Lavison, Étienne. *Recherches sur les empoisonnements pratiqués par les nègres à la Martinique*. Paris: Chez J. B. Baillière, 1844.

Schiltkamp, J. A., and J. th. de Smidt. *West Indisch Plakaatboek: Plakaten, Ordonnantiën en andere wetten, uitgevaardigd in Suriname*. 2 volumes. Amsterdam: S. Emmering, 1973.

Semedo, João Curvo. *Observaçoens medicas doutrinaes de cem casos gravissimos*. Lisbon: Na Officina de Antonio Pedroso Galram, 1727.

Snelgrave, William. *A New Account of Some Parts of Guinea, and the Slave-Trade*. London: James, John, and Paul Knapton, at the Crown in Ludgate-Street, 1734.

Stedman, John Gabriel. *Narrative of a Five Years Expedition Against the Revolted Negroes of Surinam, in Guinea, on the Wild Coast of South America; from the Year 1772, to 1777*. 2 volumes. London: J. Johnson and J. Edwards, 1796.

———. *Narrative of a Five Years Expedition Against the Revolted Negroes of Surinam: Transcribed for the First Time from the Original 1790 Manuscript*. 2nd ed. Edited by Richard Price and Sally Price. Baltimore: Johns Hopkins University Press, 2010.

Vide, D. Sebastião Monteiro. *Constituições primeiras do Arcebispado da Bahia (1707)*. São Paulo: Tipografia 2 de Dezembro, 1853.

Vigier, João. *Pharmacopea Ulyssiponense, Galenica, e Chymica, que contem os principios, diffiniçoens, e termos geraes de huma, & outre pharmacia: & hum lexicon universal dos termos Pharamaceuticos Galenicas, de que se usa neste reyno, & virtudes, & dosis dos medicamentos chymicos*. Lisbon: Na Officina de Pascoal da Sylva, Impressor de S. Magestade, 1716.

Virginia Gazette (Parks, 1736–1746), Williamsburg.

Virginia Gazette (Royle, 1762–1765), Williamsburg.

Virginia Gazette (Rind, 1774), Williamsburg.

Virginia Gazette (Purdie, 1777), Williamsburg.

Virginia Independence Chronicle (1786–1789), Richmond.

Voyages Database. 2009. *Voyages: The Transatlantic Slave Trade Database*. https://slavevoyages.org/ (accessed 5 May 2022).

Secondary

"*AHR* Forum: Entangled Empires in the Atlantic World." *American Historical Review* 112, no. 3 (June 2007): 710–799.

Ankarloo, Bengt, and Stuart Clark. *Witchcraft and Magic in Europe: The Eighteenth and Nineteenth Centuries*. London: Athlone, 1999.

Bassi, Ernesto. *An Aqueous Territory: Sailor Geographies and New Granada's Transimperial Greater Caribbean World*. Durham, NC: Duke University Press, 2016.

Bastide, Roger. *The African Religions of Brazil: Toward a Sociology of the Interpenetration of Civilizations*. Translated by Helen Sebba. Baltimore: Johns Hopkins University Press, 1978.

Bastin, Yvonne, André Coupez, and Michael Mann. *Continuity and Divergence in the Bantu Languages: Perspectives from a Lexicostatistic Study*. Tervuren, Belgium: Musée Royal de l'Afrique Central, 1999.

Baum, Robert M. "Crimes of the Dream World: French Trials of Diola Witches in Colonial Senegal." *International Journal of African Historical Studies* 37, no. 2 (2004): 201–228.

Bay, Edna. *Wives of the Leopard: Gender, Politics, and Culture in the Kingdom of Dahomey*. Charlottesville: University of Virginia Press, 1998.

Beeldsnijder, Rudi Otto. *"Om Werk Van Jullie te Hebben": Plantageslaven in Suriname, 1730–1750.* Utrecht: Instituut voor Culturel Antropologie te Utrecht, 1994.

Behar, Ruth. "Sex and Sin, Witchcraft and the Devil in Late-Colonial Mexico." *American Ethnologist* 14, no. 1 (1987): 34–54.

Bennett, Herman L. *African Kings and Black Slaves: Sovereignty and Dispossession in the Early Modern Atlantic.* Philadelphia: University of Pennsylvania Press, 2019.

Berlin, Ira. *Generations of Captivity: A History of African American Slaves.* Cambridge, MA: Harvard University Press, 2003.

———. *Many Thousands Gone: The First Two Centuries of Slavery in North America.* Cambridge, MA: Harvard University Press, 1998.

Blier, Suzanne Preston. *African Vodun: Art, Psychology, and Power.* Chicago: University of Chicago Press, 1995.

Bloch, Marc. *The Historian's Craft.* New York: Vintage, 1953.

Bostoen, Koen. "Pots, Words and the Bantu Problem: On Lexical Reconstruction and Early African History." *Journal of African History* 48, no. 2 (2007): 173–199.

Bostoen, Koen, and Inge Brinkman, eds. *The Kongo Kingdom: The Origins, Dynamics and Cosmopolitan Culture of an African Polity.* Cambridge: Cambridge University Press, 2017.

Bostoen, Koen, and Gilles-Maurice de Schryver. "Linguistic Innovation, Political Centralization and Economic Integration in the Kongo Kingdom: Reconstructing the Spread of Prefix Reduction." *Diachronica* 32, no. 2 (2015): 139–185.

Bostoen, Koen, Odjas Ndonda Tshiyayi, and Gilles-Maurice de Schryver. "On the Origin of the Royal Kongo Title *Ngangula*." *Africana Linguistica* 19 (2013): 53–83.

Breen, Benjamin Patrick. *The Age of Intoxication: Origins of the Global Drug Trade.* Philadelphia: University of Pennsylvania Press, 2019.

———. "Tropical Transplantations: Drugs, Nature, and Globalization in the Portuguese and British Empires, 1640–1755." PhD diss. University of Texas, Austin, 2015.

Brooks, George E. *Landlords and Strangers: Ecology, Society, and Trade in Western Africa, 1000–1630.* Boulder, CO: Westview, 1993.

Brown, Matthew, and Gabriel Paquette. *Connections After Colonialism: Europe and Latin America in the 1820s.* Tuscaloosa: University of Alabama Press, 2013.

Brown, Peter. *The Body and Society: Men, Women, and Sexual Renunciation in Early Christianity.* 2nd ed. New York: Columbia University Press, 2008.

Brown, Vincent. *The Reaper's Garden: Death and Power in the World of Atlantic Slavery.* Cambridge, MA: Harvard University Press, 2008.

Browne, Randy. "The 'Bad Business' of Obeah: Power, Authority, and the Politics of Slave Culture in the British Caribbean." *William and Mary Quarterly* 68, no. 3 (2011): 451–480.

———. *Surviving Slavery in the British Caribbean.* Philadelphia: University of Pennsylvania Press, 2017.

Bryson, Sasha Turner. "The Art of Power: Poison and Obeah Accusations and the Struggle for Dominance and Survival in Jamaica's Slave Society." *Caribbean Studies* 41, no. 2 (2013): 61–90.

Burkhill, H. M. *The Useful Plants of West Tropical Africa.* 6 volumes. Kew, England: Royal Botanic Gardens, 1985.

Burnard, Trevor, and John Garrigus. *The Plantation Machine: Atlantic Capitalism in French Saint-Domingue and British Jamaica.* Philadelphia: University of Pennsylvania Press, 2016.

Bush, Barbara. *Slave Women in Caribbean Society, 1650–1838.* Bloomington: Indiana University Press, 1990.

Cagle, Hugh. *Assembling the Tropics: Science and Medicine in Portugal's Empire, 1450–1700.* Cambridge: Cambridge University Press, 2018.

Calainho, Daniela Buono. *Metrópole das mandingas: Religiosidade negra e inquisição portuguesa no antigo regime.* Rio de Janeiro: Garamond, 2008.

Candido, Mariana P. *An African Slaving Port in the Atlantic World: Benguela and Its Hinterland.* Cambridge: Cambridge University Press, 2013.

Cañizares-Esguerra, Jorge, ed. *Entangled Empires: The Anglo-Iberian Atlantic, 1500–1830.* Philadelphia: University of Pennsylvania Press, 2018.

———. *Nature, Empire, and Nation: Explorations of the History of Science in the Iberian World.* Stanford: Stanford University Press, 2006.

Caraccioli, Mauro José. *Writing the New World: The Politics of Natural History in the Early Spanish Empire.* Gainesville: University of Florida Press, 2021.

Carney, Judith A., and Richard Nicholas Rosomoff. *In the Shadow of Slavery: Africa's Botanical Legacy in the Atlantic World.* Berkeley: University of California Press, 2009.

Cervantes, Fernando. *The Devil in the New World: The Impact of Diabolism in New Spain.* New Haven: Yale University Press, 1994.

Chambers, Douglas B. *Murder at Montpelier: Igbo Africans in Virginia.* Jackson: University Press of Mississippi, 2005.

Chireau, Yvonne. *Black Magic: Religion and the African American Conjuring Tradition.* Berkeley: University of California Press, 2003.

Clark, Stuart. "Inversion, Misrule and the Meaning of Witchcraft." *Past and Present,* no. 87 (1980): 98–127.

———. *Thinking with Demons: The Idea of Witchcraft in Early Modern Europe.* Oxford: Clarendon, 1997.

Collard, Franck. *The Crime of Poison in the Middle Ages.* Trans. Deborah Nelson-Campbell. Westport, CT: Praeger, 2008.

Colley, Linda. *Britons: Forging the Nation, 1707–1837.* New Haven: Yale University Press, 1992.

Cook, Harold J. *Matters of Exchange: Commerce, Medicine, and Science in the Dutch Golden Age.* New Haven: Yale University Press, 2007.

Copenhaver, Brian P. *Magic in Western Culture: From Antiquity to the Enlightenment.* Cambridge: Cambridge University Press, 2015.

Crawford, Matthew James. *The Andean Wonder Drug: Cinchona Bark and Imperial Science in the Spanish Atlantic, 1630–1800.* Pittsburgh: University of Pittsburgh Press, 2016.

Crawford, Matthew James, and Joseph M. Gabriel, eds. *Drugs on the Page: Pharmacopoeias and Healing Knowledge in the Early Modern Atlantic World.* Pittsburgh: University of Pittsburgh Press, 2019.

Davies, Owen. *Cunning-Folk: Popular Magic in English History.* London: Hambledon & London, 2003.

Davies, Owen, and Willem de Blécourt. *Beyond the Witch Trials: Witchcraft and Magic in Enlightenment Europe.* Manchester: University of Manchester Press, 2004.

Davis, Natalie Zemon. "Judges, Masters, Diviners: Slaves' Experience of Criminal Justice in Colonial Suriname." *Law and History Review* 29, no. 4 (2011): 925–984.

Dawson, Kevin. *Undercurrents of Power: Aquatic Culture in the African Diaspora.* Philadelphia: University of Pennsylvania Press, 2018.

de Almeida, Marcos Abreu Leitão. "African Voices from the Congo Coast: Languages and the Politics of Identification in the Slave Ship *Joven Maria* (1850)." *Journal of African History* 60, no. 2 (2019): 167–189.

———. "Speaking of Slavery: Slaving Strategies and Moral Imaginations in the Lower Congo (Early Times to the Late 19th Century)." PhD diss., Northwestern University, 2020.

de Barros, Juanita. "'Setting Things Right': Medicine and Magic in British Guiana, 1803–38." *Slavery & Abolition* 25, no. 1 (2004): 28–50.

de Blécourt, Willem, and Cornelie Usborne, eds. *Cultural Approaches to the History of Medicine: Mediating Medicine in Early Modern and Modern Europe.* New York: Palgrave Macmillan, 2004.

Debbasch, Yvan. "Opinion et droit: Le crime d'empoisonnement aux Iles pendant la période esclavagiste." *Revue française d'histoire d'outre-mer* 50, no. 179 (1963): 137–188.

de Kind, Jaspar, Gilles-Maurice de Schryver, and Koen Bostoen. "Pushing Back the Origin of Bantu Lexicography: The 'Vocabularium Congense' of 1652, 1928, 2012." *Lexicos* 22 (2012): 159–194.

de Luna, Kathryn M. "Affect and Society in Precolonial Africa." *International Journal of African Historical Studies* 46, no. 1 (2013): 123–150.

———. *Collecting Food, Cultivating People: Subsistence and Society in Central Africa.* New Haven: Yale University Press, 2016.

———. "Sounding the African Atlantic." *William and Mary Quarterly* 78, no. 4 (2021): 581–616.

de Luna, Kathryn M., and Jeffrey B. Fleisher. *Speaking with Substance: Methods of Language and Materials in African History.* New York: Springer, 2018.

de Mello e Souza, Laura. *The Devil and the Land of the Holy Cross: Witchcraft, Slavery, and Popular Religion in Colonial Brazil.* Translated by Diane Grosklaus Whitty. Austin: University of Texas Press, 2003.

de Schryver, Gilles-Maurice, et al. "Introducing a State-of-the-Art Phylogenetic Classification of the Kikongo Language Cluster. *Africana Linguistica* 21 (2015): 87–162.

Diniz, José de Oliveira Ferreira. *Populações indígenas de Angola.* Coimbra, Portugal: Impresa da Universidade de Coimbra, 1918.

Diof, Sylviane A. *Servants of Allah: African Muslims Enslaved in the Americas.* 15th anniv. ed. New York: New York University Press, 2013.

Ehret, Christopher. *An African Classical Age: Eastern and Southern Africa in World History, 1000 BC to AD 400.* Charlottesville: University Press of Virginia, 1998.

———. *History and the Testimony of Language.* Berkeley: University of California Press, 2011.

Eustace, Nicole, Eugenia Lean, Julie Livingston, Jan Plamper, William M. Reddy, and Barbara H. Rosenwin. "AHR Conversation: The Historical Study of Emotions." *American Historical Review* 117, no. 5 (2012): 1487–1531.

Evans-Pritchard, E. E. *Witchcraft, Oracles, and Magic Among the Azande.* Oxford: Clarendon, 1976.

Feierman, Steven, and John M. Janzen. *The Social Basis of Health and Healing in Africa.* Berkeley: University of California Press, 1992.

Ferreira, Jackson André da Silva. "Loucos e pecadores: Suicide na Bahia do século XIX." PhD diss. Universidade Federal da Bahia, 2004.

Ferreira, Roquinaldo. *Cross-Cultural Exchange in the Atlantic World: Angola and Brazil During the Era of the Slave Trade.* Cambridge: Cambridge University Press, 2012.

Ferrer, Ada. *Freedom's Mirror: Cuba and Haiti in the Age of Revolutions.* New York: Cambridge University Press, 2014.

Fett, Sharla M. *Working Cures: Healing, Health, and Power on Southern Slave Plantations.* Chapel Hill: University of North Carolina Press, 2002.

Fick, Carolyn E. *The Making of Haiti: The Saint Domingue Revolution from Below.* Knoxville: University of Tennessee Press, 1990.

Fields-Black, Edda L. *Deep Roots: Rice Farmers in West Africa and the African Diaspora.* Indianapolis: Indiana University Press, 2008.

Fleisch, Axel, and Rhiannon Stephens, eds. *Doing Conceptual History in Africa.* New York: Berghahn, 2016.

Frey, Sylvia R., and Betty Wood. *Come Shouting to Zion: African American Protestantism in the American South and British Caribbean to 1830.* Chapel Hill: University of North Carolina Press, 1998.

Friedman, Lawrence M. *A History of American Law.* 2nd ed. New York: Simon & Schuster, 1985.

Fromont, Cecile. *The Art of Conversion: Christian Visual Culture in the Kingdom of Kongo.* Chapel Hill: University of North Carolina Press, 2014.

Fuentes, Marisa. *Dispossessed Lives: Enslaved Women, Violence, and the Archive.* Philadelphia: University of Pennsylvania Press, 2016.

Games, Alison. "Cohabitation, Suriname-Style: English Inhabitants in Dutch Suriname After 1667." *William and Mary Quarterly* 72, no. 2 (2015): 195–242.

———. *Witchcraft in Early North America.* Plymouth: Rowman & Littlefield, 2010.

Garrigus, John. "'Like an Epidemic One Could Only Stop with the Most Violent Remedies': African Poisons Versus Livestock Disease in Saint Domingue, 1750–88." *William and Mary Quarterly* 78, no. 4 (2021): 617–652.

Geschiere, Peter. *The Perils of Belonging: Autochthony, Citizenship, and Exclusion in Africa and Europe.* Chicago: University of Chicago Press, 2009.

———. *Witchcraft, Intimacy, and Trust: Africa in Comparison.* Chicago: University of Chicago Press, 2013.

Ginzburg, Carlo. *The Night Battles: Witchcraft and Agrarian Cults in the Sixteenth and Seventeenth Centuries.* Translated by John and Anne C. Tedeschi. Baltimore: Johns Hopkins University Press, 1983.

Glowacki, Donna M., and Scott Van Keuren. *Religious Transformation in the Late Pre-Hispanic Pueblo World.* Tucson: University of Arizona Press, 2011.

Gokee, Cameron and Amanda L. Logan. "Comparing Craft and Culinary Practice in Africa: Themes and Perspectives," *African Archaeological Review* 31, no. 2 (2014):87–104.

Gomez, Michael. *African Dominion: A New History of Empire in Early and Medieval West Africa.* Princeton: Princeton University Press, 2018.

———. *Exchanging Our Country Marks: The Transformation of African Identities in the Colonial and Antebellum South.* Chapel Hill: University of North Carolina Press, 1998.

———. *Reversing Sail: A History of the African Diaspora.* 2nd ed. Cambridge: Cambridge University Press, 2020.

Gómez, Pablo F. *The Experiential Caribbean: Creating Knowledge and Healing in the Early Modern Atlantic.* Chapel Hill: University of North Carolina Press, 2016.

Gordon, David M. *Invisible Agents: Spirits in Central African History.* Athens: Ohio University Press, 2012.

Gordon-Reed, Annette. *The Hemingses of Monticello: An American Family.* New York: W. W. Norton, 2008.

Graf, Fritz. *Magic in the Ancient World.* Cambridge, MA: Harvard University Press, 1999.

Green, Toby. *The Rise of the Trans-Atlantic Slave Trade in Western Africa, 1300–1589.* Cambridge: Cambridge University Press, 2012.

Grollemund, Rebecca. "Nouvelles approaches en classification: Application aux langues Bantu du Nord-Ouest." PhD diss., Université Lumière Lyon 2, 2012.

Grollemund, Rebecca, Simon Branford, Koen Bostoen, Andrew Meade, Chris Venditti, and Mark Pagel. "Bantu Expansion Shows That Habitat Alters the Route and Pace of Human Dispersals." *Proceedings of the National Academy of Sciences of the United States of America* 112, no. 43 (2015): 13296–13301.

Grove, Richard H. *Green Imperialism: Colonial Expansion, Tropical Island Edens and the Origins of Environmentalism, 1600–1860.* Cambridge: Cambridge University Press, 1995.

Guthrie, Malcolm. *Comparative Bantu: An Introduction to the Comparative Linguistics and Prehistory of the Bantu Languages.* London: Gregg International, 1971.

Guyer, Jane I., and Samuel M. Eno Belinga. "Wealth in People as Wealth in Knowledge: Accumulation and Composition in Equatorial Africa." *Journal of African History* 36 (1995): 91–120.

Hall, Gwendolyn Midlo. *Social Control in Slave Plantation Societies: A Comparison of St. Domingue and Cuba.* Baltimore: Johns Hopkins University Press, 1971.

Handler, Jerome S., and Kenneth M. Bilby. *Enacting Power: The Criminalization of Obeah in the Anglophone Caribbean, 1769–2011.* Jamaica, Barbados, Trinidad and Tobago: University of the West Indies Press, 2012.

Harding, Rachel. *A Refuge in Thunder: Candomblé and Alternative Spaces of Blackness.* Bloomington: Indiana University Press, 2000.

Hawthorne, Walter. *From Africa to Brazil: Culture, Identity, and an Atlantic Slave Trade, 1600–1830.* Cambridge: Cambridge University Press, 2010.

Heine, Bernd, and Derek Nurse. *African Languages: An Introduction.* Cambridge: Cambridge University Press, 2000.

Helfield, Randa. "Poisonous Plots: Women Sensation Novelists and Murderesses of the Victorian Period." *Victorian Review* 21, no. 2 (Winter 1995): 161–188.

Herbert, Eugenia W. *Iron, Gender, and Power: Rituals of Transformation in African Societies.* Bloomington: Indiana University Press, 1993.

Heywood, Linda, and John K. Thornton. *Central Africans, Atlantic Creoles, and the Foundations of the Americas, 1585–1660.* New York: Cambridge University Press, 2007.

Hogarth, Rana A. *Medicalizing Blackness: Making Racial Difference in the Atlantic World, 1780–1840.* Chapel Hill: University of North Carolina Press, 2017.

Hunt, Nancy Rose. "The Affective, the Intellectual, and Gender History." *Journal of African History* 55, no. 3 (2014): 331–345.

Hurston, Zora Neale. *Barracoon: The Story of the Last "Black Cargo"* New York: Harper Collins, 2018.

Iannini, Christopher P. *Fatal Revolutions: Natural History, West Indian Slavery, and the Routes of American Literature.* Chapel Hill: University of North Carolina Press, 2012.

Isaac, Rhys. *Landon Carter's Uneasy Kingdom: Revolution and Rebellion on a Virginia Plantation.* Oxford: Oxford University Press, 2004.

——. *The Transformation of Virginia, 1740–1790*. 2nd ed. Chapel Hill: University of North Carolina Press, 1999.

Janzen, John M. *Lemba, 1650–1930: A Drum of Affliction in Africa and the New World*. New York: Garland, 1982.

——. "Therapy Management: Concept, Reality, Process." *Medical Anthropology Quarterly* 1, no. 1 (1987): 68–84.

Janzen, John M., and William Arkinstall. *The Quest for Therapy in Lower Zaire*. Berkeley: University of California Press, 1978.

Kananoja, Kalle. "Healers, Idolaters, and Good Christians: A Case Study of Creolization and Popular Religion in Mid-Eighteenth Century Angola." *International Journal of African Historical Studies* 43, no. 3 (2010): 443–465.

——. *Healing Knowledge in Atlantic Africa: Medical Encounters, 1500–1850*. Cambridge: Cambridge University Press, 2021.

Kieckhefer, Richard. *Magic in the Middle Ages*. Cambridge: Cambridge University Press, 2000.

Knight, Franklin W., and Peggy K. Liss. *Atlantic Port Cities: Economy, Culture, and Society in the Atlantic World, 1650–1850*. Knoxville: University of Tennessee Press, 1991.

Kodesh, Neil. *Beyond the Royal Gaze: Clanship and Public Healing in Buganda*. Charlottesville: University of Virginia Press, 2010.

——. "Networks of Knowledge: Clanship and Collective Well-Being in Buganda." *Journal of African History* 49 (2008): 197–216.

Kriger, Colleen. *Pride of Men: Ironworking in 19th Century West Central Africa*. Portsmouth, NH: Heinemann, 1999.

Landers, Jane. *Atlantic Creoles in an Age of Revolution*. Cambridge, MA: Harvard University Press, 2010.

Lane, Kris. "Taming the Master: Brujería, Slavery, and the Encomienda in Barbacoas at the Turn of the Eighteenth Century." *Ethnohistory* 45, no. 3 (1998): 477–507.

Langbein, John H. *Prosecuting Crime in the Renaissance: England, Germany, France*. Cambridge, MA: Harvard University Press, 1974.

Lara, Silvia Hunold. "Customs and Costumes: Carlos Julião and the Image of Black Slaves in Late Eighteenth-Century Brazil." *Slavery & Abolition* 23, no. 2 (2002): 123–146.

——. *Fragmentos Setecentistas: Escravidão, cultura e poder no América portuguesa*. São Paulo: Companhia das Letras, 2007.

Law, Robin. *Ouidah: The Social History of a West African Slaving Port, 1727–1892*. Athens: Ohio University Press, 2004.

Leong, Elaine. *Recipes and Everyday Knowledge: Medicine, Science, and the Household in Early Modern England*. Chicago: University of Chicago Press, 2018.

Levack, Brian P. *The Witch-Hunt in Early Modern Europe*. London: Longman, 1987.

Lewis, Laura A. *Hall of Mirrors: Power, Witchcraft, and Caste in Colonial Mexico*. Durham, NC: Duke University Press, 2003.

Lima, Tiana Andrade, Marcos André Torres de Souza, and Glaucia Malerba Sene. "Weaving the Second Skin: Protection Against Evil Among the Valongo Slaves in Nineteenth-Century Rio de Janeiro." *Journal of African Diaspora Archaeology and Heritage* 3 (2014): 103–136.

Lovejoy, Paul E., and David V. Trotman, eds. *Trans-Atlantic Dimensions of Ethnicity in the African Diaspora*. London: Continuum, 2003.

MacGaffey, Wyatt. *Kongo Political Culture: The Conceptual Challenge of the Particular*. Bloomington: Indiana University Press, 2000.

Mann, Kristen, and Edna G. Bay, eds. *Rethinking the African Diaspora: The Making of a Black Atlantic World in the Bight of Benin and Brazil*. Portland, OR: F. Cass, 2001.

McCaskie, Tom. "Unspeakable Words, Unmasterable Feelings: Calamity and the Making of History in Asante." *Journal of African History* 59, no. 1 (2018): 3–20.

Miller, Joseph C. *Way of Death: Marchant Capitalism and the Atlantic Slave Trade, 1730–1830*. Madison: University of Wisconsin Press, 1988.

Mobley, Christina. "The Kongolese Atlantic: Central African Slavery & Culture from Mayombe to Haiti." PhD diss., Duke University, 2015.

Moitt, Bernard. *Women and Slavery in the French Antilles, 1635–1848*. Bloomington: Indiana University Press, 2001.

Mollenauer, Lynn Wood. *Strange Revelations: Magic, Poison, and Sacrilege in Louis XIV's Court*. University Park: Pennsylvania State University Press, 2006.

Morgan, Philip D. *Slave Counterpoint: Black Culture in the Eighteenth-Century Chesapeake and Lowcountry*. Chapel Hill: University of North Carolina Press, 1998.

Morris, Thomas D. *Southern Slavery and the Law, 1619–1860*. Chapel Hill: University of North Carolina Press, 1996.

Mott, Luiz. *Bahia: Inquisição & Sociedade*. Salvador: EDUFBA, 2010.

———. "Feiticeiros de Angola na América Portuguesa." *Revista Pós Ciências Sociais* 5, no. 9 (2008): 1–32.

Northrup, David. *Africa's Discovery of Europe: 1450–1850*. New York: Oxford University Press, 2002.

Norton, Marcy. *Sacred Gifts, Profane Pleasures: A History of Tobacco and Chocolate in the Atlantic World*. Ithaca, NY: Cornell University Press, 2008.

Nurse, Derek and Gérard Philippson, eds.. *The Bantu Languages*. London: Routledge, 2003.

Ogundiran, Akinwumi, and Paula Saunders. *Materialities of Ritual in the Black Atlantic*. Bloomington: Indiana University Press, 2014.

Ortman, Scott G. "Conceptual Metaphor in the Archaeological Record: Methods and an Example from the American Southwest." *American Antiquity* 65, no. 4 (2000): 613–645.

Oudin-Bastide, Caroline. *L'effroi et la terreur: Esclavage, poison et sorcellerie aux Antilles*. Paris: Éditions La Découverte, 2013.

———. *Traveil, capitalism et société esclavagiste: Guadeloupe, Martinique (XVIIIe–XIXe siècle)*. Paris: Découverte, 2005.

Owens, Dierdre Cooper. *Medical Bondage: Race, Gender, and the Origins of American Gynecology*. Athens: University of Georgia Press, 2017.

Palmié, Stephan. *Wizards and Scientists: Explorations in Afro-Cuban Modernity & Tradition*. Durham, NC: Duke University Press, 2002.

Papstein, Robert Joseph. "The Upper Zambezi: A History of the Luvale People, 1000–1900." PhD diss., University of California, Los Angeles, 1978.

Parés, Luis Nicolau. *The Formation of Candomblé: Vodun History and Ritual in Brazil*. Translated by Richard Vernon. Chapel Hill: University of North Carolina Press, 2013.

Parés, Luis Nicolau, and Roger Sansi. *Sorcery in the Black Atlantic*. Chicago: University of Chicago Press, 2011.

Parrish, Susan Scott. *American Curiosity: Cultures of Natural History in the Colonial British Atlantic World*. Chapel Hill: University of North Carolina Press, 2006.

Paton, Diana. *The Cultural Politics of Obeah: Religion, Colonialism and Modernity in the Caribbean World*. Cambridge: Cambridge University Press, 2015.

——. "Witchcraft, Poison, Law, and Atlantic Slavery." *William and Mary Quarterly* 69, no. 2 (2012): 235–264.

Paton, Diana, and Maarit Forde, eds. *Obeah and Other Powers: The Politics of Caribbean Religion and Healing.* Durham, NC: Duke University Press, 2012.

Phillips, John Ed., ed. *Writing African History.* Rochester: University of Rochester Press, 2005.

Pluchon, Pierre. *Vaudou, sorciers, empoisonneurs de Saint-Domingue à Haïti.* Paris: Éditions Karthala, 1987.

Polcha, Elizabeth. "Voyeur in the Torrid Zone: John Gabriel Stedman's *Narrative of a Five Years Expedition Against the Revolted Negroes of Surinam, 1773–1838.*" *Early American Literature* 54, no. 3 (2019): 673–710.

Porter, Roy. *The Greatest Benefit to Mankind: A Medical History of Humanity.* New York: W. W. Norton, 1997.

Price, Richard. *Alabi's World.* Baltimore: Johns Hopkins University Press, 1990.

Rankin, Alisha. *The Poison Trials: Wonder Drugs, Experiment, and the Battle for Authority in Renaissance Science.* Chicago: University of Chicago Press, 2021.

Rankin, Hugh F. *Criminal Trial Proceedings in the General Court of Virginia.* Charlottesville: University Press of Virginia, 1956.

Rarey, Matthew Francis. "Assemblage, Occlusion, and the Art of Survival in the Black Atlantic." *African Arts* 51, no. 4 (2018): 20–33.

Reddy, William M. *The Navigation of Feeling: A Framework for the History of Emotions.* Cambridge: Cambridge University Press, 2001.

Reis, João José. *Divining Slavery and Freedom: The Story of Domingos Sodré, an African Priest in Nineteenth-Century Brazil.* Translated by H. Sabrina Gledhill. Cambridge: Cambridge University Press, 2015.

——. "Magia Jeje na Bahia: A invasão do calundu do pasto de cachoeira, 1785." *Revista Brasilia de Historia* 8, no. 16 (1988): 57–81.

——. *Slave Rebellion in Brazil: The Muslim Uprising of 1835 in Bahia.* Translated by Arthur Brakel. Baltimore: Johns Hopkins University Press, 1993.

Robinson, David. *Muslim Societies in African History.* New York: Cambridge University Press, 2004.

Rosenwein, Barbara. "Worrying About Emotions in History." *American Historical Review* 107, no. 3 (2002): 821–845.

Rutten, A. M. G. *Dutch Transatlantic Medicine Trade in the Eighteenth Century Under the Cover of the West India Company.* Rotterdam: Erasmus, 2000.

Santos, Vanicléia Silva. "As bolsas de mandinga no espaço Atlântico: Século XVIII." PhD diss., Universidade de São Paulo, 2008.

Savage, John. "'Black Magic' and White Terror: Slave Poisoning and Colonial Society in Early 19th Century Martinique." *Journal of Social History* 40, no. 3 (2007): 635–662.

Savitt, Todd Lee. *Medicine and Slavery: The Diseases and Health Care of Blacks in Antebellum Virginia.* Urbana: University of Illinois Press, 1978.

Schiebinger, Londa. *Plants and Empire: Colonial Bioprospecting in the Atlantic World.* Cambridge, MA: Harvard University Press, 2004.

——. *Secret Cures of Slaves: People, Plants, and Medicine in the Eighteenth-Century Atlantic World.* Stanford: Stanford University Press, 2017.

Schoenbrun, David Lee. "Conjuring the Modern in Africa: Durability and Rupture in Histories of Public Healing Between the Great Lakes of East Africa." *American Historical Review* 111, no. 5 (2006): 1403–1439.

———. *A Green Place, A Good Place: Agrarian Change, Gender, and Social Identity in the Great Lakes Region.* Portsmouth, NH: Heinemann, 1998.

———. *The Historical Reconstruction of Great Lakes Bantu Cultural Vocabulary: Etymologies and Distributions.* Cologne: Rüdiger Köppe, 1997.

———. "A Mask of Calm: Emotion and the Founding of the Kingdom of Bunyoro in the Sixteenth Century." *Comparative Studies in Society and History* 55, no. 3 (2013): 634–664.

———. "Mixing, Moving, Making, Meaning: Possible Futures for the Distant Past." *African Archaeological Review* 29, no. 2/3 (2012): 392–217.

Schwartz, Stuart B., ed. *Implicit Understandings: Observing, Reporting, and Reflecting on the Encounters Between Europeans and Other Peoples in the Early Modern Era.* Cambridge: Cambridge University Press, 1994.

———. *Sugar Plantations in the Formation of Brazilian Society: Bahia, 1550–1835.* Cambridge: Cambridge University Press, 1985.

Schwarz, Philip J. *Twice Condemned: Slaves and the Criminal Laws of Virginia, 1705–1865.* Baton Rouge: Louisiana State University Press, 1988.

Seth, Suman. *Difference and Disease: Medicine, Race, and the Eighteenth-Century British Empire.* Cambridge: Cambridge University Press, 2018.

Sharples, Jason T. "Discovering Slave Conspiracies: New Fears of Rebellion and Old Paradigms of Plotting in Seventeenth-Century Barbados." *American Historical Review* 120, no. 3 (2015): 811–843.

Shaw, Rosalind. *Memories of the Slave Trade: Ritual and the Historical Imagination in Sierra Leone.* Chicago: University of Chicago Press, 2002.

Singh, R. K., D. Singh, and A. G. Mahendrakar. "Jatropha Poisoning in Children." *Medical Journal of the Armed Forces India* 66 (January 2010): 80–81.

Slenes, Robert W. "'Malungu, ngoma vem!': Africa coberta e descoberta do Brasil." *Revista USP* 12 (1992): 48–67.

Smith, Sean Morey, and Christopher D. Willoughby, eds. *Medicine and Healing in the Age of Slavery.* Baton Rouge: Louisiana State University Press, 2021.

Snyder, Terri L. *The Power to Die: Slavery and Suicide in British North America.* Chicago: Chicago University Press, 2015.

Stanton, Lucia. *"Those Who Labor for My Happiness": Slavery at Thomas Jefferson's Monticello.* Charlottesville: University of Virginia Press, 2012.

Stephens, Rhiannon. *A History of African Motherhood: The Case of Uganda, 700–1900.* Cambridge: Cambridge University Press, 2013.

Sweet, James H. "Defying Social Death: The Multiple Configurations of African Slave Family in the Atlantic World." *William and Mary Quarterly* 70, no. 2 (2013): 251–272.

———. *Domingos Álvares, African Healing, and the Intellectual History of the Atlantic World.* Chapel Hill: University of North Carolina Press, 2011.

———. "Reimagining the African-Atlantic Archive: Method, Concept, Epistomology, Ontology." *Journal of African History* 55 (2014): 147–159.

———. *Recreating Africa: Culture, Kinship, and Religion in the African-Portuguese World, 1441–1770.* Chapel Hill: University of North Carolina Press, 2003.

Thornton, John K. *Africa and Africans in the Making of the Atlantic World*. 2nd ed. Cambridge: Cambridge University Press, 1998.

———. "Afro-Christian Syncretism in the Kingdom of Kongo." *Journal of African History* 54 (2013): 53–77.

———. "Cannibals, Witches, and Slave Traders in the Atlantic World." *William and Mary Quarterly* 60, no. 2 (April 2003): 273–294.

———. *A History of West Central Africa to 1850*. Cambridge: Cambridge University Press, 2020.

———. *The Kongolese Saint Anthony: Dona Beatriz Kimpa Vita and the Antonian Movement, 1684–1706*. Cambridge: Cambridge University Press, 1998.

Townsend, Camilla. *Annals of Native America: How the Nahuas of Colonial Mexico Kept Their History Alive*. Oxford: Oxford University Press, 2017.

———. *Malintzin's Choices: An Indian Woman in the Conquest of Mexico*. Albuquerque: University of New Mexico Press, 2006.

Trouillot Michel-Rolphe. *Silencing the Past: Power and the Production of History*. Boston: Beacon, 1995.

Turner, Sasha. "The Nameless and the Forgotten: Maternal Grief, Sacred Protection, and the Archive of Slavery." *Slavery & Abolition* 38, no. 2 (2017): 232–250.

van den Berg, Margot. "Ningretongo and Bakratongo: Race/Ethnicity and Language Variation in 18th Century Suriname," *Revue belge de philologie et d'histoire* 91, no. 3 (2013): 735–761.

Van de Veld, Mark, Koen Bostoen, Derek Nurse, and Gérard Philippson. *The Bantu Languages*. 2nd ed. New York: Routledge, 2019.

Vansina, Jan. *How Societies Are Born: Governance in West Central Africa Before 1600*. Charlottesville and London: University of Virginia Press, 2004.

———. *Paths in the Rainforests: Toward a History of Political Tradition in Equatorial Africa*. Madison: University of Wisconsin Press, 1990.

van Stipriaan, Alex. *Surinaams contrast: Roofbouw en overleven in een Caraïbsche plantage economie, 1750–1863*. Amsterdam: Centrale Huisdrukkerij Vrije Universiteit, 1991.

———. "An Unusual Parallel: Jews and Africans in Suriname in the 18th and 19th Centuries," *Studia Rosenthaliana* 31, no. ½ (1997): 74–93.

Voeks, Robert A. *Sacred Leaves of Candomblé: African Magic, Medicine, and Religion in Brazil*. Austin: University of Texas Press, 1997.

Voeks, Robert, and John Rashford, eds. *African Ethnobotany in the Americas*. New York: Springer, 2013.

von Germeten, Nicole. *Violent Delights, Violent Ends: Sex, Race, and Honor in Colonial Cartagena de Indias*. Albuquerque: University of New Mexico Press, 2013.

von Oppen, Achim. *Terms of Trade and Terms of Trust: The History and Contexts of Pre-Colonial Market Production Around the Upper Zambezi and Kasai*. Munster: Lit Verlag, 1994.

Walker, Timothy D. *Doctors, Folk Medicine and the Inquisition: The Repression of Magical Healing in Portugal During the Enlightenment*. Leiden: Brill, 2005.

Weaver, Karol K. *Medical Revolutionaries: The Enslaved Healers of Eighteenth-Century Saint Domingue*. Urbana: University of Illinois Press, 2006.

Wexler, Peter, ed. *Toxicology in the Middle Ages and Renaissance*. London: Elsevier, 2017.

White, Sophie. *Voices of the Enslaved: Love, Labor, and Longing in French Louisiana*. Chapel Hill: University of North Carolina Press, 2019.

INDEX

abolition movement, 16, 18, 66, 156–57
alchemist, 57
Amazon, 56–58, 88
amulet. *See* object, power
ancestors. *See* spirits
André (accused of poisoning, Suriname),
127–29
Angola: as an ethnic term, 76; present-day
region of, 23, 26–29, 52, 56, 59; Portuguese colony of, 37, 48–49, 57, 59, 63–64,
118, 137, 140, 148
Anselmo de Almada, Manoel, 74, 84
anthrax, 107
antidote, 35, 37, 80. *See also* theriac
Antonil, André João, 140
apothecary, 55
Arabic (language and speakers), 23, 45
archives: languages as, 92, 167; silencing in,
11–12, 150, 165; sources for this book in, 8,
11–14
arsenic, 87–89, 156, 180
Atkins, John, 44, 100
Atlantic Africa: adaptations of practices
from, 116, 120, 124, 137, 148–49; as a
source of secret knowledge, 54, 121,
140–41; diplomacy of, 6, 48, 53; history of
emotions in, 91–92, 94–95; intellectual
history and moral philosophy of, 3–4,
6–7, 11, 15–16, 38–39, 43, 45–48, 58,
67–69, 89, 91–92, 94, 118, 126, 164, 169,
178; Europeans in, 38–39, 41–47, 105;
physical geography of, 22–23, 29, 32,
40–41, 49, 51–52, 148; states, rulers,
and conflicts in, 26, 35, 53, 59, 61, 181.
See also Angola; Biafra, Bight of;
Benin, Bight of; Dahomey; Gold
Coast; Oyo; Senegambia; slave trade,
transatlantic

Atlantic world: cross-cultural interaction
in, 1–2, 4, 6, 15–16, 36–39, 44–45, 48–49,
53–58, 115, 122; entanglement in, 11, 163;
general period and region of, 9, 15, 18–19,
33, 35–36, 38–41, 45, 48, 52, 61, 70, 89;
knowledge circulation in, 7, 55, 58, 113,
158, 164, 178; literature on, 6, 12, 113, 165;
physical geography of, 9, 40; potential of
historical linguistics for the study of, 165
autochthony, 123

Bahia: court system, operations, and record
keeping of, 11, 73–74, 152, 176, 179; history
of slavery in, 10, 64, 181–83; laws of, 72, 85,
177, 179; newspapers in, 131; police in, 71,
107, 130; total poison cases in, 177. *See also*
empire, Portuguese; Inquisition
Barbados, 11, 123, 136
Barbot, Jean, 41–42, 100
Bellomont, Earl of, 99
belly: as a source of emotions, 91–92, 94–95,
106; symptoms relating to, 74, 92–95, 121,
150
Benguela, 59, 62
Benin, Bight of, 40–41, 58, 95, 106, 130, 182
Berbice, 3, 103, 125, 138, 149, 153–54, 176–79
bezoar, 34, 55
Biafra, Bight of, 40–43, 147, 183
binding. *See* tying
bioprospecting, 37, 55
bison, 56
Blom, Anthony, 99
bociɔ, 45–46, 95. *See also* object, power
bolsa de mandinga (or *bolsa*), 45, 54, 56, 68,
115–20, 122, 130. *See also* object; power
Bosman, Willem, 41–42, 44, 46–47, 100,
147–48
Boyle, Robert, 100

ACKNOWLEDGMENTS

No writer is an island. I could not have written this book or even conceived of undertaking it without an enormous amount of help. This is a project that began in office hours with my advisers at Georgetown University, who nurtured my intellectual growth in our seminars and supported me in my exploration of unusual connections in the Atlantic world. Above all, I want to thank my adviser Alison Games for her tireless reading, insightful critique, and constant encouragement from my first proposal through the final draft. Special thanks are also due to Kate de Luna for training me in the basics of historical linguistics; to David Collins, for nudging me toward anthropological approaches in the early stages of the project; and to Adam Rothman for his helpful comments and suggestions on drafts. Kate also generously read a revised full draft long after I left the nest, helping me to expand and better integrate my linguistic material: it was in that conversation that she also suggested I consider a version of the chapter reorganization that ultimately came to fruition.

A wide cast of commentators, editors, and guides aided me at all stages of this project. The first time in a new archive can be a bewildering experience, and I am grateful to numerous scholars and archivists who were generous with their time in helping me navigate each brave new world. Special thanks are due in this regard to James Sweet, Hendrick Kraay, Alexandre Dubé, and Suze Zijlstra. Ryan Kashanipour, Nikki Ferraiolo, and the rest of the crew in the Council on Library and Information Resources Mellon Fellowship for Dissertation Research in Original Sources helped me feel my way through the transition from research to the earliest stages of writing. Victoria Barnett Woods, Christopher Willoughby, and Sean Smith helped me refine draft versions of two of the dissertation chapters for edited volumes. I am also grateful for the workshop scholars who dedicated their time and offered their critiques on proposals and chapter drafts at the Summer Academy of Atlantic History, the International Center for Jefferson Studies Fellows Forum, the Huntington Library brown bag series, the Georgetown

Early Modern Global History Seminar, the Johns Hopkins University Atlantic History Workshop, and the McNeil Center for Early American Studies. Panel organizers at several conferences also gave me the opportunity to share and get feedback on my work in progress: I especially want to thank the participants in the 2018 "Medicine and Healing in the Age of Slavery" symposium at Rice University. Blind readers at the *William and Mary Quarterly* and the University of Pennsylvania Press helped me step back and see the manuscript with fresh eyes, and their thoughtful and thorough notes were crucial to the revision process.

Bob Lockhart has been a terrific editor as he encouraged me in undertaking a major overhaul of the organization of the initial manuscript. It was an exciting—though daunting—leap to reimagine the book's entire structure, made possible by Bob's firm support. I also want to thank him for his patience as career changes and the rhythms of my family life stretched out the tail end of the revision.

The globetrotting research for this project would not have been possible without the generous aid of the Council on Library and Information Resources, the McNeil Center for Early American Studies, the Social Science Research Council, the American Society for Eighteenth-Century Studies, the Huntington Foundation, the Cosmos Club Foundation, and the Robert H. Smith International Center for Jefferson Studies. Financial support from Randolph College also gave me the necessary time to revise the early manuscript drafts.

In the years since this project began, I got married, shifted career paths, and had a beautiful baby girl: I got by with *a lot* of help from my friends. At Georgetown and Randolph, Finn Macartney, Kate Steir, Anthony Eames, Jackson Perry, Kelsey Molseed, and Jess Kindler were all fonts of solidarity and celebration. Across (multiple) archives Alix Rivière and the world's greatest dog, Arya, shared many adventures with me, while Casey Schmitt was a fellow in the truest sense of the word, from Philadelphia lunches to long pandemic Zoom chats with wine. My parents and all my extended family members have cheered me on at every step of my academic career, from grade school through the PhD and beyond. Paisley the cat has provided not only constant companionship but also a generous service, keeping my proofreading skills sharp by periodically walking across the keyboard. Finally, my husband, Nick, has been my rock and true friend, supporting me with what I needed when I needed it—time together, time away at far-flung archives, and the occasional bucking up. Thank you.